Gastrointestinal Pathology

Gastrointestinal Pathology

Editor: Matilda McDonald

AMERICAN
MEDICAL PUBLISHERS
www.americanmedicalpublishers.com

AMERICAN
MEDICAL PUBLISHERS
www.americanmedicalpublishers.com

Cataloging-in-Publication Data

Gastrointestinal pathology / edited by Matilda McDonald.
p. cm.
Includes bibliographical references and index.
ISBN 978-1-63927-141-2
1. Gastrointestinal system--Diseases. 2. Gastrointestinal system--Histopathology.
3. Gastrointestinal Diseases--pathology. I. McDonald, Matilda.
RC802.9 .G37 2022
616.33--dc23

American Medical Publishers,
41 Flatbush Avenue,
1st Floor, New York,
NY 11217, USA

ISBN 978-1-63927-141-2 (Hardback)

Contents

Preface

Over the recent decade, advancements and applications have progressed exponentially. This has led to the increased interest in this field and projects are being conducted to enhance knowledge. The main objective of this book is to present some of the critical challenges and provide insights into possible solutions. This book will answer the varied questions that arise in the field and also provide an increased scope for furthering studies.

The gastrointestinal (GI) tract is responsible for the transport of food and absorption of nutrients. Gastrointestinal pathology is a sub-branch of surgical pathology that is concerned with the characterization and diagnosis of neoplastic and non-neoplastic diseases of the GI tract. The diagnostic evaluation of the GI tract or the biopsy pathology of GI tissue are essential for gastrointestinal pathology. Understanding of the clinical presentations of GI diseases, their diagnoses and treatment modalities, disease mechanism and histomorphology, etc. are vital elements of gastrointestinal pathology. The pathologic conditions of the gastrointestinal tract impair GI functions. The chief symptoms associated with the pathologies of the GI tract are gastrointestinal hemorrhage and abdominal pain. Acute abdominal pain can arise due to gastrointestinal inflammations (pancreatitis, appendicitis, cholecystitis and diverticulitis), gastrointestinal obstruction, perforation and vascular diseases (ruptured abdominal aortic aneurysm and acute ischemia). The diagnosis of upper gastrointestinal bleeding is possible with endoscopy, while the diagnosis of lower gastrointestinal bleeding requires colonoscopy or sigmoidoscopy. This book aims to shed light on some of the unexplored aspects of gastrointestinal pathology and the recent researches in this domain. The objective of this book is to give a general view of the different gastrointestinal diseases, and their management strategies. It is a vital tool for all researching or studying gastrointestinal pathology as it gives incredible insights into emerging trends and concepts.

I hope that this book, with its visionary approach, will be a valuable addition and will promote interest among readers. Each of the authors has provided their extraordinary competence in their specific fields by providing different perspectives as they come from diverse nations and regions. I thank them for their contributions.

Editor

1

Risks of hospitalization and drug consumption in children and young adults with diagnosed celiac disease and the role of maternal education

Cristina Canova[1*], Gisella Pitter[1], Jonas F. Ludvigsson[2,3], Pierantonio Romor[4], Loris Zanier[5], Renzo Zanotti[1] and Lorenzo Simonato[1]

Abstract

Background: Celiac disease (CD) may affect healthcare use in children and young adults. Socio-economic factors may act as a confounder or effect modifier. We assessed such hypotheses in a population-based birth cohort of young celiac subjects and references matched by maternal education.

Methods: The cohort included all newborns recorded in the Medical Birth Register of Friuli-Venezia Giulia Region (Italy) between 1989 and 2011. CD incident cases were identified through pathology reports, hospital discharges and copayment exemptions and matched with up to five references by sex, year of birth and maternal education. Cox regression models were used to estimate Hazard Ratios (HRs) for major causes of inpatient diagnosis and drug prescription occurring after diagnosis in CD patients compared to references, stratifying by time of first event and maternal education.

Results: We identified 1294 CD cases and 5681 references. CD cases had a higher risk of hospital admission for any cause (HR: 2.34; 95 % CI 2.08-2.63) and for all major ICD9-CM categories except obstetric complications, skin and musculoskeletal diseases, and injuries and poisoning. Prescription of all major ATC drug categories, except dermatologicals and genito-urinary medications, was significantly increased in CD subjects. For most outcomes, HRs were highest in the first year after CD diagnosis but remained significant after five or more years. HRs were similar across different categories of maternal education.

Conclusions: Diagnosed CD subjects had a higher risk of hospitalization and medication use compared to the general population, even five or more years after diagnosis, with no effect modification of maternal education.

Keywords: Celiac disease, Healthcare use, Maternal education, Birth cohort

* Correspondence: cristina.canova@unipd.it
[1]Laboratory of Public Health and Population Studies, Department of Molecular Medicine, University of Padua, via Loredan 18, 35131 Padua, Italy
Full list of author information is available at the end of the article

Background

Celiac disease (CD) is an immune-mediated small intestinal enteropathy triggered by gluten affecting approximately 0.5-1 % of the European population and frequently diagnosed during childhood [1].

Originally considered a rare malabsorption syndrome of childhood, CD is now recognized as a systemic disorder potentially affecting many organ systems beyond the gastrointestinal tract [2]. The clinical picture is variable and several complications and comorbidities can occur, including consequences of malnutrition (e.g., low bone mineral density, anemia), infections, neurological and autoimmune diseases (e.g. type I diabetes, thyroid disorders), [2, 3] and cancers such as lymphoma [4]. The only available treatment for CD is a life-long gluten-free diet. This dietary regimen is effective in controlling symptoms, however it is burdensome for the patient and his/her family and cannot prevent many complications and comorbidities of CD [2]. Moreover, children with CD, even if adherent to the gluten-free diet, often suffer from functional gastrointestinal disorders [5] and psychological disturbances [6] that may lead to impaired quality of life [7] and greater healthcare needs.

Few studies have investigated and reported an increased use of healthcare services and drugs and associated costs in adults with CD compared to the general population; [8–11] specific data regarding children and adolescents with CD are scarce. Furthermore, only one study [11] has so far assessed the long-term persistence of increased healthcare use after CD diagnosis.

Healthcare utilization pattern is affected by educational and socio-economic factors, which may reflect socio-economic differences regarding both morbidity and access to healthcare services. Currently, social determinants are emphasised as a major source of health inequalities within developed countries [12]. As far as we know, the impact of socio-economic status on healthcare utilization associated with CD has never been investigated.

Using a population-based birth cohort of subjects born between 1989 and 2011 and followed-up until the end of 2012, we examined the risk of first hospitalization and drug consumption at different time intervals from diagnosis in CD children, adolescents and young adults compared to reference individuals matched on age, gender and maternal education level. This study had three objectives: i) to assess whether children and adolescents with CD use more healthcare resources after diagnosis compared to subjects without CD of similar age, sex, and maternal education; ii) to assess whether the possible increased healthcare use is limited to the short period after CD diagnosis or persists long-term; iii) to assess whether the risk of healthcare use in CD subjects compared to unaffected subjects is modified by maternal education.

Methods

Setting and study population

We used a matched cohort design. The underlying study population consisted of 213 635 subjects (excluding abortions, stillbirths, and neonatal deaths within 30 days of birth) born in Friuli-Venezia Giulia (FVG) Region in Italy in the period 1989-2011 identified using the regional Medical Birth Register that contains socio-demographic data on the parents, details of the pregnancy, labour, and delivery, and the newborn at birth.

Italy has a tax-based National Health Service, which provides universal coverage to all Italian and European Union citizens resident in the country regardless of income, and it is organized at a regional level. FVG Region is covered by a regional integrated healthcare system developed in the 1980s with the goal of automatically collecting and pooling data on healthcare funded by the National Health Service using a unique regional identification code that has been described in detail previously [13].

The following Regional health data were used in this study (up to 2012): mortality records; pathology reports from all the pathology departments in the FVG Region, coded in the Systematized Nomenclature of Medicine (SnoMed); hospital discharge records collected during episodes of inpatient care occurring within the FVG Region or in Italy outside the Region with up to six diagnostic codes in the International Classification of Diseases ninth revision Clinical Modification (ICD9-CM); exemption from healthcare copayment coded in a national coding system; drug prescription records coded in the Anatomical Therapeutic Chemical (ATC) Classification System (available from 1995).

Ethics, consent and permissions

The study was approved by the Institutional Review Board of the University of Padua (Italy). Patients' data were completely anonymized and de-identified prior to analysis. Therefore, no informed consent and no Ethics Committee approval were required.

CD definition

We defined CD as having at least one of the following [13]: a pathology report of villous atrophy (SnoMed codes D6218, D6318, M58, M58005, M58006, and M58007); a hospital discharge record with an ICD9-CM code 5790 in any diagnosis; an exemption from healthcare copayment with code I0060 according to the Italian national coding system. In Italy, all patients with CD can obtain clinical tests and gluten-free food free of charge from the National Health Service, provided they have a CD diagnosis certified by a specialist on the basis of a biopsy report. CD onset was defined as the earliest date identifiable in the three sources of information (pathology, hospital and copayment exemption).

Follow-up

We retrieved data on hospital discharges by cause of disease according to ICD9-CM classification (17 group of causes listed in Table 1) considering the main diagnosis and drug prescriptions according to first level of ATC Classification after date of diagnosis (index date in reference individuals).

Data analysis

For each case with a CD diagnosis up to five reference individuals were selected from subjects in the Medical Birth Register alive on the date of CD diagnosis (index date), matched on gender, year of birth and maternal education levels (up to middle school; secondary school; university level). Matching was implemented to control for confounding and improve statistical efficiency and to be able to attribute the beginning of follow-up (index date) that corresponds to CD diagnosis to reference individuals. Follow-up started at 30 days after the index date (to exclude hospitalizations and prescriptions concomitant to CD diagnosis) until the earliest of: end of the study (December 31, 2012), death, migration out of the area, or first hospitalization for each group of causes/ first drug prescription for each ATC level. Concerning drug prescription outcomes, analyses were restricted to subjects with index date ≥1995 (because drug prescription data are available from that year). Cox regression models were used to estimate the Hazard Ratios (HRs) and 95 % confidence intervals (CI) for each of the healthcare use outcome in patients with CD compared to reference individuals within the same stratum. The assumption of proportional hazards was investigated by studying graphs over the log cumulative hazards function and the Shoenfeld residuals, and verified by a global test of rho. Analyses were also stratified by time of first hospital admission/drug prescription, looking at outcomes occurred between 30-365 days and >365 days after the index date. For the latter analyses only subjects with at least one year of follow-up (alive and resident in the area one year after the index date and without any hospitalization/drug prescription for each ICD9-CM/ ATC category within one year from the index date) were considered. In order to assess the possible long-term effect on healthcare use in CD individuals compared to references, we examined the risk of hospitalization and drug consumption five or more years after diagnosis. For this analysis follow-up started five years after the index

Table 1 Risks of first hospital admission according to ICD9-CM classification after date of diagnosis in CD subjects compared to matched references[a]

ICD codes	Disease category	REFERENCES ($n = 5681$)		CD ($n = 1294$)		HR (95 % CI)
		n	py	*n*	py	
001–V89	Any	1245	33072	499	5915	**2.34** (2.08–2.63)
001–139	Infectious and parasitic diseases	73	40900	44	9396	**2.79** (1.89–4.12)
140–239	Neoplasms	56	41220	27	9686	**1.89** (1.16–3.08)
240–279	Endocrine. metabolic. immunity dis.	96	40936	69	9328	**3.19** (2.32–4.40)
280–289	Dis. of the blood and blood-forming organs	23	41334	25	9614	**4.47** (2.49–8.01)
290–319	Mental disorders	60	41203	35	9618	**2.52** (1.64–3.87)
320–389	Dis. of the nervous system and sense organs	114	40681	56	9414	**2.14** (1.53–2.98)
390–459	Dis. of the circulatory system	29	41405	16	9766	**2.77** (1.49–5.18)
460–519	Dis. of the respiratory system	347	38348	121	8763	**1.59** (1.28–1.98)
520–579	Dis. of the digestive system	220	40228	232	7846	**5.59** (4.57–6.83)
580–629	Dis. of the genito-urinary system	94	40861	42	9533	**1.95** (1.32–2.86)
630–679	Complications of pregnancy and puerperium	46	41394	15	9807	1.48 (0.82–2.67)
680–709	Dis. of skin and subcutaneous tissue	55	41215	16	9722	1.22 (0.68–2.17)
710–739	Dis. of the muscoloskeletal tissue	104	41056	27	9716	0.88 (0.55–1.44)
740–779	Congenital anomalies/Perinatal conditions	90	40902	44	9482	**2.18** (1.50–3.17)
780–799	Ill-defined conditions	83	40898	55	9413	**2.94** (2.06–4.19)
800–999	Injuries and poisoning	167	41491	57	9840	1.35 (0.98–1.86)
V01–V89	Factors influencing health status	58	41092	41	9468	**2.94** (1.94–4.47)

Py person-years, *CD* celiac disease, *HR* Hazard Ratio, *CI* confidence interval, *Dis.* Disease
Figures in bold are statistically significant results (p-value <0.05)
[a]Matched by year of birth, gender and maternal education

date and only subjects alive and resident in the area at this time were included. In this analysis, we included subjects with hospitalization/drug prescription within five years from the index date.

In order to evaluate a possible modifying effect of socioeconomic status, analyses were subsequently stratified by maternal education levels.

Results

We identified 1294 subjects with CD and 5681 reference individuals. Biopsy confirmation was available for 920 (71 %) CD individuals; 179 (14 %) were instead identified by hospital discharges and copayment records, 112 (9 %) only by hospital discharge records and 83 (6 %) only by copayment records. Mean age at diagnosis (age at index date for references) was 7.2 ± 5.3 years (min 0, max 23.8 years). Analyses of drug prescriptions were restricted to 1215 CD subjects diagnosed after 1995 and 5366 matched references. 1166 CD cases (5100 references) were alive and resident in the Region one year after the index date and 777 (3316 references) 5 years after.

CD subjects were at increased risk of hospital admission for any cause (HR: 2.34; 95 % CI: 2.08-2.63) and for all major groups of causes according to ICD9-CM classification, except for complications of pregnancy and puerperium, diseases of skin and subcutaneous tissue, diseases of the musculoskeletal tissue, and injuries and poisoning (Table 1). The risk of drug prescription was also significantly increased in CD cases for all ATC categories except dermatologicals (ATC = D) and genito-urinary medications and sex hormones (ATC = G) (Table 2).

The risk of any hospital admission in CD subjects compared to references was higher during the first year after diagnosis but remained statistically significant also after the first year of follow-up (Table 3). Examining single major groups of causes, the chronological pattern was heterogeneous (Table 3): for endocrine/metabolic/immune disorders and digestive disorders HRs were higher during the first year and declined afterwards; a similar pattern was seen, although less evident, for infectious, respiratory, and congenital disorders, for ill-defined conditions and factors influencing health status. On the contrary, hospitalization for nervous/sensory disorders and genito-urinary disorders had similar HRs within one year from diagnosis and after one year. Finally, concerning blood, mental and circulatory disorders, the low number of events occurring during the first year did not allow to estimate hazard ratios. Five years after diagnosis, CD subjects still had a higher risk of being admitted to the hospital for any cause (HR: 2.03; 95 % CI: 1.71-2.41) and for infectious (HR: 2.45; 95 % CI: 1.24-4.85), endocrine/metabolic/immune (HR: 3.13; 95 % CI: 1.94-5.06), mental (HR: 1.99; 95 % CI: 1.04-3.81), nervous/sensory (HR: 2.76; 95 % CI: 1.62-4.72), circulatory (HR: 2.39; 95 % CI: 1.14-5.00), digestive (HR: 2.90; 95 % CI: 2.09-4.02), and congenital disorders (HR: 2.93; 95 % CI: 1.64-5.21), as well as for ill-defined conditions (HR: 2.62; 95 % CI: 1.50-4.61) and factors influencing health status (HR: 4.87; 95 % CI: 2.32-10.23) (Additional file 1: Table S1).

The risk of drug prescription was higher in the first year after diagnosis for all ATC groups, except for systemic anti-infectives (ATC = J) and respiratory system (ATC = R) medications, which showed a stable risk over time (Table 4). Risk estimates for cardiovascular drugs (ATC = C), genito-urinary drugs and sex hormones (ATC = G), nervous system drugs (ATC = N), and sensory organs medications (ATC = S) were significantly increased only in the first year of follow-up. Five years after diagnosis, CD subjects still had a higher risk of being prescribed most drug categories compared to their references (Additional file 2: Table S2).

Among CD cases, 160 (12.4 %) were born to graduated mothers, 648 (50.1 %) to mothers with secondary school education and 471 (36.4 %) to less educated mothers (up to middle school) (15 cases had missing information on maternal education); by study design, references showed similar distributions, because each CD case was matched to references with the same maternal education.

In the analysis stratified by maternal education level, we found no clear modifying effect of maternal education (Additional file 3: Table S3, Additional file 4: Table S4). The risks of being hospitalized for any cause among CD subjects compared to their references born to mothers with similar maternal education were: HR 2.64 (95 % CI 1.79-3.89) for university level, HR 2.33 (95 % CI 1.97-2.76) for secondary school education and HR 2.30 (95 % CI 1.92-2.75) for primary/middle school education. Neither were there any differences in HRs for specific groups of causes according to maternal education although the low number of subjects with graduated mothers did not allow precise or computable estimates in that group (Additional file 3: Table S3). Similar risks were also seen for the majority of drug prescription categories in the groups of subjects stratified by maternal education (Additional file 4: Table S4).

Discussion

In this large population-based birth cohort, we followed-up 1294 children and adolescents with CD and 5,681 peers without CD, matched by socio-demographic characteristics, for hospitalization and drug prescription after CD diagnosis. Both hospitalization and drug consumption were increased in CD cases in most disease categories and a wide range of drug classes.

A small number of previous studies have reported a greater use of medical services and drugs in CD patients

Table 2 Risks of first drug prescription according to first level of Anatomical Therapeutic Chemical (ATC) Classification after date of diagnosis in CD subjects compared to matched references[a]

ATC codes	Drug category	REFERENCES ($n = 5366$)		CD ($n = 1215$)		HR (95 % CI)
		n	py	*n*	py	
A	Alimentary tract and metabolism	537	38094	298	8054	**2.55** (2.19–2.97)
B	Blood and blood forming organs	258	40354	193	8846	**3.69** (3.02–4.50)
C	Cardiovascular system	102	40676	43	9511	**1.77** (1.22–2.57)
D	Dermatologicals	180	40060	55	9381	1.22 (0.88–1.69)
G	Genito–urinary system and sex hormones	126	40749	38	9629	1.22 (0.83–1.79)
H	Systemic hormonal preparations. excluding sex hormones and insulins	778	37614	316	8082	**2.06** (1.79–2.37)
J	Antiinfectives for systemic use	3660	17612	885	3680	**1.27** (1.17–1.39)
L	Antineoplastic and immunomodulating agents	19	41350	25	9697	**5.24** (2.82–9.73)
M	Musculo–skeletal system	170	40674	73	9436	**1.93** (1.44–2.59)
N	Nervous system	156	40703	56	9533	**1.53** (1.12–2.11)
P	Antiparasitic products. insecticides and repellents	216	40259	90	9271	**2.01** (1.56–2.60)
R	Respiratory system	2059	27958	560	6004	**1.33** (1.20–1.48)
S	Sensory organs	147	39939	51	9252	**1.42** (1.02–1.99)

Py: person-years; CD: celiac disease; HR: Hazard Ratio; CI: confidence interval
Figures in bold are statistically significant results (*p*-value <0.05)
[a]Matched by year of birth, gender and maternal education; analysis restricted to subjects with index date ≥1995 (because drug prescription data are available from that year)

Table 3 Risks of first hospital admission according to ICD9–CM classification after date of diagnosis in CD subjects compared to matched references, stratified by first outcome occurrence (30–365 days after the index date/>365 days after the index date)[a]

First outcome occurrence	30–365 days					>1 year after index date[b]				
ICD codes	REFERENCES		CD		HR (95 % CI)	REFERENCES		CD		HR (95 % CI)
	n	py	*n*	py		*n*	py	*n*	py	
001–V89	281	5260	243	1095	**4.28** (3.56–5.13)	964	27812	256	4820	**1.58** (1.36–1.85)
001–139	18	5380	17	1221	**4.38** (2.25–8.55)	55	35520	27	8176	**2.23** (1.37–3.63)
140–239	8	5384	6	1226	2.88 (0.94–8.85)	6	35836	21	8459	**1.72** (1.00–2.98)
240–279	12	5383	24	1216	**8.37** (4.12–16.99)	84	35553	45	8112	**2.42** (1.66–3.52)
280–289	7	5426	13	1309	--	16	35947	12	8392	**2.70** (1.21–6.04)
290–319	12	5476	9	1272	--	48	35819	26	8394	**2.26** (1.37–3.72)
320–389	32	5375	13	1224	1.83 (0.94–3.56)	82	35306	43	8190	**2.26** (1.54–3.32)
390–459	2	5388	0	1229	--	27	36017	16	8537	**2.99** (1.59–5.64)
460–519	66	5356	38	1213	**2.62** (1.74–3.95)	281	32991	83	7550	**1.34** (1.03–1.73)
520–579	30	5375	123	1156	**18.96** (12.52–28.70)	190	34853	109	6690	**3.07** (2.38–3.97)
580–629	23	5378	11	1226	1.92 (0.88–4.19)	71	35483	31	8307	**1.95** (1.25–3.05)
630–679	1	5388	0	1229	--	45	36006	15	8578	1.57 (0.87–2.82)
680–709	6	5385	2	1228	0.81 (0.10–6.70)	49	35830	14	8493	1.27 (0.69–2.32)
710–739	12	5384	7	1226	2.32 (0.87–6.21)	92	35672	20	8490	0.70 (0.39–1.23)
740–779	21	5381	16	1220	**3.39** (1.74–6.59)	69	35521	28	8262	**1.80** (1.14–2.85)
780–799	16	5381	18	1220	**5.43** (2.76–10.66)	67	35517	37	8193	**2.33** (1.52–3.56)
800–999	1	5389	1	1229	5.00 (0.31–79.95)	166	36102	56	8611	1.33 (0.97–1.83)
V01–V89	15	5379	15	1223	**4.18** (2.00–8.74)	43	35713	26	8245	**2.50** (1.50–4.17)

Py person–years, *CD* celiac disease, *HR* Hazard Ratio, *CI* confidence interval, Figures in bold are statistically significant results (*p*-value <0.05)
[a]Matched by year of birth, gender and maternal education; [b]excluding subjects with less than one year of follow-up for each outcome

Table 4 Risks of first drug prescription according to first level of Anatomical Therapeutic Chemical (ATC) Classification after date of diagnosis in CD subjects compared to matched references, stratified by first outcome occurrence (30–365 days after the index date/>365 days after the index date)[a]

First outcome occurrence	30–365 days					>1 year after index date[b]				
ATC codes[b]	REFERENCES		CD		HR (95 % CI)	REFERENCES		CD		HR (95 % CI)
	n	py	*n*	py		*n*	py	*n*	py	
A	131	5320	140	1129	**4.70** (3.66–6.04)	406	32774	158	6926	**1.78** (1.45–2.17)
B	48	5543	91	1534	**6.35** (2.93–13.75)	210	34991	102	7669	**2.36** (1.83–3.04)
C	18	5380	14	1222	**3.53** (1.71–7.29)	84	35296	29	8289	1.42 (0.91–2.21)
D	43	5367	17	1220	1.45 (0.79–2.64)	137	34694	38	8162	1.14 (0.77–1.68)
G	22	5375	14	1221	**2.38** (1.16–4.88)	104	35374	24	8408	0.97 (0.61–1.54)
H	209	5286	133	1157	**3.07** (2.45–3.85)	569	32328	183	6925	**1.65** (1.38–1.97)
J	1986	4300	524	941	**1.27** (1.15–1.41)	1674	13312	361	2739	**1.28** (1.10–1.49)
L	4	5386	12	1221	**12.46** (3.94–39.42)	15	35964	13	8476	**3.33** (1.52–7.29)
M	15	5383	14	1221	**3.64** (1.66–7.97)	155	35291	59	8214	**1.75** (1.27–2.41)
N	31	5368	16	1217	**2.22** (1.20–4.12)	125	35335	40	8316	1.35 (0.93–1.97)
P	44	5368	30	1211	**3.05** (1.88–4.94)	172	34891	60	8060	**1.73** (1.27–2.35)
R	808	4969	248	1097	**1.42** (1.23–1.65)	1251	22989	312	4907	**1.26** (1.09–1.45)
S	43	5368	25	1217	**2.29** (1.37–3.83)	104	34572	26	8035	1.03 (0.65–1.64)

Py: person–years; CD: celiac disease; HR: Hazard Ratio; CI: confidence interval
Figures in bold are statistically significant results (*p*-value <0.05)
[a]Matched by year of birth, gender and maternal education; analysis restricted to subjects with index date ≥1995 (because drug prescription data are available from that year); [b]excluding subjects with less than one year of follow-up for each outcome

compared to controls after diagnosis, [9–11] but only one included children and adolescents and provided a long follow-up [11]. To our knowledge, this is the first study on the long-term healthcare impact of paediatric CD conducted in Southern Europe. Healthcare use is influenced by culture and type of healthcare system, therefore it is worthwhile to conduct similar studies in different settings. Overall the results of the present study are consistent with current knowledge that childhood CD is associated with multi-organic complications and comorbidities and also with non-specific health complaints [2, 3].

For most disease and drug categories (in particular endocrine/metabolic/immune and digestive disorders and antineoplastic/immunomodulating agents), the risk of hospitalization or prescription was highest during the first year of follow-up, indicating that CD-related health problems are likelier to occur (or become recorded) shortly after diagnosis, when clinical surveillance is greatest and dietary treatment may have not yet displayed its effects. However, our findings suggest that CD-related health problems can develop also later, since for most conditions the risk of a first event after diagnosis was increased in CD subjects compared to reference individuals also after the first year of follow-up. To assess whether the increased healthcare use in CD persisted long-term, we also examined hospital admissions and drug prescriptions occurring five or more years after diagnosis; subjects who had hospital admissions or drug prescription within five years were included in this analysis. We found that even beyond five years of follow-up, the risk of hospitalization and drug prescription was greater in CD cases compared to reference individuals. Such results are consistent with a previous study conducted in the United Kingdom showing that healthcare costs in patients with CD have a peak around time of diagnosis and decline thereafter, but remain higher than in controls for up to 10 years [11]. Unlike the abovementioned study, we did not focused on costs but rather on the risk of events.

Different factors may explain why diagnosed CD children and adolescents used more healthcare resources than their references even five years after diagnosis. First of all, as in any chronic disorder, the frequent contact with the healthcare system can increase the chance of being diagnosed and subsequently treated for other conditions. In our opinion, however, surveillance bias alone cannot explain the differences we observed. Secondly, CD has been associated with non-specific health complaints such as functional gastrointestinal disorders and depressive and anxiety symptoms that can persist over time despite appropriate treatment [5, 6]. Consistently, when we examined main diagnoses and drug categories in detail, we found that anxiety and somatoform disorders (ICD9-CM 300), personality disorders (ICD9-CM 301), eating, sleep and psychogenic pain disorders (ICD9-CM 307), ill-defined symptoms concerning nutrition and abdomen (ICD9-CM 783 and 789), prescriptions of antacids (ATC

A02), psycholeptics (ATC N05), and psychoanaleptics (ATC N06) were all more common among individuals with CD. Young CD patients may also be exposed to a persistent risk of developing complications of nutritional deficiencies due to incomplete remission of gut mucosal abnormalities or to dietary restrictions [14]. This is suggested by our finding that CD subjects had a higher proportion of iron-deficiency anemia (ICD9-CM 280), thrombocytopenia (ICD9-CM 287), leukocytopenia (ICD9-CM 288), and prescription of anti-anemic preparations (ATC B03). Infectious diseases, particularly those provoked by encapsulated bacteria, may also complicate the clinical course of CD in the long term, [15] as a result of hyposplenism [16] and perhaps of altered intestinal permeability and nutritional deficiencies. We also observed a greater frequency of hospital admissions for otitis media (ICD9-CM 381), pneumonia (ICD9-CM 481, 482, 485, 486), and urinary infections (ICD9-CM 590, 599) in CD, as well as a higher consumption of systemic anti-infectives (ATC J). Finally, a greater occurrence of several diseases, mainly but not exclusively of autoimmune origin, has been described in patients with CD. Although our study was not designed to estimate the risk of specific associated conditions, we think that some of the reported risks could be partially explained by underlying comorbidities. For instance, the greater proportion of admissions for diabetes (ICD9-CM 250) and prescription of antidiabetic agents (ATC A10) and thyroid drugs (ATC H03) could reflect the acknowledged associations between CD and type I diabetes mellitus and autoimmune thyroid disorders [17]. Similarly, the well-known comorbidity between CD and chromosomal anomalies, such as Down [18] and Turner syndrome, [3] may in part explain a higher prevalence of congenital malformations in CD subjects [19]. Several neurologic and psychiatric conditions, such as epilepsy (ICD9-CM 345) [20] and autism (ICD9-CM 299), [3, 21] have been linked to CD although with inconclusive results, and may explain our finding of a higher risk of hospital admission for neurologic and mental disorders and of prescription of antiepileptic drugs (ATC N03) in CD cases. Concerning digestive disorders, most of the increased risk in CD subjects is likely due to CD itself, especially in the first year of follow-up, since intestinal malabsorption (ICD9-CM 579) was not excluded from the analysis of hospitalization outcomes. Our CD cases also had a high frequency of hospitalizations for Crohn's disease (ICD9-CM 555) and ulcerative colitis (ICD9-CM 556), both of which have been potentially linked to CD although earlier research has shown conflicting results [22–25].

Although CD is a chronic illness, many of its symptoms and effects can be reversed or controlled with a gluten-free diet [2]. Therefore, one might suppose that with a well-conducted gluten-free diet and an appropriate follow-up, the long-term outcome of CD paediatric patients would be similar to the general population ones. Our data showed that this is not the case, at least not in FVG Region. This issue deserves further investigation to confirm our findings and to assess whether the unfavorable long-term outcome of paediatric CD can be attributed only to complications and comorbidities that are not prevented by the gluten-free diet or also to an inadequate management of CD.

Socioeconomic factors in early childhood have a well-known impact on several health outcomes in adulthood, although evidence regarding early exposure impact on childhood and adolescence health is more limited [26]. Moreover, socio-economic level has been associated with the risk of developing CD in some studies, but results are conflicting [13, 27–32]. For this reason we decided to control for the possible confounding effect of socio-economic status by design matching reference individuals by maternal education. To the best of our knowledge this has never been done before. We also hypothesised that a poorer educational and socio-economic condition may adversely affect health of CD children and adolescents compared to reference individuals within the same socio-economic stratum, possibly because of a poorer adherence to gluten-free diet. However, the analyses stratified by maternal education showed similar HR of hospital admission and drug prescription across groups. These results, although limited by the low number of events particularly for the hospitalization outcomes and among the most educated mothers, do not suggest a modifying effect of maternal education on the association between CD and healthcare use, but as any novel tested hypothesis they need to be further replicated in other setting/studies.

Strengths of our study besides the matched design include the large population size, the longitudinal design with long follow-up period and the availability of objective data, with no risk of recall bias. The main limitations are due to the use itself of administrative data with the inability to directly verify the presence of CD, and obtain data on compliance with a gluten-free diet. As regards the identification of CD cases, however, we are confident that our data are accurate since 71 % of cases had a biopsy report of villous atrophy, which has been found to be highly specific (positive predictive value 95 %) for CD in a validation study [33]. Of the remaining cases, 20 % had a copayment exemption, which in Italy is based on a physician's diagnosis. Treatment with a gluten-free diet may result in decreased consumption of health care services and drugs, [10] although some studies suggested that, even after years of compliance with a gluten-free diet, CD patients have significantly impaired quality of life [11]. Moreover, we were unable to retrieve data on outpatient visits and diagnostic procedures, which would have drawn a more comprehensive picture of healthcare utilization. A further limitation is that we did not exclude from the analyses those subjects already affected by chronic disorders other than CD before the index date. Therefore, the higher healthcare use we observed in CD individuals may in part depend on comorbidities that were already present before the onset of CD. Our study should be therefore regarded as exploratory rather than confirmatory because we did not examine temporal relationships between CD onset and outcomes. The aim of this study was to describe healthcare use pattern after CD diagnosis without inferring causal relationships between CD and associated conditions.

Conclusions

Using a population-based birth cohort matched study design, we showed that young people with diagnosed CD were at increased risk of later hospitalization and medication use compared to unaffected peers from the general population independently from socio-economic status at birth. Greater healthcare consumption may be explained both by non-specific health complaints and by complications and associated conditions of CD. Whatever the mechanism, our findings show that the burden associated with paediatric CD is heavy and persists in the long term, despite the existence of an effective treatment. Further longitudinal studies should be devoted to identify factors associated to a bad prognosis of CD in the paediatric population, in order to improve the management of this disease.

Additional files

Additional file 1: Table 1. Risks of first hospital admission according to ICD9-CM classification five or more years from date of diagnosis in CD subjects compared to matched references*.

Additional file 2: Table 2. Risks of first drug prescription according to first level of Anatomical Therapeutic Chemical (ATC) Classification five or more years from date of diagnosis in CD subjects compared to matched references*.

Additional file 3: Table 3. Risks of first hospital admission according to ICD9-CM classification after date of diagnosis in CD subjects compared to matched references, stratified by maternal education*.

Additional file 4: Table 4. Risks of first drug prescription according to first level of Anatomical Therapeutic Chemical (ATC) Classification after date of diagnosis in CD subjects compared to matched references, stratified by maternal education*.

Competing interests

The authors declare that they have no competing interests.

Authors' contributions

CC conceived the idea and design of the study, carried out statistical analyses, interpreted results, and drafted the manuscript. GP participated in the design of the study, interpreted results, and drafted the manuscript. JFL participated in interpretation of results and helped to draft the manuscript. PR participated in coordination of the study and interpretation of results. LZ participated in coordination of the study and interpretation of results. RZ participated in the design of the study and interpretation of results. LS participated in coordination of the study and interpretation of results. All authors read and approved the final manuscript.

Acknowledgements

This study was financially supported by the University of Padua with a research grant to Dr. Cristina Canova [F.S. 4.18.01.05].

Author details

[1]Laboratory of Public Health and Population Studies, Department of Molecular Medicine, University of Padua, via Loredan 18, 35131 Padua, Italy. [2]Department of Medical Epidemiology and Biostatistics, Karolinska Institutet, 17177 Stockholm, Sweden. [3]Department of Pediatrics, Örebro university Hospital, Örebro 70185, Sweden. [4]Friuli-Venezia Giulia Regional Health Information System, Informatica per il Sistema degli Enti Locali (INSIEL) S.p.A., Udine, Italy. [5]Epidemiological Service, Health Directorate, Friuli Venezia-Giulia Region, Udine, Italy.

References

1. Mustalahti K, Catassi C, Reunanen A, Fabiani E, Heier M, McMillan S, et al. The prevalence of celiac disease in Europe: results of a centralized, international mass screening project. Ann Med. 2010;42:587–95.
2. Green PH, Jabri B. Coeliac disease. Lancet. 2003;362:383–91.
3. Newton KP, Singer SA. Celiac disease in children and adolescents: special considerations. Semin Immunopathol. 2012;34:479–96.
4. Tio M, Cox MR, Eslick GD. Meta-analysis: coeliac disease and the risk of all-cause mortality, any malignancy and lymphoid malignancy. Aliment Pharmacol Ther. 2012;35:540–51.
5. Turco R, Boccia G, Miele E, Giannetti E, Buonavolontà R, Quitadamo P, et al. The association of coeliac disease in childhood with functional gastrointestinal disorders: a prospective study in patients fulfilling Rome III criteria. Aliment Pharmacol Ther. 2011;34:783–9.
6. Mazzone L, Reale L, Spina M, Guarnera M, Lionetti E, Martorana S, et al. Compliant gluten-free children with celiac disease: an evaluation of psychological distress. BMC Pediatr. 2011;11:46. 2431-11-46.
7. Altobelli E, Paduano R, Gentile T, Caloisi C, Marziliano C, Necozione S, et al. Health-related quality of life in children and adolescents with celiac disease: survey of a population from central Italy. Health Qual Life Outcomes. 2013; 11:204. 7525-11-204.
8. Long KH, Rubio-Tapia A, Wagie AE, Melton LJ 3rd, Lahr BD, Van Dyke CT, et al. The economics of coeliac disease: a population-based study. Aliment Pharmacol Ther. 2010;32:261–9.
9. Roos S, Wilhelmsson S, Hallert C. Swedish women with coeliac disease in remission use more health care services than other women: a controlled study. Scand J Gastroenterol. 2011;46:13–9.
10. Ukkola A, Kurppa K, Collin P, Huhtala H, Forma L, Kekkonen L, et al. Use of health care services and pharmaceutical agents in coeliac disease: a prospective nationwide study. BMC Gastroenterol. 2012;12:136. 230X-12-136.
11. Violato M, Gray A, Papanicolas I, Ouellet M. Resource use and costs associated with coeliac disease before and after diagnosis in 3,646 cases: results of a UK primary care database analysis. PLoS One. 2012;7:e41308.
12. Marmot M, Allen J, Bell R, Bloomer E, Goldblatt P. WHO European review of social determinants of health and the health divide. Lancet. 2012;380:1011–29.
13. Canova C, Zabeo V, Pitter G, Romor P, Baldovin T, Zanotti R, et al. Association of maternal education, early infections, and antibiotic use with celiac disease: a population-based birth cohort study in northeastern Italy. Am J Epidemiol. 2014;180:76–85.
14. Penagini F, Dilillo D, Meneghin F, Mameli C, Fabiano V, Zuccotti GV. Gluten-free diet in children: an approach to a nutritionally adequate and balanced diet. Nutrients. 2013;5:4553–65.
15. Ludvigsson JF, Olen O, Bell M, Ekbom A, Montgomery SM. Coeliac disease and risk of sepsis. Gut. 2008;57:1074–80.
16. Di Sabatino A, Rosado MM, Cazzola P, Riboni R, Biagi F, Carsetti R, et al. Splenic hypofunction and the spectrum of autoimmune and malignant complications in celiac disease. Clin Gastroenterol Hepatol. 2006;4:179–86.
17. Elfstrom P, Sundstrom J, Ludvigsson JF. Systematic review with meta-analysis: associations between coeliac disease and type 1 diabetes. Aliment Pharmacol Ther. 2014;40:1123–32.
18. Marild K, Stephansson O, Grahnquist L, Cnattingius S, Söderman G, Ludvigsson JF. Down syndrome is associated with elevated risk of celiac disease: a nationwide case-control study. J Pediatr. 2013;163:237–42.

19. Wingren CJ, Agardh D, Merlo J. Congenital anomalies and childhood celiac disease in Sweden. J Pediatr Gastroenterol Nutr. 2012;55:736–9.
20. Ludvigsson JF, Zingone F, Tomson T, Ekbom A, Ciacci C. Increased risk of epilepsy in biopsy-verified celiac disease: a population-based cohort study. Neurology. 2012;78:1401–7.
21. Ludvigsson JF, Reichenberg A, Hultman CM, Murray JA. A nationwide study of the association between celiac disease and the risk of autistic spectrum disorders. JAMA Psychiatry. 2013;70:1224–30.
22. Yang A, Chen Y, Scherl E, Neugut AI, Bhagat G, Green PH. Inflammatory bowel disease in patients with celiac disease. Inflamm Bowel Dis. 2005;11: 528–32.
23. Casella G, D'Inca R, Oliva L, Daperno M, Saladino V, Zoli G, et al. Prevalence of celiac disease in inflammatory bowel diseases: An IG-IBD multicentre study. Dig Liver Dis. 2010;42:175–8.
24. Virta LJ, Kolho KL. The risk of contracting pediatric inflammatory bowel disease in children with celiac disease, epilepsy, juvenile arthritis and type 1 diabetes–a nationwide study. J Crohns Colitis. 2013;7:53–7.
25. El-Matary W, Senthilselvan A, Fedorak RN, Dieleman L, Spady D. Celiac disease in children with inflammatory bowel disease: a prospective cohort study. Am J Gastroenterol. 2013;108:455–6.
26. Spencer N, Thanh TM, Louise S. Low income/socio-economic status in early childhood and physical health in later childhood/adolescence: a systematic review. Matern Child Health J. 2013;17:424–31.
27. Kondrashova A, Mustalahti K, Kaukinen K, Viskari H, Volodicheva V, Haapala AM, et al. Lower economic status and inferior hygienic environment may protect against celiac disease. Ann Med. 2008;40:223–31.
28. Roberts SE, Williams JG, Meddings D, Davidson R, Goldacre MJ. Perinatal risk factors and coeliac disease in children and young adults: a record linkage study. Aliment Pharmacol Ther. 2009;29:222–31.
29. Olen O, Bihagen E, Rasmussen F, Ludvigsson JF. Socioeconomic position and education in patients with coeliac disease. Dig Liver Dis. 2012;44:471–6.
30. Wingren CJ, Bjorck S, Lynch KF, Ohlsson H, Agardh D, Merlo J. Coeliac disease in children: a social epidemiological study in Sweden. Acta Paediatr. 2012,101.185–91.
31. Whyte LA, Kotecha S, Watkins WJ, Jenkins HR. Coeliac disease is more common in children with high socio-economic status. Acta Paediatr. 2014; 103:289–94.
32. Zingone F, West J, Crooks CJ, Fleming KM, Card TR, Ciacci C, et al. Socioeconomic variation in the incidence of childhood coeliac disease in the UK. Arch Dis Child. 2015;100:466–73.
33. Ludvigsson JF, Brandt L, Montgomery SM, Granath F, Ekbom A. Validation study of villous atrophy and small intestinal inflammation in Swedish biopsy registers. BMC Gastroenterol. 2009;9:19.

2

Uridine stimulate laxative effect in the loperamide-induced constipation of SD rats through regulation of the mAChRs signaling pathway and mucin secretion

Ji Eun Kim[1], Jun Go[1], Ji Eun Sung[1], Hyun Ah Lee[1], Woo Bin Yun[1], Jin Tae Hong[2] and Dae Youn Hwang[1*]

Abstract

Background: Uridine (Urd), which has been reported as a major component of RNA, plays an important role in various biological process including neuroprotection, biochemical modulation and glycolysis, although its role in constipation has yet to be established. Therefore, in this study, we investigated the laxative effects of Urd on chronic constipation.

Methods: The constipation phenotypes and their related mechanisms were investigated in the transverse colons of SD rats with loperamide (Lop)-induced constipation after treatment with 100 mg/kg of Urd.

Results: The number, weight and water contents of stools were significantly higher in the Lop + Urd treated group than the Lop + Vehicle treated group, while food intake and water consumption of the same group were maintained at a constant level. The thickness of the mucosa layer, muscle and flat luminal surface, as well as the number of goblet cells, paneth cells and lipid droplets were enhanced in the Lop + Urd treated group. Furthermore, the expression of the muscarinic acetylcholine receptors M2 and M3 (mAChR M2 and M3) at the transcriptional and translational level was recovered in the Lop + Urd treated group, while some markers such as Gα and inositol triphosphate (IP3) in their downstream signaling pathway were completely recovered by Urd treatment. Moreover, the ability for mucin secretion and the expression of membrane water channel (aquaporine 8, AQP8) were increased significantly in the Lop + Urd treated group compared with Lop + Vehicle treated group. Finally, the activity of Urd was confirmed in primary smooth muscle of rat intestine cells (pRISMC) based on Gα expression and IP3 concentration.

Conclusions: The results of the present study provide the first strong evidence that Urd can be considered an important candidate for improving chronic constipation induced by Lop treatment in animal models.

Keywords: Constipation, Uridine, Loperamide, Excretion parameters, Mucin, Muscarinic acetylcholine receptors

Background

Constipation is an acute or chronic gastrointestinal disease characterized by infrequent bowel movements, hard and dry feces, incomplete bowel evacuation and difficulty during defecation [1]. Although a variety of treatments for this disease are known, the best method for treatment of constipation is making simple changes to incorporate more fiber into the diet, drink plenty of fluids, and add exercise into the patient's daily routine. In most cases, chemical drugs (laxatives) such as senna, correctol, exlax, senokot and gaviscon can be widely prescribed to help patients pass stools [2]. These drugs act as stimulants to increase bulkiness and soften stool, or as osmotic agents, enhancing water flow into the colon to promote elimination and trigger bowel movements. However, most of these agents have undesirable side effects including artery contraction, coronary spasms

* Correspondence: dyhwang@pusan.ac.kr
[1]Department of Biomaterials Science, College of Natural Resources & Life Science/Life and Industry Convergence Research Institute, Pusan National University, 50 Cheonghak-ri, Samnangjin-eup Miryang-si, Gyeongsangnam-do 627-706, Korea
Full list of author information is available at the end of the article

and myocardial infarction [3–5]. Therefore, identification of novel laxatives with no side effects has been the main focus of the constipation treatments.

Urd, which is one of the five standard nucleosides that makes up nucleic acids, is a glycosylated pyrimidine-analog consisting of uracil linked to a ribose ring [6]. After phosphorylation to nucleotides, Urd was used for the synthesis of nucleic acid and membrane constituents, as well as glycosylation [7]. Moreover, Urd is widely involved in a variety of biochemical processes including the glycolysis pathway, biochemical modulation and neuroprotection. Urd plays a role in the glycolysis pathway of galactose even if catabolic processes for the metabolism of galactose are not involved this process [8]. Furthermore, Urd has been used successfully as a biochemical modulating agent to alleviate the side effects of various anti-cancer and anti-HIV drugs, although fever and diarrhea have been considered the major factors limiting increasing the dose of Urd [9–11]. Urd is the major form of pyrimidine nucleoside taken up by the brain, and it has been suggested that it be used as a neuroprotective agent to treat epileptic and neurodegenerative diseases, including depression and Alzheimer's disease [7, 12]. Urd acts as a central nervous system (CNS) depressant, having anticonvulsant effects and inducing decreased spontaneous activity of adult male C-57 mice [13, 14] Although studies conducted to date have provided some information regarding the possibility of a correlation between intestinal bowel disease and Urd, no studies have investigated the laxative effects of Urd in the constipated animal model.

Therefore, the present study was conducted to verify the laxative activity and action mechanism of Urd in a Lop-induced constipation model. Our results provide the first scientific evidence that Urd can successfully induce laxative effects in the constipated animal model without any significant side effects.

Methods

Experimental design for animal study

Adult SD rats purchased from Samtako Inc. (Osan, Korea) were handled in the Pusan National University-Laboratory Animal Resources Center, which is accredited by the Korea Food and Drug Administration (FDA)(Accredited Unit Number-000231) and AAALAC International according to the National Institutes of Health guidelines (Accredited Unit Number; 001525). Animals were provided with *ad libitum* access to a standard irradiated chow diet (Samtako Inc.) and water. During the experiment, rats were maintained in a specific pathogen-free (SPF) state under a strict light cycle (lights on at 08:00 h and off at 20:00 h) at 23 ± 2 °C and 50 ± 10% relative humidity.

Constipation of SD rats was induced by subcutaneously injection of Lop as previously described [5, 15]. First, 8-week-old SD rats ($n = 28$) were assigned to either a non-constipation group (No group, $n = 14$) or a constipation group ($n = 14$). Constipation was induced by subcutaneous injection of Lop (4 mg/kg weight) in 0.5% Tween 20 in saline twice a day for 3 days, whereas the non-constipation group was injected with 0.5% Tween 20 in saline alone. The non-constipation group was further divided into a No treated group ($n = 7$) and a Urd treated group ($n = 7$). The No treated group was untreated during the experimental period, whereas the Urd treated group received 100 mg/kg Urd (Sigma-Aldrich Co., Saint Louis, MO, USA) at one time. Additionally, the constipation group was further divided into a Lop + Vehicle treated group ($n = 7$) and Lop + Urd treated group ($n = 7$). The Lop + Urd treated groups were orally administered 100 mg/kg body weight Urd at once, while the Lop + Vehicle treated group received the same volume of 1× PBS under the same pattern. At 24 h after Urd treatment, all SD rats were euthanized using CO_2 gas and tissue samples were acquired and stored in Eppendorf tubes at −70 °C until assay.

Analysis of food intake, water intake and body weight

Alterations in food intake, water consumption and body weight of SD rats treated with Lop + Urd were measured daily at 10:00 am throughout the experimental period using an electrical balance and a measuring cylinder. All measurements were performed three times to ensure accuracy.

Measurement of stool parameters

During all experimental periods, SD rats of all groups were bred in metabolic cages to harvest pure stools and urine without any contamination (Daejong Instrument Industry Co., LTD, Seoul, Korea). The stool number and weight were measured as previously described [15, 16]. The stools excreted from each SD rat were collected at 10:00 am. Stool samples were weighed three times per sample using an electric balance, whereas the number of stools was counted three times.

Western blotting

Total proteins were extracted from the transverse colons of subset groups (No, Urd, Lop + Vehicle and Lop + Urd treated SD rats) and pRISMCs using Pro-Prep Protein Extraction Solution (Intron Biotechnology, Inc., Seongnam, Korea). Following centrifugation at 13,000 rpm and 4 °C for 5 min, the protein concentrations were determined using a SMARTTM Bicinchoninic Acid Protein assay kit (Thermo Fisher Scientific, Inc.). Proteins (30 μg) were separated by 4–20% sodium dodecyl sulfate-polyacrylamide gel electrophoresis (SDS-PAGE) for 3 h, after which the resolved proteins were transferred to nitrocellulose membranes for 2 h at 40 V. Each membrane was then incubated separately with primary antibody, anti-mAChR M2 antibody (Alomone Labs, Jerusalem, Israel), anti-PI-3K (Cell Signaling Technology Inc., Cambridge, MA, USA), anti-p-PI3K (Cell Signaling Technology Inc.), anti-mAChR M3 antibody (Alomone Labs, Jerusalem, Israel), anti-PKC (Cell Signaling Technology Inc.), anti-p-PKC (Cell Signaling Technology Inc.), anti-Gα (Abcame, Cambridge, UK) or anti-actin (Sigma-Aldrich Co.) overnight at 4 °C. Next, the membranes were washed with washing buffer (137 mM NaCl, 2.7 mM KCl, 10 mM Na_2HPO_4, 2 mM KH_2PO_4, and 0.05% Tween 20) and incubated with horseradish peroxidase-conjugated goat anti-rabbit IgG (Zymed Laboratories, South San Francisco, CA, USA) at a dilution of 1:1000 and room temperature for 2 h. Finally, the membrane blots were developed using Chemiluminescence Reagent Plus kits (Pfizer, New York, NY, USA and Pharmacia, New York, NY, USA).

RT-PCR

Total RNA was isolated from the frozen tissue of transverse colons using RNAzol B solution (Tet-Test Inc.) according to manufacturer's protocols. After the synthesis of cDNA, genes were amplified by subjecting the samples to 28 cycles of 30 s at 94 °C, 30 s at 62 °C and 45 s at 72 °C in a Perkin-Elmer Thermal Cycler. The primer sequences used to evaluate mAChR M2 expression were as follows: sense primer, 5′-CCAGT ATCTC CAAGT CTGGT GCAAG G-3′, antisense primer, 5′-GTTCT TGTAA CACAT GAGGA GGTGC-3′. The primer sequences used to evaluate mAChR M3 expression were as follows: sense primer, 5′-GTCAC TTCTG GTTCA CCACC AAGAG C-3′, antisense primer, 5′-GTGTT CACCA GGACC ATGAT GTTGT AGG-3′. The primer sequences used to evaluate AQP8 expression were as follows: sense primer, 5′-GTAGT ATGGA CCTAC GTGAG ATCAA GG-3′, antisense primer, 5′-AGAAC CTTTC CTCTG GACTC ACCAC C-3′. The primer sequences used to evaluate MUC2 expression were as follows: sense primer, 5′-GCTGC TCATT GAGAA GAACG ATGC-3′, antisense primer, 5′-CTCTC CAGGT ACACC ATGTT ACCAG G-3′. The sequences of the β-actin sense and antisense primers were 5′-TGGAA TCCTG TGGCA TCCAT GAAAC-3′ and 5′-TAAAA CGCAG CTCAG TAACA GTCCG-3′, respectively. The PCR products were quantified using 1% agarose gels and a Kodak Electrophoresis Documentation and Analysis System 120.

Histopathological analysis

Transverse colons collected from No, Urd, Lop + Vehicle and Lop + Urd treated SD rats were fixed with 10% formalin for 48 h, embedded in paraffin wax, and then sectioned into 5 μm thick slices that were stained with hematoxylin and eosin (H&E, Sigma-Aldrich Co.). Morphological features of these sections were observed by light microscopy, after which the mucosa thickness, muscle thickness, flat luminal surface thickness, number of goblet cells and number of lipid droplets were measured using Leica Application Suite (Leica Microsystems, Switzerland).

For mucin staining, transverse colons collected from SD rats that had been cotreated with Lop + Urd were fixed with 10% formalin for 48 h, embedded in paraffin wax, and then sectioned into 4 μm thick slices that were subsequently deparaffinized with xylene and rehydrated. Next, the tissue sections on the slides were rinsed with distilled water and stained with an Alcian Blue Stain kit (IHC WORLD, Woodstock, MD, USA). Finally, the morphological features in the stained colon sections were observed by light microscopy.

Ultrastructure analysis using transmission electron microscopy (TEM)

The transverse colons collected from SD rats of subset groups were fixed in 2.5% glutaraldehyde in 1× PBS buffer, washed, dehydrated with ascending concentrations of ethanol, incubated in 1% OsO_4 for 1 h at room temperature, and then embedded in Epon812 media (Polysciences Inc., Eppelheim, Germany). Ultra-thin sections (70 nm) were subsequently collected on holey formvar coated grids, contrasted with uranyl acetate and lead citrate, and examined by TEM (Hitachi, Tokyo, Japan) at 4000× magnification.

Measurement of IP3 concentration

The levels of IP3 were determined using an IP3 ELISA kit (Cusabio Biotech Co., Ltd., Wuhan, China) according to the manufacturer's instructions. Briefly, the pRISMCs (5×10^7) were washed and homogenized in ice-cold PBS (pH 7.2–7.4) with a glass homogenizer (Sigma-Aldrich Co.). The cell lysates were then centrifuged at 1000 rpm for 5 min at room temperature, after which the supernatant was collected for analysis. An anti-IP3 detection antibody was added and incubated at 37 °C for 60 min, after which substrate solution was added and the samples were incubated for 15 min at 37 °C. The reaction was terminated following the addition of stop solution and the plates were read at an absorbance of 450 nm using a Molecular Devices VERSA max Plate reader (Molecular Devices, Sunnyvale, CA, USA).

Treatment and preparation of pRISMC

pRISMCs used in this study were prepared from intestines of infant rats (3 days old)($n = 3$) as previously described, with some modification [17]. Moreover, the purity of the pRISMCs population was confirmed by RT-

PCR analysis with some modification as previously described [18]. Amplification was conducted in a Perkin-Elmer Thermal Cycler using the following cycles: 30 s at 94 °C, 30 s at 62 °C, and 45 s at 72 °C. The primer sequences for target gene expression identification were as follows: Myh11 (myosin-smooth muscle cells marker), sense primer: 5′-GCAAC TGAGC AATGA GCTGG TCAC-3′, anti-sense primer: 5′-CTGCT CCTTG TACTG CTCCA CCATC-3′; PGP9.5 (neuronal cell marker), sense primer: 5′-TACTT CATGA AGCAG ACCAT CG-3′, anti-sense primer: 5′-CTGCA GCAGA GAGTC CTCTG AACTG-3′; β-actin, sense primers; 5′-TGG AAT CCT GTG GCA TCC ATG AAA C-3′, anti-sense primer: 5′-TAA AAC GCA GCT CAG TAA CAG TCC G-3′. The final PCR products were separated on 1.2% agarose gel and then visualized by ethidium bromide staining. Among the two markers, only Myh11, indicating myosin-smooth muscle cells, was detected at high levels, while PGP9.5, indicating neuronal cells, was found at an extremely low level (Fig. 6a).

To treat Urd, pRISMCs were seeded at a density of 1×10^7 cells/10 ml in 100 mm-diameter culture dishes, then grown with 20 μM Lop in a 37 °C incubator. After 12 h, cells were removed from the culture media with Lop and incubated with 100 μM Urd or 1× PBS for another 12 h. Next, cells harvested from 100 mm diameter culture dishes were used to determine the IP3 concentration and for western blot analysis.

Statistical analysis

One-way ANOVA (SPSS for Windows, Release 10.10, Standard Version, Chicago, IL, USA) was used to determine the variance and identify significant differences between the No treated group and others groups, as well as between the Vehicle treated group and Urd treated group within the constipation group. All values are presented as the means ± standard deviation (SD). A p <0.05 was considered significant.

Results

Effect of Urd administration on feeding behavior and excretion parameters

To investigate whether Urd administration could affect the feeding behavior and excretion parameters of constipated rats, alterations in food intake, water consumption, stool number, and weight and water contents of stools were measured in Lop-induced constipated SD rats after Urd administration. As shown Table 1, no significant alterations in body weight, food intake or water consumption were observed. However, the decreases in the number, weight and water contents of stools in the Lop + Vehicle treated group were almost recovered in the Lop + Urd treated groups relative to those in the No and Urd treated group, although there were a few differences in the recovery rate. The opposite pattern was observed for the urine volume (Table 1).

Effect of Urd administration on histological structure of the transverse colon

We investigated whether Urd treatment could induce alterations in the histological structure of the transverse colon. To accomplish this, alterations in the histological parameters indicating laxative effects were measured in the H&E stained transverse colons of subset groups. The Urd treated group showed a similar structure as the No treated group. A significant decrease in the thickness of mucosa, muscle and flat luminal surface was observed in the Lop + Vehicle treated group relative to the No treated group and the Urd treated group. However, these levels dramatically increased by 283, 219 and 39% following Lop + Urd cotreatment when compared with the Lop + Vehicle treated group (Fig. 1 and Table 2). Furthermore, the number of goblet cells, crypt of lieberkuhn and enterocytes were 41, 54 and 34% lower in the Lop + vehicle treated group than the No treated group, respectively (Table 2). However, these levels were recovered in the Lop + Urd treated groups, although not

Table 1 Measurement of body weight, feeding behavior, stools and urine secretion in Lop-induced constipated SD rats

Contents	No	Urd	Lop	
			Vehicle	Urd
Body weight (g)	270 ± 11.1	267 ± 14.5	261 ± 18.7	254 ± 17.4
Feeding behavior				
Food intake (g/day)	18.3 ± 2.2	18.4 ± 1.5	16.4 ± 1.9	16.1 ± 2.0
Water consumption (ml/day)	14.3 ± 2.1	15.7 ± 2.1	13.3 ± 4.1	15.7 ± 1.9
Stool				
Stool number (ea)	64.7 ± 9.5	65.7 ± 9.7	38.0 ± 13.1*	67.5 ± 12.2#
Stool weight (g)	8.8 ± 1.0	9.0 ± 1.5	5.2 ± 2.2*	10.0 ± 2.2#
Water content (%)	35.3 ± 3.1	35.9 ± 3.2	14.6 ± 0.8*	30.8 ± 3.4#
Urine volume (ml/day)	13 ± 1.6	13.3 ± 1.2	20.7 ± 1.7*	15.3 ± 1.7#

Data represent the means ± SD from three replicates. *$p < 0.05$ compared to the No treated group. #$p < 0.05$ compared to the Lop + Vehicle treated group.
Urd; uridine, Lop; loperamide

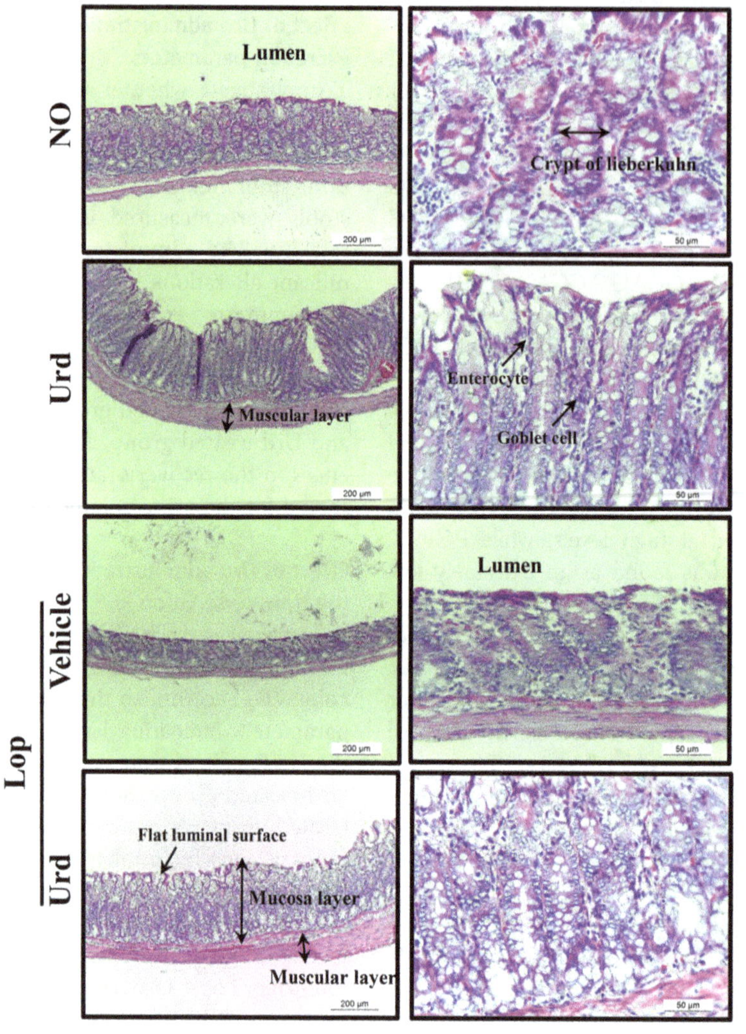

Fig. 1 Alteration of histological structures in Lop-induced constipated rats. H&E stained sections of transverse colon rats from the No, Urd, Lop + Vehicle or Lop + Urd treated group were observed at 100× (left column) and 200× (right column) using a light microscope. Five to six rats per group were assayed in triplicate by H&E

Table 2 Histopathological alterations in constipated SD rats after Urd treatment

Contents	No	Urd	Lop	
			Vehicle	Urd
Mucosa layer thickness (μm)	394 ± 35.2	415 ± 21.3	105 ± 12.5*	402 ± 23.5#
Muscle thickness (μm)	89.3 ± 6.5	92.3 ± 7.6	28.3 ± 4.3*	90.2 ± 6.6#
Flat luminal surface thickness (μm)	16.1 ± 3.2	15.4 ± 2.3	10.6 ± 1.1*	14.8 ± 2.0#
Number of goblet cells (ea)	85.6 ± 8.5	88.4 ± 6.7	51.2 ± 5.5*	72.6 ± 9.8#
Number of crypt of lieberkuhn (ea)	12.5 ± 2.6	14.2 ± 1.5	5.8 ± 1.1*	11.2 ± 2.1#
Number of enterocytes (ea)	125.2 ± 8.6	117.8 ± 7.7	82.3 ± 9.2*	102.4 ± 7.8#

*$p < 0.05$ compared with the non-constipation group. #$p < 0.05$ compared with the Lop + Vehicle treated constipation group. Urd; uridine, Lop; loperamide

completely to those of the No treated group (Fig. 1 and Table 2).

Effect of Urd administration on ultrastructure of the transverse colon

Based on the above histopathological alterations, we examined whether Urd administration could accompany alterations in the ultrastructure of the transverse colon. To accomplish this, ultrastructural changes were observed in thin tissue section of the transverse colon using TEM analysis. In the No treated group and the Urd treated group, the Crypt of Lieberkuhn was clearly observed as a ring structure in which enterocytes, goblet cells, and paneth cells surrounded a lumen at the center. Following Lop treatment, the ultrastructure of the crypt changed dramatically. The number of paneth cells and lipid droplets was also higher in the Lop + Vehicle treated group than in the No-treated group. However, their levels were significantly recovered or they disappeared from around the cryp lumen in the Lop + Urd treated group. The decrease in the average size and number of goblet cells in the Lop + Vehicle treated group was also enhanced in the Lop + Urd treated group (Fig. 2).

Correlation between the laxative effects of Urd and downstream signaling pathway of mAchRs

We next investigated the molecular mechanism of the laxative effects of Urd in the constipation model. To accomplish this, the mRNA and protein of mAChRs M2 and M3 were measured in the transverse colon of the Lop + Urd treated group using specific primers and antibodies. A similar alteration pattern in the mRNA and proteins of mAChRs M2 and M3 was observed in the subset group. The levels of these two receptors were lower in the Lop + Vehicle treated group than the No treated group and the Urd treated group. However, their levels rapidly increased by 303 and 395% in the Lop + Urd treated group (Fig. 3).

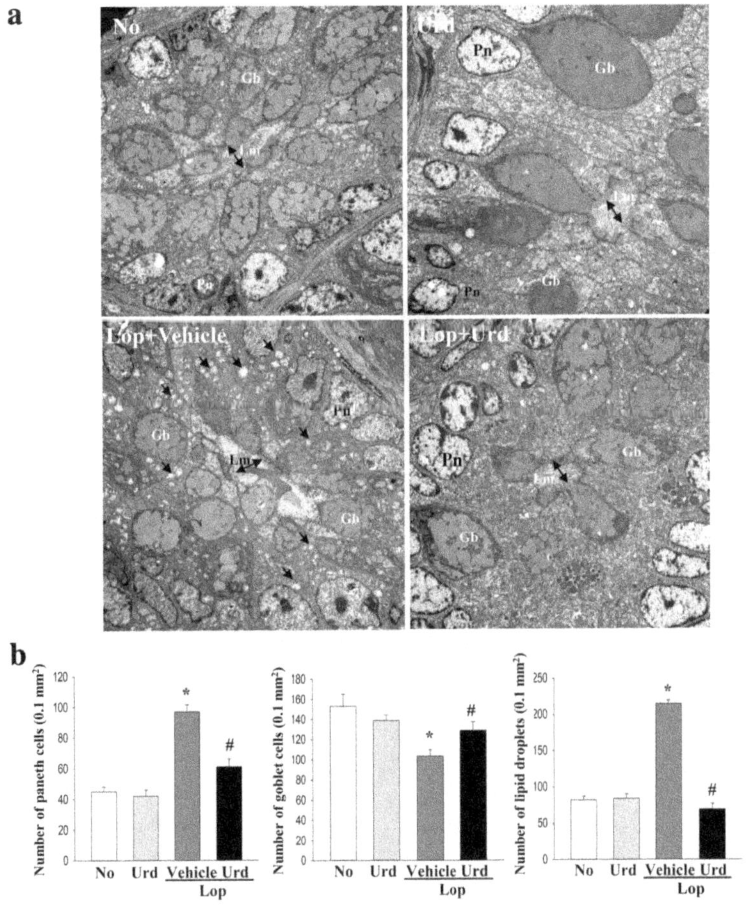

Fig. 2 Ultrastructure image of transverse colon. **a** The ultrastructure of the crypt in the No, Urd-, Lop + Vehicle and Lop + Urd treated group was viewed by TEM at 4000x magnification. **b** The number of paneth cells, lipid droplets and goblet cells was measured using Leica Application Suite (Leica Microsystems, Switzerland). Five to six rats per group were assayed in triplicate by TEM analysis. The arrow indicates a lipid droplet distributed around the lumen of the crypt. Data represent the mean ± SD from three replicates. *, $p < 0.05$ compared to the No treated group. #, $p < 0.05$ compared to the Lop + Vehicle treated group. Lm, lumen of crypt; Gb, goblet cells; Pn, paneth cells

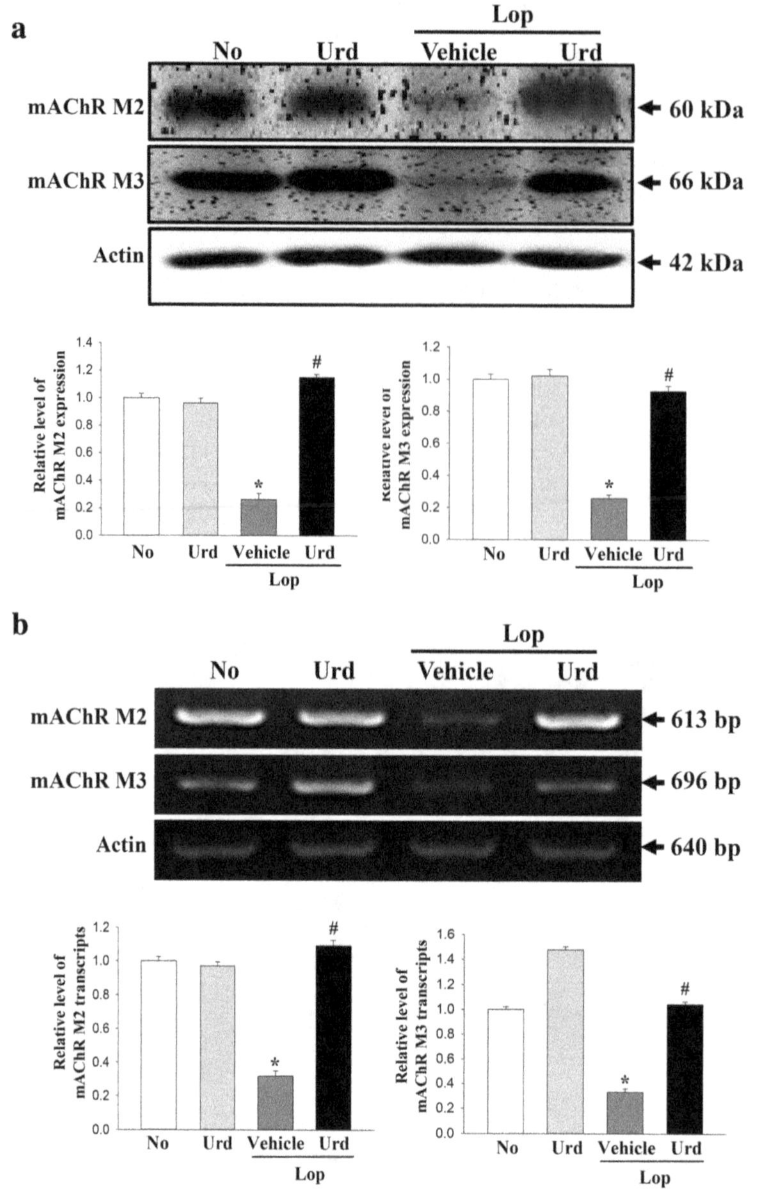

Fig. 3 Expression of mAChRs transcript and protein in the transverse colon. **a** The expression of mAChR M2 and M3 proteins was measured by Western blot analysis using HRP-labeled anti-rabbit IgG antibody. **b** The levels of mAChR M2 and M3 transcripts in the total mRNA of transverse colons were measured by RT-PCR using specific primers. After the intensity of each band was determined using an imaging densitometer, the relative levels of mAChR M2 and M3 were calculated based on the intensity of actin. Five to six rats per group were assayed in triplicate by western blot and RT-PCR assays. Data represent the means ± SD of three replicates. *, $p < 0.05$ compared to the No treated group. #, $p < 0.05$ compared to the Lop + Vehicle treated group

Significant alterations in the expression of downstream of mAChR were also observed. The overall change in all experimental groups was very similar to the changes in the expression of PKC, p-PKC, PI3K and p-PI3K proteins. Specifically, these levels were dramatically increased by 2900 and 300%, respectively, in the Lop + Vehicle treated group relative to the No and Urd treated group. However, their levels significantly recovered in Lop + Urd treated groups, even though the rate of decrease varied (Fig. 4).

Effect of Urd administration on regulation of the ability to secrete mucin

To determine if Urd treatment could enhance the ability to secrete mucin in the transverse colon, the levels of mucin were observed in tissue sections of the transverse

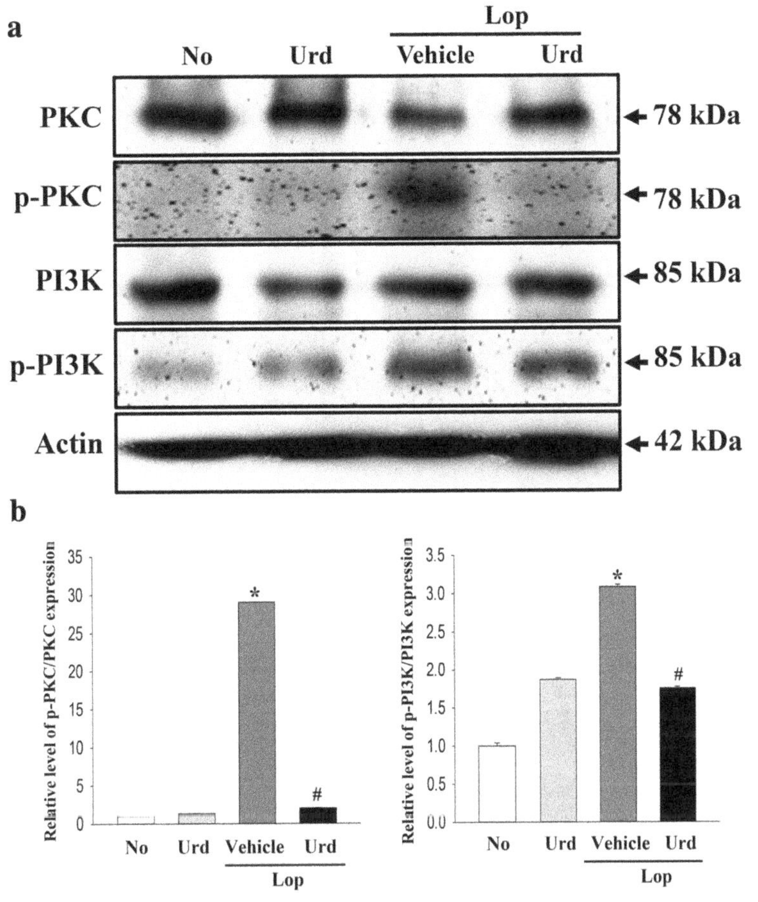

Fig. 4 Expression of key proteins in the mAChR M2 and M3 downstream signaling pathway. The expression of several related proteins including PKC, p-PKC, PI3K and p-PI3K was measured by Western blot analysis using HRP-labeled anti-rabbit IgG antibody. After the intensity of each band was determined using an imaging densitometer, the relative levels of four proteins were calculated based on the intensity of actin protein. Five to six rats per group were assayed in triplicate by Western blotting. Data represent the means ± SD of three replicates. *, $p < 0.05$ compared to the No treated group. #, $p < 0.05$ compared to the Lop + Vehicle treated group

colon stained with Alcian blue. In the No treated group and the Urd treated group, the region stained with dark blue indicating mucin was concentrated into the crypt in the mucosa layer of the transverse colon. The level of mucin was decreased in the Lop + Vehicle treated group and dramatically increased in the Lop + Urd treated group (Fig. 5a). A similar pattern was also detected in the expression level of MUC2 mRNA. The decrease in the level of this gene in the Lop + Vehicle treated group was significantly increased by 165% in the Lop + Urd treated group. Furthermore, we investigated whether mucin secretion induced by Urd treatment was accompanied by altered expression of a membrane water channel by measuring the level of AQP8 mRNA in the transverse colon of subset groups. The level of AQP8 mRNA was very similar to that of MUC2 mRNA. These values decreased by 90.5% in the Lop + Vehicle relative to the No treated group, but AQP8 mRNA was dramatically increased in the Lop + Urd treated groups (Fig. 5b).

Confirmation of Urd effects in pRISMC

Finally, we confirmed the laxative effect of Urd in pRISMCs collected from the transverse colon. The expression of Gα protein was 42% higher in the Lop + Vehicle treated group than the No treated group. However, these levels were dramatically decreased after Lop + Urd treatment (Fig. 6b). Additionally, significant alterations were observed upon analysis of the IP3 concentration. The decrease in IP3 in the Lop + Vehicle treated group was significantly recovered after Lop + Urd treatment (Fig. 6c).

Discussion

Herbal plants and natural products have recently received increased attention as novel therapeutic drugs for

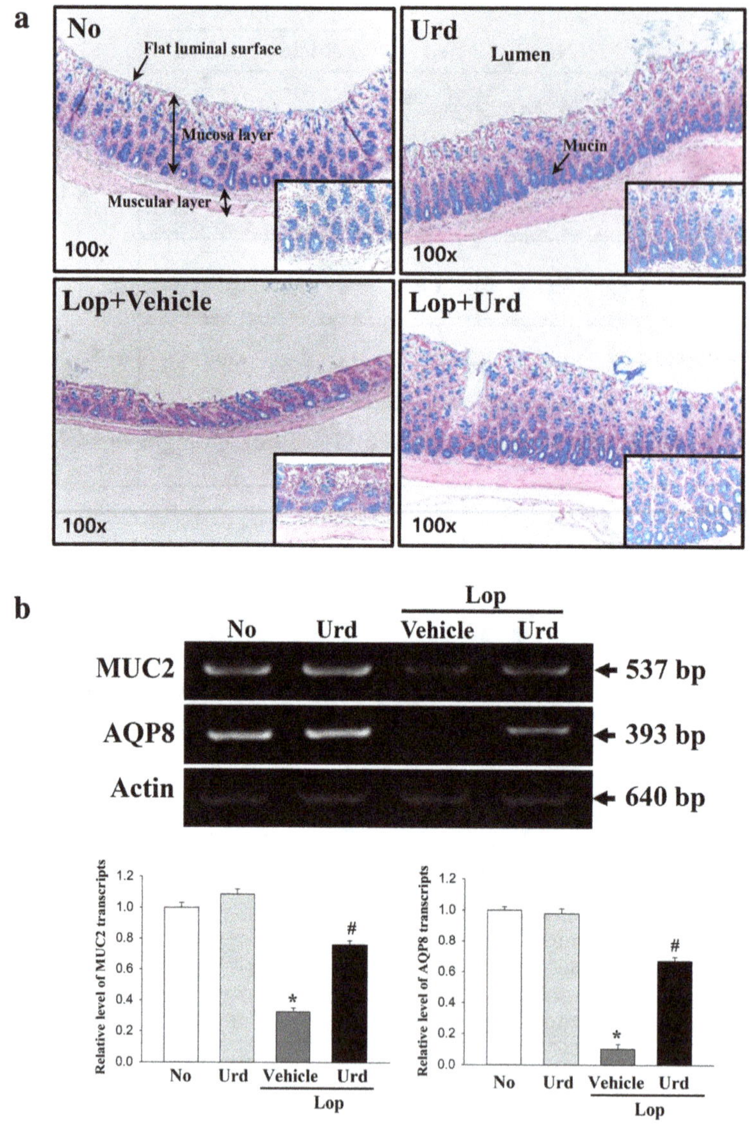

Fig. 5 Detection of mucin secretion and membrane water channel expression. **a** Mucin secreted from crypt layer cells was stained with alcian blue at pH 2.5 and their images were observed at 100x magnification. The high magnification image (200x) is presented in the right corner of each figure. Five to six rats per group were assayed in triplicate by alcian blue staining. **b** The levels of MUC2 and AQP8 transcripts in the total mRNA of transverse colons were measured by RT-PCR using specific primers. After the intensity of each band was determined using an imaging densitometer, the relative levels of MUC2 and AQP8 mRNA were calculated based on the intensity of actin as an endogenous control. Five to six rats per group were assayed in triplicate by RT-PCR assays. Data represent the means ± SD of three replicates. *, $p < 0.05$ compared to the No treated group. #, $p < 0.05$ compared to the Lop + Vehicle treated group

the treatment of constipation and its related diseases because they show a significant possibility for the prevention and treatment of inflammation related diseases [16, 19, 20]. Some studies have been focused on the identification of key compounds involved in constipation although they did not report key compounds with laxative effects. In an effort to identify drugs for the treatment of constipation, we investigated the therapeutic effects of Urd on Lop-induced constipated SD rats because Urd have been detected from extracts of several medicinal plants that have therapeutic effects against some human diseases. These included the aqueous extract of *Isatis indigotica*, which has anti-cancer and anti-viral effects [21, 22], and the extract of *Longan arillus*, which has anxiolytic-like effects [23]. In addition, Urd was detected in the alkaloid extract of *Pinelliae pedatisecta*, which has anti-cancer effects [24]. The results of the present study clearly demonstrated that Urd may induce laxative effects, including elevation of stool excretion and the recovery of histological changes induced by Lop injection in the transverse colon. Our data are the first to demonstrate that the laxative effects of Urd are tightly

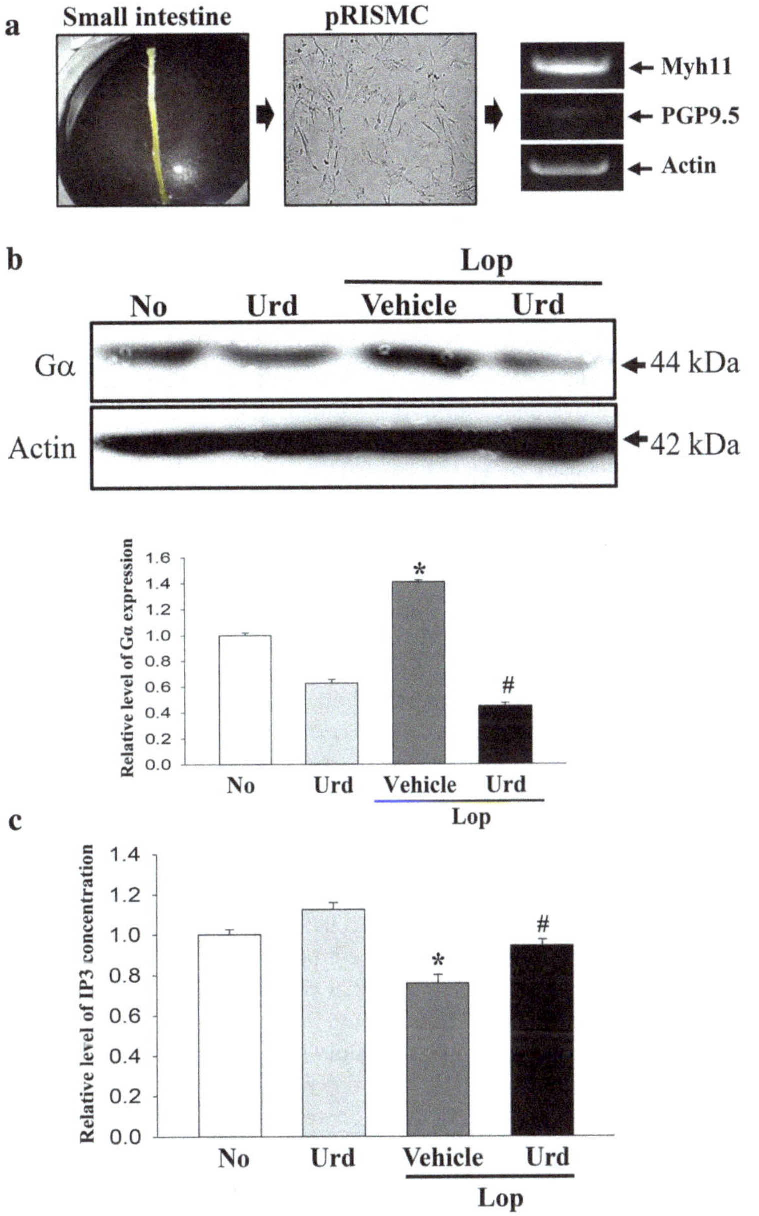

Fig. 6 Detection of Gα expression and IP3 concentration in pRISMC. **a** pRISMCs were collected from the small intestines of infant rats and confirmed by RT-PCR analysis using specific primers. **b** Total cell lysate protein was extracted from Lop-pretreated pRISMC after treatment with the Urd. The levels of Gα expression were detected using specific antibodies. The actin level is also shown as an endogenous control. The band intensity of the three proteins was determined using an imaging densitometer and the relative level of each protein was calculated based on the intensity of actin protein as an endogenous control. **b** After treatment with Lop for 12 h, pRISMC were further incubated with Urd as described in the materials and methods. The IP3 concentration in the total cell lysate was measured using an ELISA kit that could detect IP3 at 5 pg/ml to 1000 pg/ml. Data represent the means ± SD of three replicates. *, $p < 0.05$ compared to the No treated group. $^{\#}$, $p < 0.05$ compared to the Lop + Vehicle treated group

correlated with down-regulation of the mAChRs signaling pathway, up-regulation of the mucin secretion ability and water content capacity in the transverse colon.

Neurobiological roles of Urd have been investigated in many pharmacological studies, but none of these have provided direct evidence of a relationship between Urd and intestinal function [6]. Urd can bypass the blood brain barrier by binding one of two transporters, high affinity transporter (1–50 μM range) and low affinity transporter (100–800 μM range) [25, 26]. Urd also mediates as a novel neurotransmitter via purinergic receptor (P2 receptor) in response to extracellular purine and pyrimidines when it is not providing a substrate for phosphatidylcholine synthesis [27, 28]. It can also induce the creation of membrane and dendrites of neuronal cells through enhancement of phosphatidylcholine levels in the brain as well as neuronal differentiation and outgrowth via activation of NGF signaling [29, 30]. Furthermore, administration of some drugs containing uridine and uridine-5-monophosphate enhanced dopamine output from activated neurons by 11.6–20.5% and improved spatial short term memory, recognition, recall, attention and executive function [30]. Although the above studies suggested that Urd can be potentially used as laxative compounds, there are however, no direct scientific evidence on the therapeutic effect of Urd for chronic constipation. Therefore, the results of the present study provide the first evidence that the laxative effects of Urd may correlate with neuronal functions of the transverse colon. However, more studies are needed to elucidate the molecular mechanism responsible for the effects of Urd against chronic constipation.

Alterations in excretion factors such as number, weight and water contents of stools in Lop-injected rats were dramatically recovered by treatment with herbal medicines such as *Aloe ferox Mill.*, *Liriope platyphylla* and *Mareya micrantha Mull.* [5, 15, 20]. However, the rate of increase varied in each group treated with different herbal medicine. The stool weight was enhanced by 176–272% in rats treated with the aqueous extract of *Mareya micrantha*, while it was increased by 71–143% in the case of *Aloe ferox Mill.* treatment [15, 20]. Moreover, an increase of 52–80% and 86% in the number of stools was measured in the group treated with the aqueous-methanol extract of *Fumaria parviflora* and aqueous extract of *L. platyphylla* (AEtLP) [5, 31]. In our study, the number, weight and water content of stools increased by 77.6, 92.3 and 110.9%, respectively, in the Lop + Urd treated group when compared with the Lop + Vehicle treated group. These findings were similar to those observed for in animals treated with several herbal medicines, although the level of each parameter extended in broad range.

Stool excretion, histopathological structure of colon, mucin secretion and mAChR expression are considered to be important factors for evaluation of constipation symptoms and therapeutic effects of some drugs [5, 15, 16, 32]. However, in the most studies conducted to date, the laxative effects were measured using stool excretion parameters, including number, weight, and water content, as well as histopathological features of the colon including thickness of the villus layer, crypt layer and muscle layer after the administration of various plant extracts [15, 20]. In this study, similar results were detected in the above parameters, although the alteration rate varied in each group. Therefore, these results indicate that Urd administration could improve Lop-induced constipation through stimulation of stool and urine excretion, recovery of the histopathological structure, and mucin secretion. OUr study also investigated the molecular mechanism responsible for the mAChR signaling pathway and mucin secretion in constipated SD rats treated with Urd. The results regarding the effects of Urd on the mAChR signaling pathway and mucin secretion provide basic information that will be useful to future studies of the causes of constipation and selection of targets for constipation treatment.

IP3 can also be considered one of the factors related to bowel movements because it induces increases in intracellular Ca^{2+} levels through a release from the sarcoplasmic reticulum [33]. Smooth muscle tone in the intestine is controlled by phosphorylation of the regulatory light chain (MLC) of myosin II. Ca^{2+}/CaM-dependent myosin light chain kinase and myosin phosphatase regulated this process to control the velocity and force of actomyosin cross-bridging [34]. Therefore, we measured the IP3 level in pRISMC to investigate the effects of Urd response to Lop treatment. The results of the present study suggest that Urd may play an important role in pRISMCs collected from the small intestine of infant rats treated with Lop and that its effects are tightly correlated with those of laxatives that improve chronic constipation.

AQP, which is one of the membrane water channels that control water content in various cells, is connected to several diseases including congenital cataracts and nephrogenic diabetes insipidus [35]. Among several subtypes of AQPs distributed in the intestinal epithelial cells, AQP8 is primarily expressed in the absorptive epithelial cells and localized normally in colonic epithelial cells [36, 37]. The expression of AQP8 was observed as three major patterns based on their pathological condition. In most cases, the expression of this gene is downregulated in experimental colitis [38], inflammatory bowel diseases [38], diarrhea-predominant bowel syndrome (D-IBD) [39], melanosis coli [40], rotavirus-induced diarrhea [41] and ulcerative colitis [42]. However, AQP8 mRNA and protein levels were significantly enhanced in the colon of ulcerative colitis [43] and paraneoplastic normal tissues [44]. Furthermore, AQP8 was not expressed in the colonic mucosa of slow transit constipation rats treated with diphenoxylate solution [45]. In the present study, the level of AQP8 mRNA was significantly decreased in the Lop + Vehicle treated group when compared with the No treated group. This pattern was very similar to that of several bowel diseases, although the decrease rate varied. However, the level of AQP8 in the Lop treated group differed from that of the constipation induced by diphenoxylate solution. It is likely that the observed differences between studies can be attributed to the disease induction mechanism of the compound; however, more studies are needed to understand what other factors determine AQP8 expression.

Lop used in this study is widely applied to induce chronic constipation, including the extension of stool evacuation time and the delay of intestinal luminal transit SD rats and ICR mice through inhibition of water secretion [46] and smooth movement in the intestinal wall [47, 48]. However, this animal model induced by Lop injection could only simulate slow transit constipation among three afflictions categorized in human patients based on assessment of colonic transit and anorectal function; normal transit or irritable bowel syndrome, pelvic floor dysfunction (functional defecatory disorders) and slow transit constipation [49–51]. Therefore, the present study has some limits and restrictions to the clinical translation of results obtained from Lop induced rats to human conditions.

Alterations in endogenous metabolites were also examined in the serum of Lop-induced constipation rats. Among 35 endogenous metabolites, four amino acids (alanine, glutamate, glutamine and glycine) and six endogenous metabolites related to the glycolysis pathway (acetate, glucose, glycerol, lactate, succinate and taurine) were dramatically decreased after Lop treatment [52]. These results provide a possibility that Urd can rescue the Lop-induced constipation by interfering with the balance of metabolites because Urd plays a role in the glycolysis pathway of galactose [53]. However, additional studies are needed to determine if this is the case.

Conclusions

The results of the present study provide the first strong evidence that Urd could induce the recovery of pathological symptoms including excretion parameters, histological structure, ultrastructure mucin secretion and water homeostasis in Lop-induced constipation SD rats. Our results also provide information that will help elucidate the laxative mechanism of Urd on the downstream signaling pathway and expression of mAChRs.

Abbreviations

AQP8: Aquaporine 8; IP3: Inositol triphosphate; Lop: Loperamide; mAChR: Muscarinic acetylcholine receptors; mAChRs: Muscarinic acetylcholine receptors; PI-3K: Phosphoinositide 3-kinase; pRISMC: Primary smooth muscle of rat intestine cells; TEM: Transmission electron microscope; Urd: Uridine

Acknowledgments

We thank Jin Hyang Hwang, the animal technicians, for directing the animal care and use at the Laboratory Animal Resources Center in Pusan National University.

Funding

The experimental design, the preparation of sample, the analysis of animals and the interpretation of results data for this research was mainly supported by Basic Science Research Program through the National Research Foundation of Korea (NRF) funded by the Ministry of Education (2014R1A1A2058360).

Authors' contributions

JEK, JG, JES, HAL, WBY and DYH participated in the design of the study, sample preparation, animal experiments and data analyses. JTH helped with data analysis and manuscript preparation. All authors read and approved the final manuscript.

Competing interests

The authors declare that they have no competing interest.

Author details

[1]Department of Biomaterials Science, College of Natural Resources & Life Science/Life and Industry Convergence Research Institute, Pusan National University, 50 Cheonghak-ri, Samnangjin-eup Miryang-si, Gyeongsangnam-do 627-706, Korea. [2]College of Pharmacy, Chungbuk National University, Chungju 361-763, Korea.

References

1. Walia R, Mahajan L, Steffen R. Recent advances in chronic constipation. Curr Opin Pediatr. 2009;21:661–6.
2. Voderholzer WA, Schatke W, Muhldorfer BE, et al. Clinical response to dietary fiber treatment of chronic constipation. Am J Gastroenterol. 1997;92:95–8.
3. Lembo A, Camilleri M. Chronic constipation. N Engl J Med. 2003;349:1360–8.
4. Busti AJ, Murillo JR, Jr CB. Tegaserod-induced myocardial infarction: case report and hypothesis. Parmacotherapy. 2004;24:526–31.
5. Kim JE, Lee YJ, Kwak MH, et al. Aquous extracts of *Liriope platyphylla* induced significant laxative effects on loperamide-induced constipation of SD rats. BMC Complement Altern Med. 2013;13:333.
6. Gasser T, Moyer JD, Handschumacher RE. Novel single-pass exchange of circulating uridine in rat liver. Science. 1981;213(4509):777–8.
7. Dobolyi A, Juhasz G, Kovacs Z, et al. Uridine function in the central nervous system. Curr Top Med Chem. 2011;11:1058–67.
8. Berg JM, Tymoczko JL, Stryer L. Biochemistry: Glycogen Metabolism. 5th ed. New York: W H Freeman; 2002. Chapter 21.
9. Van Groeningen CJ, Peters GJ, Pinedo HM. Modulation of fluorouracil toxicity with uridine. Semin Oncol. 1992;19:148–54.
10. Van Groeningen CJ, Peters GJ, Pinedo HM. Reversal of 5-fluorouracil-induced toxicity by oral administration of uridine. Ann Oncol. 1993;4:317–20.
11. Van Groeningen CJ, Peters GJ, Nadal JC, et al. Clinical and pharmacologic study of orally administered uridine. J Natl Cancer Inst. 1991;83:437–41.
12. Kimura T, Kimura T, Miki M, et al. Possible existence of a novel receptor for uridine analogues in the central nervous system using two isomers, N3-(S)-(+)- and N3-(R)-(-)-alpha-hydroxy-beta-phenethyluridines. Biol Pharm Bull. 2001;24:729–31.
13. Krooth RS, Hsiao WL, Lam GF. Effects of natural pyrimidines and of certain related compounds on the spontaneous activity of the mouse. J Pharmacol Exp Ther. 1978;207:504–14.
14. Roberts CA. Anticonvulsant effects of uridine: comparative analysis of metrazol and penicillin induced foci. Brain Res. 1973;55:291–308.
15. Wintola OA, Sunmonu TO, Afolayan AJ. The effect of Aloe ferox Mill. in the treatmentet of loperamide-induced constipation in Wistar rats. BMC Gastroenterol. 2010;10:95.
16. Lee HY, Kim JH, Jeung HW, et al. Effects of *Ficus carica* paste on loperamide-induced constipation in rats. Food Chem Toxicol. 2012;50:895–902.
17. Kim BJ. Shengmaisan refulates pacemaker potentials in interstitial cells of cajal in mice. J Pharmacopuncture. 2013;16:36–42.
18. Parajuli SP, Choi SO, Lee J, et al. The inhibitory effects of hydrogen sulfide on pacemaker activity of interstitial cells of cajal from mouse small intestine. Korean J Physiol Pharmacol. 2010;14:83–9.
19. Kakino M, Izuta H, Ito T, et al. Agarwood induced laxative effects via acetylcholine receptors on loperamide-induced constipation in mice. Biosci Biotechnol Biochem. 2010;74:1550–5.
20. Meite S, Bahi C, Yeo D, et al. Laxativeactivities of *Mareya micrantha (Benth.) Müll. Arg. (Euphorbiaceae)* leaf aqueous extract in rats. BMC Complement Altern Med. 2010;10:7–10.

21. Liu R, Yuan B, Liu Z, et al. Identification of 5 constituents of the aqueous extract of *Isatis indigotica* by HPLC-MS2. Zhong Yao Cai. 2005;28(9):772–4.
22. Zou P, Hong Y, Koh HL. Chemical fingerprinting of *Isatis indigotica* root by RP-HPLC and hierarchical clustering analysis. J Pharm Biomed Anal. 2005;38(3):514–20.
23. Okuyama E, Ebihara H, Takeuchi H, et al. Adenosine, the anxiolytic-like principle of the Arillus of *Euphoria longana*. Planta Med. 1999;65(2):115–9.
24. Wang R, Wen Y, Yang L, et al. Chemical constituents of rhizoma *Pinelliae pedatisecta*. Zhongguo Zhong Yao Za Zhi. 1997;22(7):421–3. 447-8.
25. Cornford EM, Oldendorf WH. Independent blood-brain barrier transport systems for nucleic acid precursors. Biochim Biophys Acta. 1975;394(2):211–9.
26. Pastor-Anglada M, Felipe A, Casado FJ. Transport and mode of action of nucleoside derivatives used in chemical and antiviral therapies. Trends Pharmacol Sci. 1998;19(10):424–30.
27. Burnstock G. Physiology and pathophysiology of purinergic neurotransmission. Physiol Rev. 2007;87(2):659–797.
28. Illes P, Alexandre RJ. Molecular physiology of P2 receptors in the central nervous system. Eur J Pharmacol. 2004;483(1):5–17.
29. Spires-Jones TL, Meyer-Luehmann M, Osetek JD, et al. Impaired spine stability underlies plaque-related spine loss in an Alzheimer's disease mouse model. Am J Pathol. 2007;171(4):1304–11.
30. Neary JT, Rathbone MP, Cattabeni F, et al. Trophic actions of extracellular nucleotides and nucleosides on glial and neuronal cells. Trends Neurosci. 1996;19(1):13–8.
31. Rehman N, Mehmood MH, Al-Rehaily AJ, et al. Species and tissue-specificity of prokinetic, laxative and spasmodic effects of *Fumaria parviflora*. BMC Complement Altern Med. 2012;12:16.
32. Sheehan JK, Carlstedt I. Models for the macromolecular structure of mucus glycoproteins. Spec Publ R Soc Chem. 1989;74:256–75.
33. Hofmann F. Smooth muscle tone regulation. In: Offermanns S, Rosenthal W, editors. Encyclopedic Reference of Molecular Pharmacology. Heidelberg: Springer; 2004. p. 870–5.
34. Somlyo AP, Somlyo AV. Ca2+ sensitivity of smooth muscle and nonmuscle myosin II: modulated by G proteins, kinases, and myosin phosphatase. Physiol Rev. 2003;83:1325–58.
35. Yamamoto T, Kuramoto H, Kadowaki M. Downregulation in aquaporin 4 and aquaporin 8 expression of the colon associated with the induction of allergic diarrhea in a mouse model of food allergy. Life Sci. 2007;81(2):115–20.
36. King LS, Agre P. Pathophysiology of the aquaporin water channels. Annu Rev Physiol. 1996;58:619–48.
37. Ma T, Verkman AS. Aquaporin water channels in gastrointestinal physiology. J Physiol. 1999;517:317–26.
38. Te Velde AA, Pronk I, de Kort F, et al. Glutathione peroxidase 2 and aquaporin 8 as new markers for colonic inflammation in experimental colitis and inflammatory bowel diseases: an important role for H_2O_2. Eur J Gastroenterol Hepatol. 2008;20:555–60.
39. Wang JP, Hou XH. Expression of aquaporin 8 in colonic epithelium with diarrhoea-predominant irritable bowel syndrome. Chin Med J. 2007;120:313–6.
40. Liu J, Tian DA, Wang JP, Liu J, Tian DA, Wang JP, et al. Expression of aquaporin 8 and its relationship with melanosis coli. Chin Med J (Engl). 2011;124:3061–5.
41. Cao M, Yang M, Ou Z, et al. Involvement of aquaporins in a mouse model of rotavirus diarrhea. Virol Sin. 2014;29:211–7.
42. Min SB, Le-Carlson M, Singh N, et al. Video capsule endoscopy impacts decision making in pediatric IBD: a single tertiary care center experience. Inflamm Bowel Dis. 2013;19:2139–45.
43. Zahn A, Moehle C, Langmann T, et al. Aquaporin-8 expression is reduced in ileum and induced in colon of patients with ulcerative colitis. World J Gastroenterol. 2007;13:1687–95.
44. Wang W, Li Q, Yang T, et al. Expression of AQP5 and AQP8 in human colorectal carcinoma and their clinical significance. World J Surg Oncol. 2012;10:242.
45. Zhi H, Yuan WT. Expression of aquaporin 3, 4, and 8 in colonic mucosa of rat models with slow transit constipation. Zhonghua Wei Chang Wai Ke Za Zhi. 2011;14:459–61.
46. Hughes S, Higgs NB, Turnberg LA. Loperamide has antisecretory activity in the human jejunum in vivo. Gut. 1984;25:931–5.
47. Sohji Y, Kawashima K, Shimizu M. Pharmacological studies of loperamide, an anti-diarrheal agent. II. Effects on peristalsis of the small intestine and colon in guinea pigs (author's transl). Nihon Yakurigaku Zasshi. 1978;74:155–63.
48. Yamada K, Onoda Y. Comparison of the effects of T-1815, yohimbine and naloxone on mouse colonic propulsion. J Smooth Muscle Res. 1993;29:47–53.
49. Bharucha AE. Constipation. Best Pract Res Clin Gastroenterol. 2007;214:709–31.
50. Shimotoyodome A, Meguro S, Hase T, et al. Decreased colonic mucus in rats with loperamide-induced constipation. Comp Biochem Physiol A Mol Integr Physiol. 2000;126:203–12.
51. Yang ZH, Yu HJ, Pan A, et al. Cellular mechanisms underlying the laxative effect of flavonol naringenin on rat constipation model. PLoS One. 2008;3:3348.
52. Kim JE, Lee YJ, Kwak MH, et al. Metabolomics approach to serum biomarker for loperamide-induced constipation in SD rats. Lab Anim Res. 2014;30(1):35–43.
53. Berg JM, Tymoczko JL, Stryer L. Biochemistry: glycolysis is an energy-conversion pathway in many organisms. 5th ed. New York: W H Freeman; 2002.

3

Risk prediction models for colorectal cancer in people with symptoms

Tom G. S. Williams[1], Joaquín Cubiella[2], Simon J. Griffin[3], Fiona M. Walter[3] and Juliet A. Usher-Smith[3*]

Abstract

Background: Colorectal cancer (CRC) is the fourth leading cause of cancer-related death in Europe and the United States. Detecting the disease at an early stage improves outcomes. Risk prediction models which combine multiple risk factors and symptoms have the potential to improve timely diagnosis. The aim of this review is to systematically identify and compare the performance of models that predict the risk of primary CRC among symptomatic individuals.

Methods: We searched Medline and EMBASE to identify primary research studies reporting, validating or assessing the impact of models. For inclusion, models needed to assess a combination of risk factors that included symptoms, present data on model performance, and be applicable to the general population. Screening of studies for inclusion and data extraction were completed independently by at least two researchers.

Results: Twelve thousand eight hundred eight papers were identified from the literature search and three through citation searching. 18 papers describing 15 risk models were included. Nine were developed in primary care populations and six in secondary care. Four had good discrimination (AUROC > 0.8) in external validation studies, and sensitivity and specificity ranged from 0.25 and 0.99 to 0.99 and 0.46 depending on the cut-off chosen.

Conclusions: Models with good discrimination have been developed in both primary and secondary care populations. Most contain variables that are easily obtainable in a single consultation, but further research is needed to assess clinical utility before they are incorporated into practice.

Keywords: Colorectal cancer, Risk, Model, Symptoms, Prediction

Background

Colorectal cancer (CRC) is the third most common cancer worldwide and the fourth leading cause of cancer-related death [1]. Detecting the disease at an early stage improves outcomes [2]. Whilst screening has been successful in reducing the incidence and mortality of CRC by increasing the proportion diagnosed at an early stage and facilitating removal of pre-neoplastic lesions [3–5], the majority of cancers are still diagnosed after symptomatic presentation [6]. Three previous meta-analyses have shown that individual symptoms, such as rectal bleeding and change in bowel habit, are associated with CRC, but are also common in populations without cancer and so have poor sensitivity for CRC [7–9]. Consequently, identifying which patients from primary care should be referred for diagnostic investigation remains challenging.

Several approaches have been developed to improve the appropriateness of referrals for investigation of symptoms suggestive of CRC and reduce delays in diagnosis. The NHS in England introduced the two-week wait (2WW) referral system in 2000, followed by the NICE suspected cancer referral guidelines in 2005 which have been recently updated [10]. A number of evaluations have shown that the 2WW referral system for suspected CRC has variable sensitivity and low specificity and does not improve diagnostic accuracy [9, 11–16]. In

* Correspondence: jau20@medschl.cam.ac.uk
[3]The Primary Care Unit, Department of Public Health and Primary Care, University of Cambridge, Cambridge CB1 8RN, UK
Full list of author information is available at the end of the article

recent years, several predictive models have been developed to identify people at higher risk of CRC among those with symptoms. These have the potential to improve the consistency and quality of clinical decision-making. However, their strengths, weaknesses and relative performance are uncertain, and few direct comparisons have been made. The aim of this review was to systematically identify and compare the performance of models that predict the risk of undiagnosed prevalent primary CRC for symptomatic individuals.

Methods

We performed a systematic literature review following an a priori established study protocol (available on request) that followed the PRISMA guidelines (see Additional file 1 for the PRISMA checklist).

Search strategy

We used a combination of subject headings including 'colorectal cancer', 'risk/risk factor/risk assessment/chance' and 'prediction/model/score' to conduct an electronic literature search within Medline and EMBASE. The search period ran from January 2000 to March 2014 (see Additional file 2 for the complete search strategy for Medline and EMBASE). We subsequently hand searched the reference lists of all included papers. We also considered for inclusion papers published before 2000 describing the development of models that were validated in included papers.

Study selection

To be included, studies had to be published as a primary research paper in a peer-reviewed journal and either describe, validate or assess the impact of a risk model that allowed identification of people at higher risk of CRC or CRC and advanced colorectal neoplasia. The risk model had to feature two or more risk factors, including symptoms, for prevalent undiagnosed colorectal cancer at the level of the individual. In addition, a quantitative measure of model performance was required. Conference proceedings, papers not in English, and studies of a specific patient group, for example immunosuppressed patients or patients with a past history of CRC, were excluded.

One reviewer (JUS) screened the titles and abstracts of papers identified by the Medline and EMBASE searches to exclude studies that were clearly not relevant. A second reviewer (TGSW) independently assessed a random selection of 10 % of the papers at title and abstract level and both reviewers (TGSW and JUS) independently assessed all the full text of papers if a definite decision to reject could not be made based on title and abstract alone. All reviewers met to discuss discrepancies and reach a consensus decision on inclusion or exclusion.

Data extraction and synthesis

Two reviewers (TGSW and JC) extracted data from each paper using a standardised form. Discrepancies were examined and resolved by a third reviewer (JUS). We extracted information on the components of each risk model and potential sources of bias. These included: study design and participants; methods of model development; and variables included in the risk model. The methods of studies published for each risk model was also classified according to the TRIPOD guidelines (1a-Development only; 1b-Development and validation using resampling; 2a-Random split-sample development and validation; 2b-Non-random split-sample development and validation; 3-Development and validation using separate data; 4-Validation study) [17]. Where multiple models were described within the same study, each model was included separately.

Reported measures of discrimination (area under the receiver operating characteristic curve (AUROC)), accuracy (sensitivity and specificity), calibration and utility were used to compare the performance of different risk models and thresholds in development and validation populations. Numerical values for the AUROC were used to compare discrimination and the sensitivity and specificity to compare the accuracy, of different models and thresholds. For those papers in which sensitivity and specificity were not reported explicitly, where possible we calculated the values from data provided in the paper. Figures were produced using RevMan version 5.3 and where multiple studies reported the sensitivity and specificity of the same model at the same threshold, the combined values were calculated using Meta-DiSc version 1.4.

Quality assessment

Quality assessment was performed at the same time as data extraction. Since our review included studies with different designs we used a checklist based on the Critical Appraisal Skills Programme guidelines for case-control and cohort studies [18] as an initial framework, and then classified each study as high, medium or low quality. No studies were excluded based on quality assessment alone.

Results

Included studies

After duplicates were removed, the search identified 12,808 papers of which 12,765 were excluded at title and abstract level. A further 29 were excluded after full-text assessment by at least two reviewers (TGSW and JUS). There was complete agreement among researchers throughout the screening process. The most common reasons for exclusion were that the papers did not report a statistical measure of model performance ($n = 9$), only evaluated one predictor ($n = 6$), or were conference abstracts

($n = 4$). Three additional papers were identified through citation searching, including one published prior to 2000 which was included as it had been externally validated in one of the papers identified through the literature search. In total we included 18 papers describing 15 risk prediction models in the review (Fig. 1). Only one paper assessed the impact of one of the models in practice [19].

A summary of the quality assessment of each of the 18 papers is given in Table 1. Eleven were assessed as high quality, four as medium quality and three as low quality. The studies assessed as low quality were two cross-sectional studies recruiting patients presenting to either primary or secondary care with rectal bleeding [20, 21], and the single study assessing model impact [19].

Risk model development and validation

Table 1 also summarizes the methods used to develop and validate the models. Of the 15 included models, nine were developed in primary care populations [21–27] and six in secondary care [20, 28–32]. Most ($n = 11$) had CRC as a single outcome, whilst two in secondary care predicted CRC combined with advanced adenoma (a polyp measuring 10 mm or bigger, or a polyp of any size with a villous histology [20]) or pre-malignant adenomas [28]. The remaining two reported CRC risk alongside the risk of cancers of several other sites [26, 27].

Most models were developed from either cross sectional ($n = 6$), prospective cohort ($n = 4$) or case-control studies ($n = 4$), with one developed based on clinical experience [30]. Four used self-administered questionnaires or interviews conducted by non-medically trained staff to gather information. The remaining 11 models required the input of a health-care worker. Nine of the 15 models have been validated: one using bootstrap resampling [32]; two using a random split-sample [26, 27]; and six in external populations [21, 24, 25, 30]. Details of the methods and study populations for the validation studies are also given in Table 1.

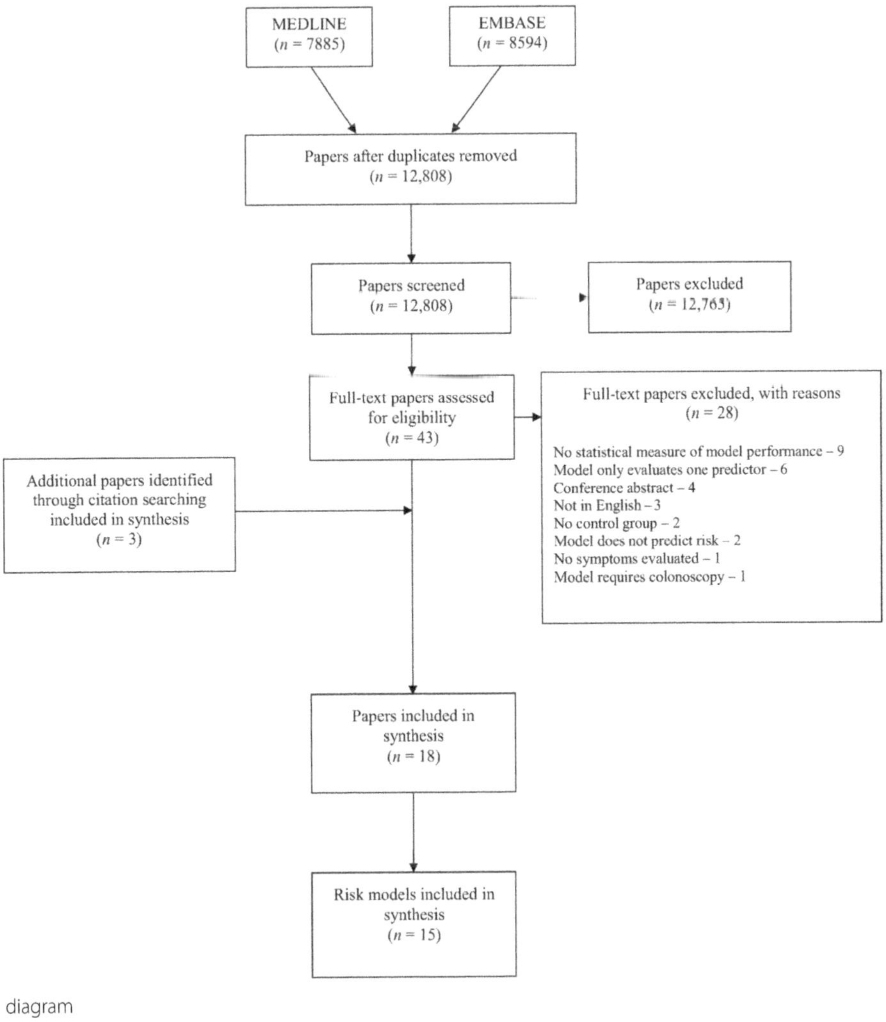

Fig. 1 PRISMA flow diagram

Table 1 Summary of quality assessment and study design for the 18 included papers

Author, date, country, setting	Quality[f]	Outcome	Data collection	Selection of variables	Identification of study population		Identification of outcome cases	Exclusions	Study population	
Model development; Case-control studies										
					Cases	Controls			Cases	Controls
Hamilton, 2005, UK, primary care [22]	M	CRC	Primary care records from 21 practices	Occurring in at least 2.5 % of cases or controls	>40 years with primary CRC	5 controls per case matched for sex, general practice and age and alive at point of case diagnosis	Cancer registry at one hospital	Unobtainable records, no consultations in 2 years before diagnosis, previous CRC, residence outside Exeter at time of diagnosis.	349	1,744
Hamilton, 2009, UK, primary care [23]	M	CRC	THIN database	Literature review	> 30 years with CRC	Up to 7 controls without CRC matched for practice, sex and age	Diagnosis of CRC within study period	< 2 years of full electronic records before date of case diagnosis.	5,477	38,314
Model development and external validation; Case-control study										
					Cases	Controls			Cases	Controls
Marshall, 2011, UK, primary care [24]	H	CRC	BB equation development and CAPER Score external validation							
			See Hamilton, 2009 [23]					As in Hamilton, 2009 plus patients with severe anaemia (Hb < 10 g/dl), rectal bleeding, abnormal rectal examination or positive FOBT, or without any of abdominal pain, weight loss, diarrhoea or constipation	117	433
		CRC	CAPER Score development and BB equation external validation							
			See Hamilton, 2005 [22]							
Model development and random split-sample internal validation; Cohort studies										
									Included	Cases (% of included)
Hippisley-Cox, 2012, UK, primary care (QCancer® (colon)) [25]	H	CRC	QResearch database	'Established predictor variables' and red flag symptoms	30–84 year-old patients registered with practices between 1/1/2000 and 30/09/2010 and without CRC		Incident cancer diagnosis in the 2 years after cohort entry recorded in GP records or ONS cause-of-death record	History of CRC, recorded red flag symptom[f] in the 12 months preceding the study date, or missing Townsend deprivation score.	Development F: 1,172,670 M:1,178,382 Internal validation F: 616,361 M: 620,240	 F:4,798 (0.2 %) M:4,798 (0.2 %) F: 2603 (0.2 %) M:2603 (0.2 %)

Table 1 Summary of quality assessment and study design for the 18 included papers *(Continued)*

Hippisley-Cox, 2013 (female), UK, primary care (QCancer® (combined)) [26]	H	CRC and 11 other cancers[a]	QResearch database	Previous study, and literature review	25–89 year-old patients registered with practices between 1/1/2000 and 1/04/2012 and without CRC	Incident cancer diagnosis in the 2 years after cohort entry recorded in GP records or ONS cause-of-death record	Recorded red flag symptom[f] in the 12 months before the study entry date, or missing Townsend deprivation score.	Development 1,240,864 Internal validation 679,174	 2607 (0.18 %) 1725 (0.25 %)
Hippisley-Cox, 2013 (male), UK, primary care (QCancer® (combined)) [27]	H	CRC and 9 other cancers[b]	QResearch database	Previous study, and literature review	25–89 year-old patients registered with practices between 1/1/2000 and 1/04/2012 and without CRC	Incident cancer diagnosis in the 2 years after cohort entry recorded in GP records or ONS cause-of-death record	Recorded red flag symptom[f] in the 12 months before the study entry date, or missing Townsend deprivation score.	Development 1,263,071 Internal validation 667,603	 3250 (0.26 %) 1356 (0.2 %)
Model development; Cross-sectional studies									
								Included	Cases (% of included)
Adelstein, 2010, Australia, secondary care [32]	H	CRC	Self-administered questionnaire	Not reported	Patients > 18 years old scheduled for colonoscopy at hospitals	Complete colonoscopy and histology	Completion of questionnaire > 6 months before colonoscopy, advanced adenoma[c], incomplete colon evaluation	7,736	159 (2.1 %)
Adelstein, 2011, Australia, secondary care [31]	H	CRC	See Adelstein 2010 [32]				Completion of questionnaire > 6 months before colonoscopy, adenoma[d], incomplete colon evaluation	6943	159 (2.3 %)
Fijten, 1995, Netherlands, primary care [21]	L	CRC	Patient and doctor questionnaires, and blood sample	Literature review	Patients presenting to 83 GP practices with overt rectal bleeding or a history of visible rectal blood loss in previous 3 months.	Medical record review coded using the International Classification of Primary Care for diagnostic classification	Patients aged <18 or >75, pregnancy, urgent admission to hospital or follow-up not available.	290	9 (3.4 %)
Hurst, 2007, UK, secondary care [28]	M	CRC or pre-malignant adenomas	Proforma-based history, examination and blood sample	Not reported	All adult patients referred to a specialist colorectal clinic	Patients tracked until a definitive diagnosis was reached	Patients not further investigated after initial consultation or who did not attend follow up	300	95 (31.7 %)

Table 1 Summary of quality assessment and study design for the 18 included papers *(Continued)*

Lam, 2002, Hong Kong, secondary care [20]	L	CRC or significant neoplasia[e]	Questionnaire conducted by non-medically trained interviewers	Not reported	New patients attending surgical department for rectal bleeding	Rigid sigmoidoscopy and proctoscopy, followed by barium enema or colonoscopy at the physician's discretion	Refusal for colonoscopy or barium enema	174	29 (16.7 %)
Mahadavan, 2011, UK, secondary care [29]	M	CRC	Self-administered questionnaire, history, faecal, blood and rectal samples	Not reported	All patients >40 years referred to a surgical clinic via the 2ww[g] system for colorectal cancer	Incident diagnosis of CRC within 6 months of study entry from primary care or hospital records confirmed histologically	Previous confirmed IBD, GI cancer, investigation of the bowel within the last 6 months or absent rectal sampling result	714	72 (10.1 %)
Model development and external validation; Cross-sectional study									
								Included	Cases (% of included)
Selvachandran, 2002, UK, secondary care (WNS) [30] [h]	H	CRC	Self-administered questionnaire	Not reported	Patients referred by GPs with symptoms suggestive of distal colonic or anorectal disease	Not reported (all patient's received endoscopy)	Not reported	2,268	95 (4.2 %)
Model external validation; Cohort study									
		Model(s) validated						Included	Cases (% of included)
Collins, 2012, UK, primary care [33]	H	QCancer® (colon) (female and male) [25]	THIN database	N/A	30–84 year-old patients registered with practices between 1/1/2000 and 30/09/2010 and without CRC	Incident cancer diagnosis of CRC in the 2 years after cohort entry	Patients with a history of CRC, a recorded red flag symptom[f] in the 12 months preceding the study date, registered <12 months with practice or with invalid dates	Female: 1,075,775	Female: 1,676 (0.15 %)
								Male: 1,059,765	Male: 2,036 (0.19 %)
Model external validation; Cross-sectional studies									
		Model(s) Validated						Included (% of eligible)	Cases (% of included)
Ballal, 2009, UK, secondary care [35]	H	WNS [30]	Self-administered questionnaire	N/A	Patients with colorectal symptoms referred by GPs	A combination of rigid sigmoidoscopy, flexible sigmoidoscopy, colonoscopy or barium enema	Patients thought (on the basis of the referral) most likely to have right-sided CRC, or but did not attend for investigation	3,457	186 (5.4 %)

Table 1 Summary of quality assessment and study design for the 18 included papers *(Continued)*

Hodder, 2005, UK, secondary care [34]	H	WNS [30], Fijten 1995 [21]	Self-administered questionnaire	N/A	Patients referred from primary care with colorectal symptoms	Secondary care investigations - minimum flexible sigmoidoscopy	Not reported	3,302	156 (4.7 %)
Rai, 2008, UK, secondary care [11]	H	WNS [30]	Self-administered questionnaire	N/A	GP referral with any of: lower bowel-related symptoms, unexplained iron deficiency anaemia, positive FOBT, or palpable rectal/ abdominal mass	Follow up during course of hospital investigations until a final diagnosis made	Patients admitted hospital as an emergency and subsequently diagnosed with CRC	1,422	83 (5.84 %)
Model utility; cohort study									
		Model used				Outcome measures		Included	Interviews
Hamilton, 2013, UK, primary care [19]	L	Hamilton 2005 [22]	GP usage and outcomes from practices and local trusts; qualitative interviews	Not reported	Risk assessment tools (RATs) supplied to 614 GPs at 164 practices for 6 months; interviews with GP cancer network leads and sample of GP users from practices with differing patient demographics.	Number of 2WW referrals and colonoscopies for patients >40; symptoms used in RATs; qualitative interview data.	RATs performed on patients <40; RATs that did not identify the reported symptoms.	1433	23 GP responders

CRC colorectal cancer, *ONS* office of national statistics, *FOBT* faecal occult blood test, *IBD* Inflammatory bowel disease, *Hb* haemoglobin, *WNS* Weighted Numerical Score developed by Selvachandran 2002 [30], *RAT* risk assessment tool

[a]Lung, gastro-oesophageal, pancreatic, renal tract, haematological, breast, ovarian, uterine, cervical and other cancer

[b]Lung, gastro-oesophageal, pancreatic, renal tract, haematological, prostate, testicular, and other cancer

[c]Adenoma with significant (> 25 %) villous features, or high grade dysplasia, including carcinoma-in-situ, or size 10 mm or larger

[d]Adenoma of any size or histology

[e]Polyp 10 mm or larger, or a polyp of any size with a villous histology

[f]rectal bleeding, weight loss, abdominal pain, loss of appetite

[g]2WW - Two week wait

[h]The method of developing the WNS is copyrighted and incompletely reported

Variables included in the risk models

We categorized risk factor variables into five types: demographic, personal and family medical history, symptoms, signs, and investigations (Table 2). Seventeen variables were included in three or more models: four demographic variables (age, sex, smoking, alcohol); family history of CRC; eight symptoms (rectal bleeding, change in bowel habit, diarrhoea, constipation, abdominal pain, weight loss, loss of appetite, mucous in the stool); abnormal rectal examination; and three investigations (haemoglobin, mean cell volume, faecal occult blood testing). All models included symptoms, four included only symptoms [22–24], and most also included age ($n = 11$) and sex ($n = 9$). The choice of variable in each model was often influenced by the study design. For example, the Hamilton et al. 2005 risk model [22] and the CAPER score [24] were developed from case-control studies using primary care records and include symptoms plus additional signs and investigations without any demographic information or personal or family medical history. In contrast, the models developed by Adelstein [31, 32] from patient-completed questionnaires include symptoms plus demographic information and personal or family medical history.

Performance of risk models

Accuracy

Sensitivity and specificity were reported for 11 of the 15 models in either development populations ($n = 5$), in random split-sample internal validation ($n = 2$), random split-sample internal validation and external populations ($n = 2$) or in external populations ($n = 2$); for four models these were provided for multiple thresholds. These values are summarized in Fig. 2 in which models are divided into those developed (and validated) in primary care, and those developed (and validated) in secondary care.

At all selected risk thresholds the seven models developed in primary care populations achieved high specificity (range 0.90–0.98), whilst the sensitivity ranged from 0.25 for the QCancer® (colon) model [25] with the threshold set at the top 1 % in internal validation, to 1.00 for the Fijten et al. model developed from a cohort of patients presenting to primary care practices in the Netherlands with rectal bleeding that contained only nine CRC cases [21]. Information on sensitivity and specificity of three models developed in primary care was reported in external cohorts: the CAPER score [24] and the two QCancer® (colon) models for male and female individuals [33]. Whilst all three models had similarly high specificity, the QCancer® (colon) models had higher sensitivity at all thresholds used for external validation and performed better in males then females.

Only one model developed in secondary care, the Weighted numerical scoring system (WNS) [30], has been externally validated. Four studies reported the sensitivity and specificity at four different thresholds (a score of 40, 50, 60 or 70). As expected, the lowest threshold of 40 had the highest pooled sensitivity (0.96 (95 % C.I. 0.93–0.97), $n = 4$ studies) and the lowest pooled specificity (0.40 (95 % C.I. 0.39–0.41), $n = 4$ studies), whilst the threshold of 70 had values comparable to those in primary care with a lower sensitivity of 0.64 (95 % C.I. 0.53–0.74) ($n = 3$) and higher specificity of 0.82 (95 % C.I. 0.81–0.83) ($n = 3$).

Discrimination

The discriminatory performance of 11 of the 16 models was reported as the AUROC. As shown in Fig. 3, these range from 0.83 to 0.97 in model development populations, 0.89 to 0.91 in internal validation studies, and 0.76 to 0.92 in external validation studies. The highest discriminatory performance (AUROC 0.97) was achieved by the model developed by Fijten et al. in patients presenting to primary care practices in the Netherlands with rectal bleeding [21]. However, in an external validation study of the model in secondary care the discrimination fell to 0.78 [34]. The models demonstrating the best discrimination in external validation studies were the BB equation developed by Marshall et al. using a case-control design in the The Health Improvement Network (THIN) database of English primary care records [24] and the QCancer® (colon) male and female models developed from a cohort within the QResearch database of English primary care records [25].

Other performance measures and utility

Three models reported performance as positive predictive values (PPVs): the model by Lam et al. with a combined outcome of CRC or a polyp measuring 1 cm or bigger or any size with a villous histology derived in Hong Kong from a secondary care population in which PPVs ranged from 4.5 to 33.6 % [20], and the models developed by Hamilton et al. in the UK from primary care populations with PPVs ranging from 0.42 to 11 % [22], and from 0.04 to 4.5 % [23].

No studies reported numerical measures of calibration but Hippisley-Cox et al. 2012 showed plots of observed and predicted risk for the male and female QCancer® (colon) models in internal validation and these show overall good calibration [25].

Only one study assessed the utility of a risk model in practice: the risk score developed by Hamilton et al. 2009 [23] was assessed alongside a risk score for lung cancer in 165 UK general practices [19]. Paper, mouse-mat and desktop easel forms displaying the risk models were provided for a six month period. During this time there was an increase in cancer diagnostic activity, urgent referrals and cancer diagnoses when compared with the previous six months but as it was not a trial it is not possible to say whether these changes were due to the use of the risk model.

Table 2 Variables included in risk models and TRIPOD classification of studies examining model performance

Author, year	TRIPOD level[a]	Demographic variables					Personal and Family Medical History		Symptoms				
		Age	Sex	Smoking	Alcohol	Other	Family history of GI cancer	Other	Rectal bleeding	Change in bowel habit	Diarrhoea	Constipation	Abdominal pain
Models predicting gastrointestinal cancers and neoplasms													
Adelstein, 2010 [32]	1b	•	•					Colonoscopy in last 10 years; history of diverticular disease, NSAID use, or aspirin use.	•				•
Adelstein, 2011 [31]	1a	•	•	•		Educat on level.		Colonoscopy in last 10 years; history of colorectal polyps, IBS, NSAID use or aspirin use.	•				
Fijten, 1995 [21]	1a, 4	•							•[d]	•			
Hamilton, 2005 [22]	1a								•		•		•
Hamilton, 2009 [23]	1a								•	•	•	•	•
Hippisley-Cox, 2012 (Male) [25]	2a, 4	•	N/A		•		•		•	•			•
Hippisley-Cox, 2012 (Female) [25]	2a, 4	•	N/A				•		•				•
Hurst, 2007 [28]	1a	•	•	•									•
Lam, 2002 [20]	1a	•							•[e]				
Mahadavan, 2011 [29]	1a	•	•						•				
Marshall, 2011 (BB equation) [24]	3								•	•	•[f]	•[f]	•[f]
Marshall, 2011 (CAPER score) [24]	4										•	•	•
Selvachandran, 2002 (WNS) [30] [c]	4, 4, 4, 4	•	•					'Family history', 'relevant medical history'.	•	•			
Models predicting cancers of multiple organ systems alongside colorectal cancer													
Hippisley-Cox, 2013 (Male) [27]	2a	•	N/A	•	•	BMI; Townsend depr vation score.	•	History of chronic pancreatitis, type 2 diabetes, or COPD; family history of prostate cancer.	•	•		•	•
Hippisley-Cox, 2013 (Female) [26]	2a	•	N/A	•	•	BMI; Townsend deprivation score.	•	History of chronic pancreatitis, type 2 diabetes, COPD, or endometrial hyperplasia/polyps; family history of breast cancer or ovarian cancer.	•	•		•	•

Table 2 Variables included in risk models and TRIPOD classification of studies examining model performance *(Continued)*

Author, year	Symptoms				Signs		Investigations			
	Weight loss	Loss of appetite	Mucous	Other	Abnor mal rectal examination	Other	Haemoglobin[b]	MCV	FOBT	Other
Models predicting gastrointestinal cancers and neoplasms										
Adelstein, 2010 [32]			•	Anaemia[b].						
Adelstein, 2011 [31]			•	Anaemia[b]; fatigue.						
Fijten, 1995 [21]										
Hamilton, 2005 [22]	•				•	Abdominal tenderness	•		•	Blood glucose
Hamilton, 2009 [23]	•						•	•		
Hippisley-Cox, 2012 (Male) [25]	•	•					•			
Hippisley-Cox, 2012 (Female) [25]	•	•					•			
Hurst, 2007 [28]	•									sMMP-9
Lam, 2002 [20]			•							
Mahadavan, 2011 [29]								•	•	eDNA; CEA
Marshall, 2011 (BB equation) [24]	•				•	Abdominal mass	•	•	•	
Marshall, 2011 (CAPER score) [24]	•				•	Abdominal mass			•	
Selvachandran, 2002 (WNS) [30] [c]	•	•		Tenesmus; urgency; incomplete emptying; perianal symptoms; 'abdominal symptoms'; tiredness.						
Models predicting cancers of multiple organ systems alongside colorectal cancer										
Hippisley-Cox, 2013 (Male) [27]	•	•		Abdominal distension; heartburn; indigestion; dysphagia, haematemesis; haematuria; haemoptysis; neck lump; Night sweats; testicular lump; testicular pain; first occurrence of a venous thromboembolism; bruising; cough; impotence; nocturia; urinary frequency; urinary retention.			•			
Hippisley-Cox, 2013 (Female) [26]	•	•		Abdominal distension; heartburn; indigestion; dysphagia; haematemesis; rectal bleeding; haematuria; haemoptysis; neck lump; weight loss; night sweats; breast lump; breast pain; nipple discharge or breast skin changes; inter-menstrual bleeding; post-menopausal bleeding; post-coital bleeding; first occurrence of a venous thromboembolism; bruising; cough.			•			

[a]Types of prediction model studies for each model defined according to the TRIPOD [17] guidelines. 1a – Development only; 1b – Development and validation using resampling; 2a – Random split-sample development and validation; 2b – Nonrandom split-sample development and validation; 3 – Development and validation using separate data; 4 – Validation study

[b]If anaemia was defined by a haemoglobin value, it was considered an investigation. Self-report of anaemia in the absence of a blood test was considered a symptom

[c]Selvachandran 2002 [30] describes a copyrighted model, the Weighted Numerical Score (WNS) that is incompletely reported

[d]specifically blood mixed with/on stool

[e]specifically rectal bleeding independent of straining or defaecation, blood clots, or dark red blood

[f]in addition to documentation of these symptoms, prescriptions used as a proxy. Laxative prescriptions taken to indicate constipation, anti-diarrhoeal prescriptions diarrhoea, and antispasmodic prescriptions abdominal pain

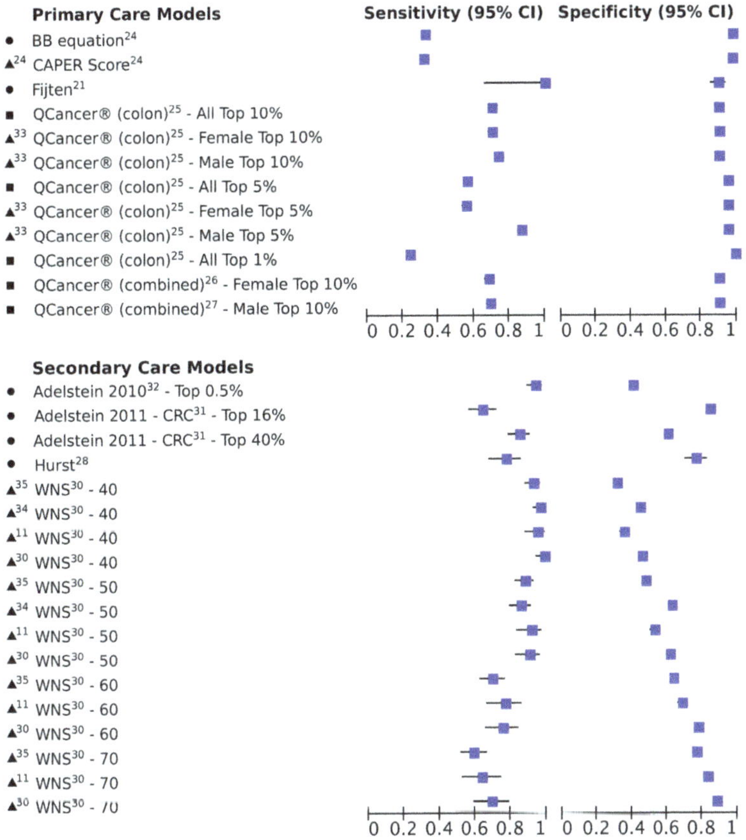

Fig. 2 Sensitivities and specificities of risk prediction models at reported thresholds. • indicates performance in a development population, ■ in an internal validation, and *black triangle* in an external validation (referenced). CRC – colorectal cancer. WNS – weighted numerical score

Comparison with existing guidelines

Although the aim of this review was not to assess the performance of referral guidelines for CRC, five papers [11, 24, 30, 34, 35] simultaneously compared the performance of risk models with that of published guidelines.

Four compared the sensitivity and specificity of the WNS to UK national or regional guidelines (Fig. 4): in three [11, 30, 34] a threshold of 50 or 60 in the WNS had a higher sensitivity and specificity than the guidelines, and in the fourth [35] a threshold of 60 had similar performance to both the NICE consultation guidelines published in 2004 [36] and the 2000 Department of Health [37] guidelines.

Figure 4 also shows Marshall et al.'s [24] study which compared the BB equation and CAPER score to three variations of NICE guidance in the UK THIN primary care database. They found the sensitivity and specificity of both risk models to be similar to the NICE 2005 guidelines [38]; however the authors also report the discrimination and show that both models outperformed the NICE guidelines with AUROCs of 0.83 (BB Equation) and 0.79 (CAPER Score), compared to 0.65 for the best performing interpretation of NICE guidelines. The same study [24] also compared the discrimination of the BB equation, CAPER score and NICE guidelines in a primary care case-control study with participants recruited from 21 practices in the UK. Again, the AUROCs achieved by the BB Equation (0.92) and CAPER Score (0.91) were significantly higher than the best performing interpretation of NICE guidelines (0.76).

Discussion

Strengths and weaknesses

The main strengths of this review are the broad search strategy and the systematic approaches used to identify studies and extract data. However, as with all systematic reviews, our conclusions are limited by the quality of published research. The included studies were heterogeneous in design, setting and duration of follow-up. Additionally, although we only included risk models with published performance data, two only provided positive predictive values, only six have been validated in external populations, and only one has been assessed for clinical utility or impact. This tendency for research into risk prediction tools to focus on model development rather than validation and impact is well documented [39, 40]. Nevertheless, it limits the conclusions that can be made about the potential role of these risk models in clinical practice.

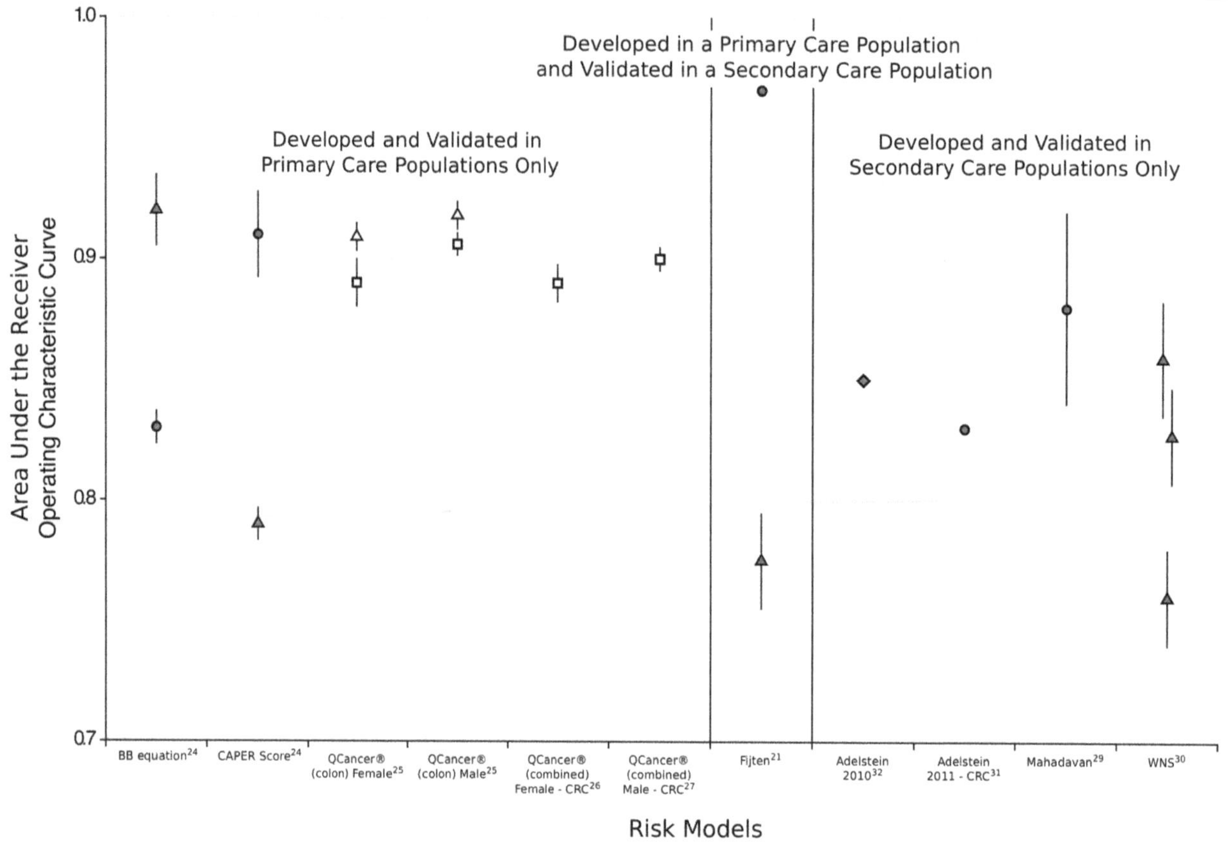

Fig. 3 Area Under the Receiver Operating Characteristic curve of risk prediction models. ● indicates performance in a development population, *black diamond* in bootstrap resampling, ■ in an internal validation, and *black triangle* in an external validation (referenced). Point colours correspond to study design; *red* represents case-control, *green* cross-sectional and *yellow* cohort studies. CRC– colorectal cancer. WNS – weighted numerical score

Comparison between risk models

Where data on discrimination and accuracy was reported there is little to distinguish between the models developed and validated in primary care. The four QCancer® models [25–27] were developed and validated using prospective cohort designs within two large UK primary care record databases, QResearch (development) and THIN (validation). All contain a combination of demographic, symptom, and investigation variables routinely recorded in electronic medical records, and all have AUROCs above 0.89 in either split-sample or external validation, and sensitivities around 0.7 with specificities over 0.95. The BB equation was also developed in the THIN database but using a case-control design [24] and has been validated in a dataset of paper-based primary care records from 21 English primary care practices, whilst the CAPER score was developed from those same primary care records and validated in the THIN database [24]. Both the BB equation and CAPER score performed better in the primary care record dataset, achieving comparable AUROCs and sensitivity and specificity to the QCancer® models. As Marshall et al. [24] describe, reasons for this may include the fact that clinical features of colorectal cancer were identified from both paper and electronic records and included analysis of free text in the primary care record dataset. The use of case-control designs instead of cohort studies for both the development and validation of these risk models, however, means that these measures may not accurately reflect their performance in population based cohorts due to the wide dispersion of risk factors in the cases and controls and the restricted distribution of matched variables.

Additionally none of these models have been validated outside data routinely collected by General practitioners (GPs). It is known that some symptoms are more likely to be recorded by a GP in patients in whom cancer is suspected. For example, patients coded as having a change in bowel habit are at greater risk than those with diarrhoea or constipation [41]. As a result of this coding bias it is likely that the recorded symptoms used in these models overestimate the significance of those symptoms in the presenting population. Whilst all these models in primary care can therefore accurately discriminate between patients in whom GPs have or have not chosen to routinely record these symptoms and could be used to identify those

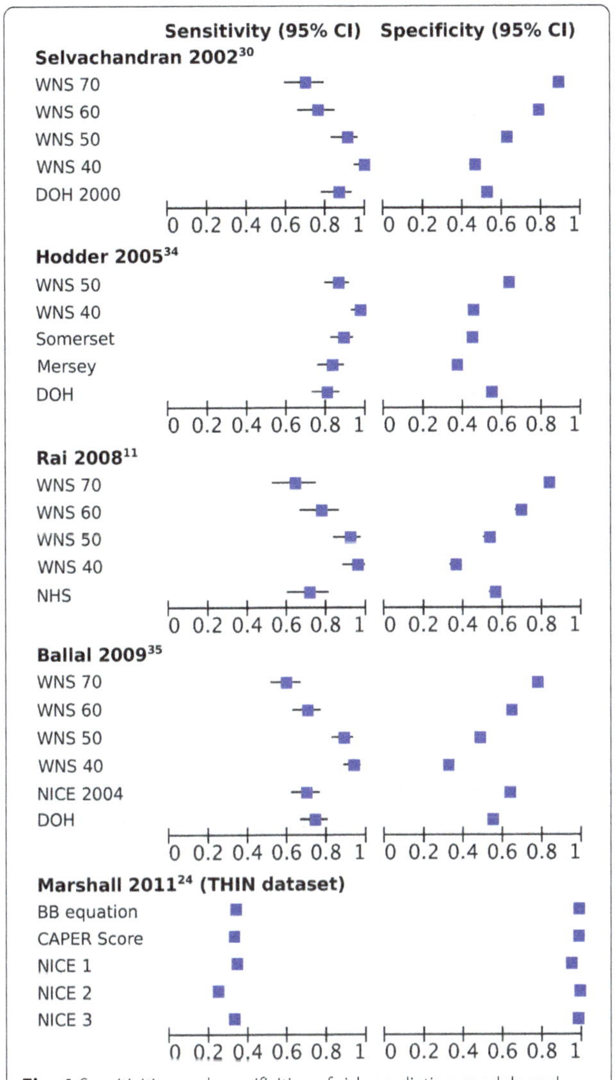

Fig. 4 Sensitivities and specificities of risk prediction models and guidelines within the same population. Highlighted boxes indicate guidelines. In NICE 1, 2 and 3 a score of 1 was given for fulfilling any of the NICE high-risk criteria and a score of 100 for a positive faecal occult blood test (FOBT), abnormal rectal examination or abdominal mass. For NICE 1 a single consultation with diarrhoea or change in bowel habit (CIBH) was assumed to indicate a 6 week change. For NICE 2 two consultations for diarrhoea between 35 and 119 days apart were taken to indicate a change in bowel habit for > 6 weeks (CIBH coding not used). For NICE 3 two consultations for diarrhoea between 35 and 119 days apart, or a single consultation with CIBH, were taken to indicate a change in bowel habit for > 6 weeks. WNS – Weighted Numerical Score developed by Selvachandran et al. 2002 with cut-offs of 40, 50, 60 or 70. DOH – Department of Health

in whom further investigation or referral is necessary, how they perform in the consultation setting when GPs are having to decide whether the patient in front of them does or does not have a given symptom is not known.

Models developed and validated in secondary care settings were instead all based on cross-sectional studies of patients referred with symptoms of CRC with data collected using patient and/or physician questionnaires at the time of investigation. All have similar discrimination (AUROC 0.8 to 0.9) in development populations, but the only model to be externally validated is the WNS developed by Selvachandran et al. [30]. This has been validated in four separate populations with a prevalence of CRC of around 5 %. The AUROCs range from 0.76 [35] to 0.86 [30] and sensitivity and specificity from 0.96 and 0.40 to 0.64 and 0.82. A low threshold, with a high sensitivity, could therefore be used to identify those in whom further investigation is not required. However, all the patients included in these studies had already been assessed as high risk by primary care physicians so the score would be likely to perform less well in an un-referred primary care population, therefore validation in that setting is required.

Implications for clinicians and policy makers

The risk models identified in this review have the potential to improve the diagnosis of CRC by helping clinicians to identify those patients presenting with symptoms of possible CRC in whom further investigation and referral is most appropriate. The potential advantages of risk prediction models in this context are that they can include combinations of symptoms and other risk factors, and different thresholds for action can be used. For example, a threshold with high sensitivity and high specificity could be used to define a high risk patients that require urgent referral, whilst one with very high sensitivity and low specificity could be used to identify those who do not require further investigation at that time.

Sackett and Haynes [42] identified four questions which must be addressed before incorporating diagnostic tests into clinical practice, however. The first three are concerned with test performance: whether test results are different between those with and without the condition; whether patients with certain test results are more likely to have the target disorder; and whether the test results distinguish patients with and without the target disorder. This review shows that risk models for CRC do exist which meet these criteria, with the best performing having sensitivities above 0.7, specificities above 0.9 and AUROCs over 0.9 in external validation studies.

Most contain variables that are easily obtainable in a single consultation and so could relatively easily be incorporated into practice. Whether any of them are any better than a clinician's assessment is, however, uncertain. In the only study to compare a risk model with clinical judgement [30] the WNS was compared to the specialist clinical assessment of a comprehensive questionnaire-gathered history and there was no significant difference in discrimination. There is more evidence to suggest that the models are better than previous referral guidelines. Although not the primary aim of this review, in all cases where models were compared with guidelines the predictive models showed better discrimination and equal or better accuracy [11, 24, 30, 34, 35].

Unanswered questions and future research

This review also cannot answer Sackett and Hayne's fourth question - whether patients undergoing the diagnostic test fare better than similar untested patients. No studies have sought to address that. Before incorporating any of these risk models into practice, further research is therefore needed to validate the most promising models in clinical settings in comparison to clinical judgement and current referral guidelines, and to assess the impact of the use of these risk models in practice. Further work is also needed to consider whether CRC alone or in combination with advanced colorectal neoplasia or adenoma is the most appropriate outcome. This review focused on risk prediction models for CRC and only two models, which both reported only limited performance data and have not been validated, included advanced colorectal neoplasia or adenoma in addition to CRC [20, 28]. It is, therefore, not possible from this review alone to know how the performance of models predicting the combined outcome of advanced colorectal neoplasia and CRC compares to those with CRC as a single outcome. One study, however, reported the performance of risk models for CRC, advanced adenoma, or adenomas 6–9 mm in diameter separately within the same population [31]. The discrimination for the CRC model was substantially better (AUROC 0.87 compared to 0.70 and 0.67 for advanced adenoma and adenomas 6–9 mm in diameter respectively). This probably reflects the fact that many adenomas are asymptomatic and so identified less well by risk prediction models developed in symptomatic populations. The discriminatory performance for advanced adenoma in this symptomatic population is comparable with risk models developed for asymptomatic individuals [43]. This suggests that models with a combined outcome of advanced colorectal neoplasia and CRC may identify those with CRC less well than models with CRC as a single outcome. However, it is widely accepted that CRC arises from the adenoma-carcinoma sequence and so identification of patients with advanced colorectal neoplasia has the potential to reduce future incidence of invasive CRC. The choice of outcome(s) therefore depends on the purpose for which the risk models are to be used. If the priority is identification of patients with prevalent CRC, then a risk model including CRC as the sole outcome is likely to have the greatest discrimination and accuracy and allow targeting of referrals and further investigations most effectively. If the priority is instead to identify both prevalent CRC and those patients at high risk of developing CRC in the future, then a risk model including advanced colorectal neoplasia would be more appropriate.

The introduction of a two-step process into the recently updated NICE referral guidelines [44], in which the referral decision for individuals at intermediate risk is made based on the result of testing for occult blood in faeces, also provides an opportunity for research into incorporating other pre-referral tests into risk models. These include faecal immunochemical tests [16] and potentially more specialised tests, such as exfoliated DNA and carcinoembryonic antigen (CEA), which were of predictive value in secondary care developed models.

From work in other disease areas [45–49] we know that uncertainty about how to account for risk factors perceived to be important but not included in the tools, and the perception that clinical judgement is as good as or better than risk tools, contribute to the low uptake of risk models. Practical issues such as lack of time, poor knowledge or understanding of the tools, and poor computer software also restrict model use. Additionally, a recent study using simulated consultations with risk prediction tools for cancer has shown that clinicians may interpret symptoms inconsistently, leading to inaccurate and unreliable cancer risk assessment, and GPs were reluctant to use the tools for fear of alarming their patients if the risk information is presented too explicitly [50]. Research is therefore also needed to understand how best to incorporate risk prediction models into routine practice, including communication of risk information to patients, and to address the barriers to their use.

Conclusions

To our knowledge this is the first systematic review of risk prediction models for CRC in symptomatic populations. We have shown that 15 models have been developed across both primary and secondary care populations. Many of these have good discrimination (AUROC > 0.85) and most contain variables that are easily obtainable in a single consultation. However, only six have been validated in external populations, and only one model has been assessed for clinical utility in a single before and after study with no control group. Further research is therefore needed before they can be incorporated into routine clinical practice.

Abbreviations

2WW, Two-week wait referral system; AUROC, Area under the receiver operating characteristic curve; BB equation, The Bristol-Birmingham equation; CEA, Carcinoembryonic antigen; CIBH, Change in bowel habit; CRC, Colorectal cancer; DOH, Department of Health; FOBT, Faecal occult blood test; GP, General practitioner; Hb, Haemoglobin; IBD, Inflammatory bowel disease; NICE, National Institute for Clinical Excellence; ONS, Office of National Statistics; PPV, Positive predictive value; THIN, The Health Improvement Network; WNS, Weighted numerical scoring system

Acknowledgements
We thank Isla Kuhn, Reader Services Librarian, University of Cambridge Medical Library, for her help developing the search strategy.

Funding
JUS is funded by a National Institute of Health Research (NIHR) Clinical Lectureship and FMW by an NIHR Clinician Scientist award. JC has received a twinning grant for a stay in the University of Cambridge through the European Commission supported "BIOCAPS" project (FP-7-REGPOT 2012-2013-1, Grant agreement no. FP7- 316265). The views expressed in this publication are those of the authors and not necessarily those of the NHS, the NIHR or the Department of Health. All researchers were independent of the funding body and the study sponsors and funder had no role in study design; data collection, analysis and interpretation of data; in the writing of the report; or decision to submit the article for publication.

Authors' contributions
All authors were involved in the design of the study. TGSW screened papers for inclusion, extracted data, analysed the results and jointly drafted the first version of the manuscript. JUS performed the initial search, screened the papers for inclusion, reviewed extracted data, analysed the results and jointly drafted the first version of the manuscript. JC extracted data, analysed the results and critically revised the manuscript, and FMW and SG analysed the results and critically revised the manuscript. JUS is guarantor for the study. All authors read and approved the final manuscript.

Competing interests
All authors have completed the Unified Competing Interest form at http://www.icmje.org/conflicts-of-interest/ (available on request from the corresponding author) and declare that (1) they have no support from or relationships with companies that might have an interest in the submitted work in the previous 3 years; (2) their spouses, partners, or children have no financial relationships that may be relevant to the submitted work; and (3) they have no non-financial interests that may be relevant to the submitted work.

Author details
[1]School of Clinical Medicine, University of Cambridge, Cambridge, UK. [2]Department of Gastroenterology, Complexo Hospitalario Universitario de Ourense, Instituto de Investigación Biomédica Ourense-Vigo-Pontevedra, Ourense, Spain. [3]The Primary Care Unit, Department of Public Health and Primary Care, University of Cambridge, Cambridge CB1 8RN, UK.

References
1. Ferlay J, Soerjomataram II, Dikshit R, Eser S, Mathers C, Rebelo M, et al. Cancer incidence and mortality worldwide: sources, methods and major patterns in GLOBOCAN 2012. Int J Cancer. 2014;136:E359–86.
2. Cancer Research UK. By stage at diagnosis. London: Cancer Research UK; 2009. Available from: http://www.cancerresearchuk.org/health-professional/cancer-statistics/statistics-by-cancer-type/bowel-cancer/survival#heading-Three.
3. Garborg K, Holme Ø, Løberg M, Kalager M, Adami HO, Bretthauer M. Current status of screening for colorectal cancer. Ann Oncol. 2013;24:1963–72.
4. Cotterchio M, Manno M, Klar N, McLaughlin J, Gallinger S. Colorectal screening is associated with reduced colorectal cancer risk: A case-control study within the population-based ontario familial colorectal cancer registry. Cancer Causes Control. 2005;16:865–75.
5. Edwards BK, Ward E, Kohler BA, Eheman C, Zauber AG, Anderson RN, et al. Annual report to the nation on the status of cancer, 1975-2006, featuring colorectal cancer trends and impact of interventions (risk factors, screening, and treatment) to reduce future rates. Cancer. 2010;116(3): 544–73. doi:10.1002/cncr.24760.
6. Mansouri D, McMillan DC, Crearie C, Morrison DS, Crighton EM, Horgan PG. Temporal trends in mode, site and stage of presentation with the introduction of colorectal cancer screening: a decade of experience from the West of Scotland. Cancer: Br. J; 2015.
7. Ford AC, Veldhuyzen van Zanten SJO, Rodgers CC, Talley NJ, Vakil NB, Moayyedi P. Diagnostic utility of alarm features for colorectal cancer: systematic review and meta-analysis. Gut. 2008;57:1545–53.
8. Astin M, Griffin T, Neal RD, Rose P, Hamilton W. The diagnostic value of symptoms for colorectal cancer in primary care. Br J Gen Pract. 2011;61(586):e231–43.
9. Jellema P, van der Windt DAWM, Bruinvels DJ, Mallen CD, van Weyenberg SJB, Mulder CJ, et al. Value of symptoms and additional diagnostic tests for colorectal cancer in primary care: systematic review and meta-analysis. BMJ. 2010;340:c1269. doi:10.1136/bmj.c1269.
10. National Institute for Health and Care Excellence. NICE Guidelines [NG12] Suspected cancer: recognition and referral [Internet]. Available from: https://www.nice.org.uk/guidance/ng12. Accessed 28 Aug 2015.
11. Rai S, Ballal M, Thomas WM, Miller AS, Jameson JS, Steward WP. Assessment of a patient consultation questionnaire-based scoring system for stratification of outpatient risk of colorectal cancer. Br J Surg. 2008;95:369–74.
12. Chohan DPK, Goodwin K, Wilkinson S, Miller R, Hall NR. How has the "two-week wait" rule affected the presentation of colorectal cancer? Colorectal Dis. 2005;7:450–3.
13. Thorne K, Hutchings HA, Elwyn G. The effects of the Two-Week Rule on NHS colorectal cancer diagnostic services: a systematic literature review. BMC Health Serv Res. 2006;6:43.
14. Shabbir J, Vijayan V, Silavant M, Fowler AL, Cook TA, Lucarotti ME. Two week rule referral for patients with colorectal cancer below the age of 50; Are we being ageist? Surg. 2009;7:276–81. Royal College of Surgeons of Edinburgh and Royal College of Surgeons in Ireland.
15. Zafar A, Mak T, Whinnie S, Chapman MAS. The 2-week wait referral system does not improve 5-year colorectal cancer survival. Colorectal Dis. 2012;14:e177–80.
16. Cubiella J, Salve M, Díaz-Ondina M, Vega P, Alves MT, Iglesias F, et al. Diagnostic accuracy of faecal immunochemical test for colorectal cancer in symptomatic patients: comparison with NICE and SIGN referral criteria. Colorectal Dis. 2014.
17. Collins GS, Reitsma JB, Altman DG, Moons KGM. Transparent Reporting of a multivariable prediction model for Individual Prognosis Or Diagnosis (TRIPOD): The TRIPOD Statement. Ann Intern Med. 2015;162:55–63.
18. Critical Appraisal Skills Programme. Available from http://www.casp-uk.net/#!casp-tools-checklists/c18f8
19. Hamilton W, Green T, Martins T, Elliott K, Rubin G, Macleod U. Evaluation of risk assessment tools for suspected cancer in general practice: a cohort study. Br J Gen Pract. 2013;63:e30–6.
20. Lam DIY, Choy CLY, Lam SCW, Kwok SPY. Age and symptoms as a triage method for per-rectal bleeding. Ann Coll Surg Hong Kong. 2002;6:77–82.
21. Fijten GH, Starmans R, Muris JW, Schouten HJ, Blijham GH, Knottnerus JA. Predictive value of signs and symptoms for colorectal cancer in patients with rectal bleeding in general practice. Fam Pract. 1995;12:279–86.
22. Hamilton W, Round A, Sharp D, Peters TJ. Clinical features of colorectal cancer before diagnosis: a population-based case-control study. Br J Cancer. 2005;93:399–405.
23. Hamilton W, Lancashire R, Sharp D, Peters TJ, Cheng K, Marshall T. The risk of colorectal cancer with symptoms at different ages and between the sexes: a case-control study. BMC Med. 2009;7:17.
24. Marshall T, Lancashire R, Sharp D, Peters TJ, Cheng KK, Hamilton W. The diagnostic performance of scoring systems to identify symptomatic colorectal cancer compared to current referral guidance. Gut. 2011;60:1242–8.
25. Hippisley-Cox J, Coupland C. Identifying patients with suspected colorectal cancer in primary care: Derivation and validation of an algorithm. Br J Gen Pract. 2012;62:29–37.
26. Hippisley-Cox J, Coupland C. Symptoms and risk factors to identify women with suspected cancer in primary care: derivation and validation of an algorithm. Br J Gen Pract. 2013;63:e11–21.
27. Hippisley-Cox J, Coupland C. Symptoms and risk factors to identify men with suspected cancer in primary care: derivation and validation of an

algorithm. Br J Gen Pract. 2013;63:e1–10.
28. Hurst NG, Stocken DD, Wilson S, Keh C, Wakelam MJO, Ismail T. Elevated serum matrix metalloproteinase 9 (MMP-9) concentration predicts the presence of colorectal neoplasia in symptomatic patients. Br J Cancer. 2007;97:971–7.
29. Mahadavan L, Loktionov A, Daniels IR, Shore A, Cotter D, Llewelyn AH, et al. Exfoliated colonocyte DNA levels and clinical features in the diagnosis of colorectal cancer: a cohort study in patients referred for investigation. Colorectal Dis. 2012;14:306–13.
30. Selvachandran SN, Hodder RJ, Ballal MS, Jones P, Cade D. Prediction of colorectal cancer by a patient consultation questionnaire and scoring system: A prospective study. Lancet. 2002;360:278–83.
31. Adelstein B-A, Macaskill P, Turner RM, Katelaris PH, Irwig L. The value of age and medical history for predicting colorectal cancer and adenomas in people referred for colonoscopy. BMC Gastroenterol. 2011;11:97.
32. Adelstein BA, Irwig L, MacAskill P, Turner RM, Chan SF, Katelaris PH. Who needs colonoscopy to identify colorectal cancer? Bowel symptoms do not add substantially to age and other medical history. Aliment Pharmacol Ther. 2010;32:270–81.
33. Collins GS, Altman DG. Identifying patients with undetected colorectal cancer: an independent validation of QCancer (Colorectal). Br J Cancer. 2012;107:260–5.
34. Hodder RJ, Ballal M, Selvachandran SN, Cade D. Pitfalls in the construction of cancer guidelines demonstrated by the analysis of colorectal referrals. Ann R Coll Surg Engl. 2005;87:419–26.
35. Ballal MS, Selvachandran SN, Maw A. Use of a patient consultation questionnaire and weighted numerical scoring system for the prediction of colorectal cancer and other colorectal pathology in symptomatic patients: A prospective cohort validation study of a Welsh population. Color Dis. 2010;12:407–14.
36. National Institute for Health and Care Excellence. Referral guidelines for suspected cancer, Draft for first consultation. 2004.
37. Department of Health. Referral Guidelines for Suspected Colorectal Cancer. NHS Exec. Heal. Serv. Circ. 2000;19.
38. National Institute for Health and Care Excellence. Referral guidelines for suspected cancer (CG27). 2005.
39. Moons KGM, Kengne AP, Grobbee DE, Royston P, Vergouwe Y, Altman DG, et al. Risk prediction models: II. External validation, model updating, and impact assessment. Heart. 2012;98:691–8.
40. Toll DB, Janssen KJM, Vergouwe Y, Moons KGM. Validation, updating and impact of clinical prediction rules: a review. J Clin Epidemiol. 2008;61:1085–94.
41. Jones R, Latinovic R, Charlton J, Gulliford MC. Alarm symptoms in early diagnosis of cancer in primary care: cohort study using General Practice Research Database. BMJ. 2007;334:1040.
42. Sackett DL, Haynes RB. The architecture of diagnostic research. BMJ. 2002; 324:539–41.
43. Usher-Smith JA, Walter FM, Emery J, Win AK, Griffin SJ. Risk prediction models for colorectal cancer: a systematic review. Cancer Prev Res (Phila). 2015;9(1):13–26. doi:10.1158/1940-6207.
44. National Institute for Health and Care Excellence. Suspected cancer : recognition and referral (NG12). 2015.
45. Van Steenkiste B, Van Der Weijden T, Stoffers HEJH, Grol R. Barriers to implementing cardiovascular risk tables in routine general practice. Scand J Prim Health Care. 2004;22:32–7.
46. Bonner C, Jansen J, McKinn S, Irwig L, Doust J, Glasziou P, et al. General practitioners' use of different cardiovascular risk assessment strategies: a qualitative study. Med J Aust. 2013;199:485–9.
47. Torley D, Zwar N, Comino EJ, Harris M. GPs' views of absolute cardiovascular risk and its role in primary prevention. Aust Fam Physician. 2005;34:503–4. 507.
48. Müller-Riemenschneider F, Holmberg C, Rieckmann N, Kliems H, Rufer V, Müller-Nordhorn J, et al. Barriers to routine risk-score use for healthy primary care patients: survey and qualitative study. Arch Intern Med. 2010;170:719–24.
49. Schmieder RE, Goebel M, Bramlage P. Barriers to cardiovascular risk prevention and management in Germany-an analysis of the EURIKA study. Vasc Health Risk Manag. 2012;8:177–86.
50. Chiang PPC, Glance D, Walker J, Walter FM, Emery JD. Implementing a QCancer risk tool into general practice consultations: an exploratory study using simulated consultations with Australian general practitioners. Br J Cancer. 2015;112:1–7.

4

Patients with longstanding ulcerative colitis in remission do not have more irritable bowel syndrome-like symptoms than controls

D. Lundgren[1*], J. Rutegård[2], V. Eklöf[3], R. Palmqvist[3] and P. Karling[1]

Abstract

Background: Irritable bowel syndrome (IBS) is more common in patients with ulcerative colitis (UC) than expected. The prevalence of IBS in patients with UC with longstanding disease is not known. We investigated the prevalence of IBS-like symptoms in patients with UC in remission and longstanding disease in comparison to control subjects.

Methods: Sixty-eight patients with UC and 33 patients with hereditary familiar colon cancer and who underwent colonoscopy surveillance were included. Faecal calprotectin (FC), Gastrointestinal Symptoms Rating Scale-Irritable Bowel Syndrome (GSRS-IBS) and Hospital Anxiety and Depression scale were fulfilled prior to endoscopy. UC in remission was define by steroid-free clinical remission, a Mayo Score ≤ 1 on endoscopy, a FC ≤ 200 μg/g and no significant active inflammation on colon biopsies.

Results: Fifty-five UC patients met the criteria for being in remission. The median disease duration was 17 years. The patients with UC in remission tended to have lower scores on total GSRS-IBS score (6 vs 10.5; $p = 0.062$) and lower or equal scores on all specific IBS symptoms in comparison to controls. There was a moderate but significant correlation between diarrhoea scores and FC levels (in the span ≤ 200 μg/g) (rs 0.38; $p = 0.004$) in the UC in remission group.

Conclusion: Patients with UC with longstanding disease and in remission do not have more IBS symptoms than controls. In UC patients in remission the FC level in the lower span showed a moderate correlation to symptoms of diarrhoea.

Keywords: Irritable bowel syndrome, Inflammatory bowel disorder, Ulcerative Colitis

Background

Ulcerative colitis (UC) is a chronic inflammatory bowel disease affecting the colon and rectum with an annual incidence of 9–20 per 100 000 in the western population [1, 2]. The natural history of UC is episodic with quiescent periods interspersed with active flare-ups. Although most patients have a decrease in symptoms over time [3] UC is a lifelong condition with potentially negative impacts on the quality of life [4]. Even in patients with UC in objective remission gastrointestinal symptoms are common. A meta-analysis showed that approximately 30% of patients with UC in remission reported irritable bowel syndrome (IBS)-like symptoms [5], which is more than twice as high as the prevalence in a normal population [6]. However there is some evidence that IBS-like symptoms in patients with UC may be due to inflammatory activity that is not apparently seen on endoscopy. For example, UC patients in remission with IBS-like symptoms had higher levels of calprotectin in faeces than patients without IBS symptoms [7]. Most studies investigating the occurrence of IBS-like symptoms in patients with UC in remission have defined remission using either clinical or endoscopic scores [5], and only a few studies have investigated IBS-like symptoms in patients using more strict criteria for remission (based on endoscopic and faecal markers) [8]. A faecal calprotectin (FC) cut-off level of 50–150 μg/g helps to discriminate patients with functional gastrointestinal

* Correspondence: david.lundgren@vll.se
[1]Department of Public Health and Clinical Medicine, Division of Medicine, Umeå University, SE-90187 Umeå, Sweden
Full list of author information is available at the end of the article

disease from those patients with inflammatory bowel disorder (IBD) [9, 10].

To date, we lack a consensus on how to define remission in patients with UC using faecal markers. A FC of approximately 120–200 μg/g has been suggested [11–13].

The patients included in previous studies investigating IBS-like symptoms in patients with UC have either had a short duration of the disease or there has been a mixture of patients with short and long duration [5, 8, 14]. Currently, there is a lack of data in the literature regarding what happens over time with IBS symptoms in patients with UC. Do patients with longstanding UC continue to have significant IBS-like symptoms? The primary aim of this study was to compare the prevalence of functional gastrointestinal symptoms including IBS-like symptoms in patients with UC in remission (with a more accurate assessment of remission) and longstanding disease with control subjects. Secondary aims were to investigate whether low-grade inflammation (in the span of a FC < 200 μg/L) correlates with IBS-like symptoms, and to determine whether symptoms of anxiety and depression have an impact on IBS-like symptoms.

Methods

Patients and control subjects

Between May 2007 to February 2013 all patients with UC who underwent a surveillance colonoscopy at the endoscopy unit at Umeå University hospital were invited to participate in the study ($n = 216$). At our clinic all patients with an extensive UC are invited to enter a surveillance colonoscopy program for ten years after diagnosis with the aim to detect dysplasia and early cancer. Control subjects were recruited from patients who underwent a surveillance colonoscopy due to hereditary familiar colon cancer.

Both patients and controls were sent an informed consent, questionnaires and a faecal calprotectin test 4–6 weeks before the planned colonoscopy.

Questionnaires

The Gastrointestinal Symptom Rating Scale-IBS (GSRS-IBS) was used to evaluate IBS-like symptoms. GSRS-IBS is a validated self-assessment instrument for assessing IBS symptoms and it consists of 13 items, each using a Likert scale (0–6 points) spanning from no symptoms to very severe symptoms [15, 16]. The items are grouped into symptom clusters for abdominal pain (two items), bloating (three items), constipation (two items), diarrhoea (four items) and satiety (two items).

In addition to the GSRS-IBS, the study subjects provided information about concurrent medications, previous operations and filled in the Hospital Anxiety and Depression Scale (HADS). HADS is a validated instrument originally designed to screen for symptoms of anxiety and depression among patients with somatic disease [17, 18]. It consists of 7 four-point Likert items each for anxiety and depression. We used the HADS because it exhibits high sensitivity in detecting symptoms of anxiety and depression, it is thoroughly validated, it is easy to fill in, and we have used it in previous research addressing the relationship between anxiety and depression with gastrointestinal symptoms [19].

Faecal Calprotectin (FC)

Calprotectin is a calcium and zinc binding protein. It is mainly found in the cytoplasm of neutrophils but is also an abundant protein in monocytes and macrophages [20]. FC is resistant to bacterial degradation and is stable in stool at room temperature up to 7 days. FC correlates well with gut inflammation and is an established marker used for screening and for monitoring patients with IBD [21, 22]. In the present study the samples for FC were sent to the accredited Department of Laboratory Medicine, Clinical Chemistry, Umeå University Hospital, and were analysed using the CALPRO® Calprotectin ELISA Test (ALP) according to the manufacturer (Calpro AS, Norway). The study participants were asked to collect the stool sample the day before the bowel preparations for the colonoscopy were scheduled.

Colonoscopy

The colonoscopy was performed as clinical routine and by different endoscopists. At least 18 biopsies from a minimum of nine locations were taken in each patient, and the specimens were judged by experienced pathologists. All endoscopists and pathologists were blinded by the outcome of questionnaires and the level of the FC.

Definition of UC remission

The patients were defined as being in remission if all of the following four criteria were met: no present flare-up or steroid treatment, a Mayo Score ≤ 1 on endoscopy [23], a FC ≤ 200 μg/g, and no significant active inflammation on colon biopsies. No significant active inflammation on colon biopsies was defined as inactive (no granulocytic reaction was found either in epithelial or stromal compartments) or mild (existence of pericryptitis and eventually a few granulocytes in crypt, and/or surface epithelium) [24]. Records from the departments of medicine, surgery and endoscopy units were checked to confirm UC diagnosis, to establish clinical remission and to confirm that the colonoscopy was performed in the surveillance program. The records of the control subjects were searched to exclude a coincident gastrointestinal disease (including a change in bowel habits the year before the endoscopy) and that the colonoscopy was performed in the surveillance program.

Exclusion

During the study period 216 patients with UC were in the surveillance program, and 80 patients accepted to participate in the study. Eleven patients were excluded due to missing FC tests, one patient was excluded due to a recent liver transplantation, and 13 patients did not meet the criteria for being in remission thus resulting in 55 patients with UC for analysis (Fig. 1). Forty-two control subjects accepted to participate in the study and 9 of these were excluded due to missing FC tests, thus resulting in 33 control subjects for the analysis.

Statistical analysis

SPSS (version 22) was used for data analysis. Student *t*-test was used for parametric comparisons. Mann-Whitney U non-parametric test was used to evaluate differences between groups. The Spearman non-parametric test was used to evaluate correlations. All tests were 2-sided and with a 5% significance level.

Results

Basal characteristics

Table 1 shows the basal characteristics of patients and controls and the Montreal classification [25] for the patients. In comparison to the control subjects, there were significantly fewer women among the patients with UC in remission. The patients with UC in remission had low levels of FC but still significantly higher FC levels than the control subjects.

IBS-like symptoms in patients with UC and controls

There was no difference in the total GSRS-IBS scores between patients with UC in remission and controls (Table 2). Symptoms of constipation were significantly higher in the controls in comparison to the UC patients in remission but there were no differences in the other symptom clusters.

Correlations between faecal calprotectin and IBS-like symptoms

There was no significant correlation between FC levels and total GSRS-IBS score in patients with UC in remission (Table 3). When analysing the different symptom clusters there was a significant correlation between FC and symptoms of diarrhoea in the patients with UC in remission. In the control group there were no statistically significant correlations between FC and total GSRS-IBS scores or any of the symptom clusters in the control group.

Correlation between IBS-like symptoms and symptoms of anxiety/depression

There were significant correlations between total GSRS-IBS score and both HADS subscores (anxiety and depression) in the patients with UC in remission (Table 4). The strongest correlation was between anxiety and bloating followed by anxiety-constipation, depression-satiety and anxiety-diarrhoea. In the control subjects there were no significant correlations between GSRS-IBS scores and HADS scores, although there were borderline significant correlations between anxiety-bloating and anxiety-satiety.

Discussion

IBS-like symptoms are common in patients with UC with active and inactive disease [5]. However, the present study shows that patients with longstanding disease in remission do not have more IBS symptoms than control subjects. The IBSEN study described the natural course of UC during a five year period after diagnosis, and found that a majority of the patients had a decrease in disease activity over time [3]. Our study may indicate that IBS-like symptoms also diminish over time. Although poorly described in most previous studies, the disease duration in UC patients in

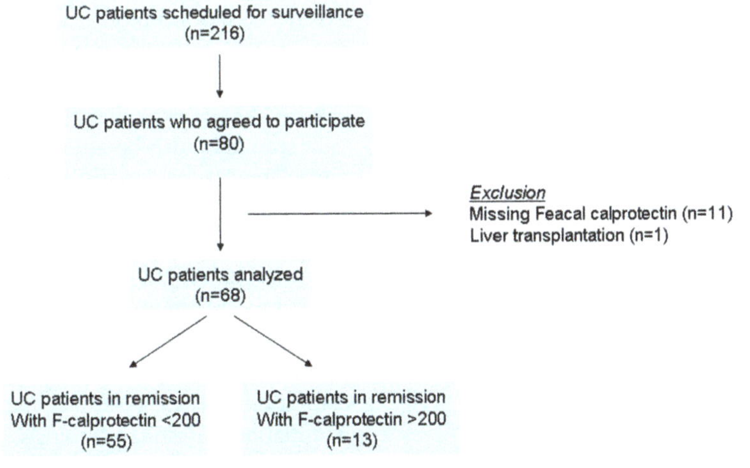

Fig. 1 Flow diagram for the selection of the patients with ulcerative colitis

Table 1 Basal characteristics: Patients with ulcerative colitis in remission and controls

	Ulcerative colitis in remission ($n = 55$)	Controls ($n = 33$)	*p*-value
Mean age years (SD)	49 (14.2)	52 (10.2)	0.27
Women	45%	60%	0.03*
Median disease duration in years (IQR)	17.5 (17)		
Montreal classification:			
A1	18%		
A2	67%		
A3	15%		
E1	0%		
E2	20%		
E3	80%		
5-ASA	85%		
Immune modulators	20%		
Biologics	2%		
Median fecal calprotectin µg/g (IQR)	37 (42)	21 (18)	<0.02*

*Statistically significant
Ulcerative colitis in remission was defined by steroid-free clinical remission, a Mayo Score ≤1 on endoscopy, a fecal calprotectin ≤200 µg/g and no significant active inflammation on colon biopsies

remission with IBS-like symptoms has been similar to those without IBS-like symptoms. The reported mean duration of UC disease in previous studies is between 3 and 12 years [7, 8, 14, 26–28], which is shorter than the median disease duration in our UC patients. Another explanation to the low scores on IBS-like symptoms among patients with UC in remission in our study could be the rigorous criteria we used for defining remission. In previous studies there has been a wide heterogeneity for criteria defining remission. A combination of clinical judgement and endoscopic scores to define remission are commonly used [7, 8, 14, 26, 28–33]. In our study, in addition to endoscopy and clinical judgement, we also included a low FC level and the presence of no significant inflammation on the biopsy from the colon to define remission. Perhaps the reported high frequency of IBS in patients with UC in previous studies could partly be explained by the presence of low-grade bowel inflammation. For example, Keohane et al. [7] described that patients with UC in remission and IBS-like symptoms had much higher FC levels than the patients without IBS-like symptoms (591 µg/g vs 229 µg/g). Also Berril et al. [28] found a trend toward a higher median FC in UC patients in clinical remission with IBS-type symptoms. Interestingly, the present study also showed that even in the lower span of FC (≤200 µg/g) there was a moderate significant correlation between FC and symptoms of diarrhoea. One can therefore argue that even in the presence of low-grade inflammation there could be reasons to optimize treatment in patients with UC (especially if they report diarrhoea symptoms).

Table 2 Irritable bowel syndrome-like symptoms and symptoms of anxiety/depression in patients with ulcerative colitis versus control subjects

	Ulcerative colitis in remission ($n = 55$)	Controls ($n = 33$)	*p*-value
Median GSRS-IBS scores			
Total score	6.0	10.5	0.062
Abdominal pain	0.5	0.5	0.57
Bloating	1.0	1.0	0.19
Diarrhoea	0.5	0.5	0.38
Constipation	0.0	0.5	0.048*
Satiety	0.0	0.0	0.14
Median HADS scores			
Anxiety	4.0	4.0	0.52
Depression	2.0	2.0	0.99

*Statistically significant
For the specific IBS symptoms the table presents the total score for each cluster divided by number of items for each cluster
Ulcerative colitis in remission was defined by steroid-free clinical remission, a Mayo Score ≤ 1 on endoscopy, a fecal calprotectin ≤ 200 µg/g and no significant active inflammation on colon biopsies.
GSRS-IBS Gastrointestinal symptoms rating scale for irritable bowel syndrome, *HADS* Hospital anxiety and depression scale

Table 3 Correlations between irritable bowel syndrome-like symptoms and faecal calprotectin in patients with ulcerative colitis and in control subjects

	Ulcerative colitis in remission ($n = 55$) rs (*p*-value)	Controls ($n = 33$) rs (*p*-value)
Total GSRS-IBS score	0.214 (0.124)	0.190 (0.115)
Abdominal pain	0.003 (0.985)	0.084 (0.641)
Bloating	0.140 (0.308)	0.008 (0.967)
Diarrhoea	0.380 (0.004)*	0.050 (0.782)
Constipation	−0.028 (0.839)	0.142 (0.431)
Satiety	0.107 (0.443)	0.210 (0.241)

*Statistically significant
Ulcerative coitis in remission was defined by steroid-free clinical remission, a Mayo Score ≤ 1 on endoscopy, a fecal calprotectin ≤ 200 µg/g and no significant active inflammation on colon biopsies.
GSRS-IBS Gastrointestinal symptom rating scale for irritable bowel syndrome

There could also be alternative explanations to the reported low scores on IBS in patients with longstanding UC. The low degree of symptoms could be due to the adaption at the gut and at the central level leading to "a normalizing of gut discomfort" or down-regulation of gut stimuli as times goes on. In 30–50% of patients with IBS the symptoms decrease or disappear with time [34].

The pathogenesis of IBS is unknown and is probably complex involving multiple mechanisms. Low grade inflammation, intestinal dysbiosis, altered intestinal permeability, visceral hypersensitivity and brain-gut interplay between psychological distress and gut signals have been

Table 4 Correlations between irritable bowel syndrome-like symptoms and symptoms of anxiety/depression in patients with ulcerative colitis in remission and in control subjects

	HADS-Anxiety		HADS-Depression	
	Ulcerative colitis in remission ($n = 55$) rs (p-value)	Controls ($n = 33$) rs (p-value)	Ulcerative colitis in remission ($n = 55$) rs (p-value)	Controls ($n = 33$) rs (p-value)
Total GSRS-IBS score	0.327 (0.019)*	0.244 (0.194)	0.294 (0.036)*	0.263 (0.160)
Abdominal pain	0.121 (0.394)	0.306 (0.094)	0.148 (0.294)	0.294 (0.109)
Bloating	0.403 (0.003)*	0.347 (0.060)	0.243 (0.079)	0.287 (0.125)
Diarrhoea	0.299 (0.029)*	0.135 (0.470)	0.267 (0.054)	0.207 (0.263)
Constipation	0.380 (0.005)*	-.072 (0.699)	0.258 (0.062)	−0.059 (0.753)
Satiety	0.225 (0.109)	0.333 (0.067)	0.354 (0.010)*	0.182 (0.327)

*Statistically significant
Ulcerative colitis in remission was defined by steroid-free clinical remission, a Mayo Score ≤ 1 on endoscopy, a fecal calprotectin ≤ 200 μg/g and no significant active inflammation on colon biopsies. GSRS-IBS = Gastrointestinal symptom rating scale for irritable bowel syndrome.
HADS Hospital anxiety and depression scale

proposed to be possible mechanisms [35]. In both patients with IBS and in patients with UC in remission there is a relationship between gut symptoms and symptoms of anxiety and depression [27, 31, 32]. In the present study we could nearly confirm an overall correlation of both anxiety and depression scores with IBS scores in the patients with UC in remission.

There are some limitations in our study. Firstly, only 80 out of 216 patients contacted accepted to participate in the study. An unknown number of patients contacted were missed due to reduced personal staff in the summer months at the endoscopy unit. A resistance and inconvenience with leaving a stool sample before the bowel preparation could be a cause for drop-out in some subjects. Secondly, in our study we used the GSRS-IBS questionnaire, which only focuses on symptoms during the last week, and has its major role in screening for IBS-like symptoms in different populations. For a strict IBS diagnosis the Rome III questionnaire is recommended. However, it has been argued that the GSRS-IBS is more sensitive than the Rome III and therefore tends to overestimate the prevalence of IBS [32]. Thirdly, the colonoscopies in our study were performed as clinical routine, and therefore are not rigorously standardized. In addition, the endoscopists may have gotten information from the patients regarding present GI-symptoms and were therefore not sufficiently blinded to the patients' symptoms.

It is well known that there are sex differences in IBS symptoms with it being more common in women [36]. For example, women report more constipation and somatic discomfort than men. Also, there are sex differences in autonomic and anti-nociceptive responses to visceral stimuli [37]. In our study there were significantly more women in the control group than in the patient group which may have influenced the results towards a higher IBS score in the control subjects. The significantly higher scores of symptoms of constipation in the control group may be contributed to the female dominance in the control group. However, the GSRS-IBS score among the controls in the present study is representative and is similar to that seen in control subjects in other studies [38].

Conclusions

In conclusion, patients with UC in remission using strict criteria for remission and with longstanding disease do not have more IBS-like symptoms than controls. A moderate correlation exists between FC levels and diarrhoea symptom scores also in UC patients in remission.

Abbreviations

FC: Faecal calprotecitn; GSRS-IBS: Gastrointestinal symptoms rating scale-irritable bowel syndrome; HADS: Hospital anxiety depression scale; IBS: Irritable bowel syndrome; UC: Ulcerative colitis

Acknowledgements

The authors extend thanks to the staff on the Endoscopic unit at Umeå University hospital, Umeå, Sweden.

Funding

From the Västerbotten county council.

Authors' contributions

DL, the main author: participated in designing the study, collecting the data, performing statistical analyses, interpreting the results, and writing the manuscript. JR: contributed to designing the study, interpreting the results, and critical revision of the manuscript. VE: contributed to collecting the data and critical revision of the manuscript. RP: contributed to designing the study, interpreting the results, and critical revision of the manuscript. PK: contributed to designing the study, collecting the data, performing statistical analyses, interpreting the results, and writing the manuscript. All authors have read and approved the final manuscript.

Competing interests

The authors declare that they have no competing interests.

Author details

[1]Department of Public Health and Clinical Medicine, Division of Medicine, Umeå University, SE-90187 Umeå, Sweden. [2]Department of Surgery and Perioperative Science, Surgery, Umeå University, SE-90187 Umeå, Sweden. [3]Department of Medical Biosciences, Pathology, Umeå University, SE-90187 Umeå, Sweden.

References

1. Sjöberg D, Holmström T, Larsson M, Nielsen AL, Holmquist L, Ekbom A, Rönnblom A. Incidence and natural history of ulcerative colitis in the Uppsala Region of Sweden 2005–2009 - results from the IBD cohort of the Uppsala Region (ICURE). J Crohns Colitis. 2013;7:351–7.
2. Ordás I, Eckmann L, Talamini M, Baumgart DC, Sandborn WJ. Ulcerative colitis. Lancet. 2012;380:1606–19.
3. Henriksen M, Jahnsen J, Lygren I, Sauar J, Kjellevold Ø, Schulz T, Vatn MH, Moum B, IBSEN Study Group. Ulcerative colitis and clinical course: results of a 5-year population-based follow-up study (the IBSEN study). Inflamm Bowel Dis. 2006;12:543–50.
4. Hjortswang H, Ström M, Almer S. Health-related quality of life in Swedish patients with ulcerative colitis. Am J Gastroenterol. 1998;93:2203–11.
5. Halpin SJ, Ford AC. Prevalence of symptoms meeting criteria for irritable bowel syndrome in inflammatory bowel disease: systematic review and meta-analysis. Am J Gastroenterol. 2012;107:1474–82.
6. Lovell RM, Ford AC. Global prevalence of and risk factors for irritable bowel syndrome: a meta-analysis. Clin Gastroenterol Hepatol. 2012;10:712–21.
7. Keohane J, O'Mahony L, O'Mahony S, Quigley EM, Shanahan F. Irritable bowel syndrome-type symptoms in patients with inflammatory bowel disease: a real association or reflection of occult inflammation? Am J Gastroenterol. 2010;105:1789–94.
8. Jelsness-Jørgensen LP, Bernklev T, Moum B. Calprotectin is a useful tool in distinguishing coexisting irritable bowel-like symptoms from that of occult inflammation among inflammatory bowel disease patients in remission. Gastroenterol Res Pract. 2013;2013:620707. doi:10.1155/2013/620707.
9. Tibble JA, Sigthorsson G, Foster R, Forgacs I, Bjarnason I. Use of surrogate markers of inflammation and Rome criteria to distinguish organic from nonorganic intestinal disease. Gastroenterology. 2002;123:450–60.
10. Licata A, Randazzo C, Cappello M, Calvaruso V, Butera G, Florena AM, Peralta S, Cammà C, Craxi A. Fecal calprotectin in clinical practice: a noninvasive screening tool for patients with chronic diarrhea. J Clin Gastroenterol. 2012;46:50–8.
11. García-Sánchez V, Iglesias-Flores E, González R, Gisbert JP, Gallardo-Valverde JM, González-Galilea A, Naranjo-Rodríguez A, de Dios-Vega JF, Muntané J, Gómez-Camacho F. Does fecal calprotectin predict relapse in patients with Crohn's disease and ulcerative colitis? J Crohns Colitis. 2010;4:144–52.
12. Scaioli E, Scagliarini M, Cardamone C, Liverani E, Ugolini G, Festi D, Bazzoli F, Belluzzi A. Clinical application of faecal calprotectin in ulcerative colitis patients. Eur J Gastroenterol Hepatol. 2015;27:1418–24.
13. Yamaguchi S, Takeuchi Y, Arai K, Fukuda K, Kuroki Y, Asonuma K, Takahashi H, Saruta M, Yoshida H. Fecal calprotectin is a clinically relevant biomarker of mucosal healing in patients with quiescent ulcerative colitis.J Gastroenterol Hepatol. 2015;25. doi: 10.1111/jgh.13061.
14. Fukuba N, Ishihara S, Tada Y, Oshima N, Moriyama I, Yuki T, Kawashima K, Kushiyama Y, Fujishiro H, Kinoshita Y. Prevalence of irritable bowel syndrome-like symptoms in ulcerative colitis patients with clinical and endoscopic evidence of remission: prospective multicenter study. Scand J Gastroenterol. 2014;49:674–80.
15. Wiklund IK, Fullerton S, Hawkey J, Jones RH, Longstreth GF, Mayer EA, Peacock RA, Wilson IK, Naesdal J. An irritable bowel syndrome-specific symptom questionnaire: development and validation. Scand J Gastroenterol. 2003;9:947–54.
16. Dimenäs E, Glise H, Hallerbäck B, Hernqvist H, Svedlund J, Wiklund I. Quality of life in patients with upper gastrointestinal symptoms. An improved evaluation of treatment regimens? Scand J Gastroenterol. 1993;28:681–7.
17. Zigmond AS, Snaith RP. The hospital anxiety and depression scale. Acute Psychiatr Scand. 1983;67:361–70.
18. Bjelland I, Dahl AA, Haug TT, Neckelmann D. The validity of the hospital anxiety and depression scale. An update literature review. J Psychosom Res. 2002;52:69–77.
19. Karling P, Norrback KF, Adolfsson R, Danielsson Å. Gastrointestinal symptoms are associated to hypothalamic-pituitary-adrenal axis suppression in healthy individuals. Scand J Gastroenterol. 2007;42:1294–301.
20. Walsham NE, Sherwood RA. Fecal calprotectin in inflammatory bowel disease. Clin Exp Gastroenterol. 2016;9:21–9.
21. Røseth AG, Fagerhol MK, Aadland E, Schjønsby H. Assessment of the neutrophil dominating protein calprotectin in feces. A methodologic study. Scand J Gastroenterol. 1992;27:793–8.
22. Tøn H, Brandsnes, Dale S, Holtlund J, Skuibina E, Schjønsby H, Johne B. Improved assay for fecal calprotectin. Clin Chim Acta. 2000;292:41–54.
23. Samaan MA, Mosli MH, Sandborn WJ, Feagan BG, D'Haens GR, Dubcenco E, Baker KA, Levesque BG. A systematic review of the measurement of endoscopic healing in ulcerative colitis clinical trials: recommendations and implications for future research. Inflamm Bowel Dis. 2014;20:1465–71.
24. Riley SA, Mani V, Goodman MJ, Dutt S, Heard ME. Microscopic activity in ulcerative colitis: what does it mean? Gut. 1991;32:174–8.
25. Satsangi J, Silverberg MS, Vermeire S, Colombel JF. The Montreal classification of inflammatory bowel disease: controversies, consensus and implications. Gut. 2006;55:749–53.
26. Ansari R, Attari F, Razjouyan H, Etemadi A, Amjadi H, Merat S, Malekzadeh R. Ulcerative colitis and irritable bowel syndrome: relationships with quality of life. Eur J Gastroenterol Hepatol. 2008;20:46–50.
27. Jonefjäll B, Strid H, Ohman L, Svedlund J, Bergstedt A, Simrén M. Characterization of IBS-like symptoms in patients with ulcerative colitis in clinical remission. Neurogastroenterol Motil. 2013;25:756–e578. doi:10.1111/nmo.12163.
28. Berrill JW, Green JT, Hood K, Campbell AK. Symptoms of irritable bowel syndrome in patients with inflammatory bowel disease: examining the role of sub-clinical inflammation and the impact on clinical assessment of disease activity. Aliment Pharmacol Ther. 2013;38:44–51.
29. Isgar B, Harman M, Kaye MD, Whorwell PJ. Symptoms of irritable bowel syndrome in ulcerative colitis in remission. Gut. 1983;24:190–2.
30. Simrén M, Axelsson J, Gillberg R, Abrahamsson H, Svedlund J, Björnsson ES. Quality of life in inflammatory bowel disease in remission: the impact of IBS-like symptoms and associated psychological factors. Am J Gastroenterol. 2002;97:389–96.
31. Minderhoud IM, Oldenburg B, Wismeijer JA, van Berge Henegouwen GP, Smout AJ. IBS-like symptoms in patients with inflammatory bowel disease in remission; relationships with quality of life and coping behavior. Dig Dis Sci. 2004;49:469–74.
32. Mikocka-Walus AA, Turnbull DA, Andrews JM, Moulding NT, Holtmann GJ. The effect of functional gastrointestinal disorders on psychological comorbidity and quality of life in patients with inflammatory bowel disease. Aliment Pharmacol Ther. 2008;28:475–83.
33. Barratt SM, Leeds JS, Robinson K, Shah PJ, Lobo AJ, McAlindon ME, Sanders DS. Reflux and irritable bowel syndrome are negative predictors of quality of life in coeliac disease and inflammatory bowel disease. Eur J Gastroenterol Hepatol. 2011;23:159–65.
34. El-Serag HB, Pilgrim P, Schoenfeld P. Systemic review: natural history of irritable bowel syndrome. Aliment Pharmacol Ther. 2004;19:861–70.
35. Chey WD, Kurlander J, Eswaran S. Irritable bowel syndrome: a clinical review. JAMA. 2015;313:949–58.
36. Mayer EA, Berman S, Chang L, Naliboff BD. Sex-based differences in gastrointestinal pain. Eur J Pain. 2004;5:451–63.
37. Fillingim RB, Maixner W. Gender differences in the responses to noxious stiumuli. Pain Forum. 1995;4:209–21.
38. Karling P, Danielsson A, Adolfsson R, Norrback KF. No difference in symptoms of irritable bowel syndrome between healthy subjects and patients with recurrent depression in remission. Neurogastroenterol Motil. 2007;11:896–904.

5

A simple scoring model for advanced colorectal neoplasm in asymptomatic subjects aged 40–49 years

Yoo Mi Park[1,2†], Hee Sun Kim[2†], Jae Jun Park[1*], Su Jung Baik[2], Young Hoon Youn[1], Jie-Hyun Kim[1] and Hyojin Park[1]

Abstract

Background: Limited data are available for advanced colorectal neoplasm in asymptomatic individuals aged 40–49 years. We aimed to identify risk factors and develop a simple prediction model for advanced colorectal neoplasm in these persons.

Methods: Clinical data were collected on 2781 asymptomatic subjects aged 40–49 years who underwent colonoscopy for routine health examination. Subjects were randomly allocated to a development or validation set. Logistic regression analysis was used to determine predictors of advanced colorectal neoplasm.

Results: The prevalence of overall and advanced colorectal neoplasm was 20.2 and 2.5% respectively. Older age (45–49 years), male sex, positive serology of *Helicobacter pylori*, and high triglyceride and low high-density lipoprotein (HDL) levels were independently associated with an increased risk of advanced colorectal neoplasm. BMI (body mass index) was not significant in multivariable analysis. We developed a simple scoring model for advanced colorectal neoplasm (range 0–9). A cutoff of ≥4 defined 43% of subjects as high risk for advanced colorectal neoplasm (sensitivity, 79%; specificity, 58%; area under the receiver operating curve = 0.72) in the validation datasets.

Conclusion: Older age (45–49 years), male sex, positive serology of *H. pylori*, high triglyceride level, and low HDL level were identified as independent risk factors for advanced colorectal neoplasm.

Keywords: Adenoma, Colonoscopy, Colorectal neoplasm, Risk assessment, Screening

Background

Colorectal cancer (CRC) is one of the most prevalent cancers with a high incidence in Western countries [1]. The incidence of CRC has increased approximately 2–4 times in the past decades in many Asian countries [2, 3]. Because most CRC develops through the adenoma–carcinoma sequence [4], CRC can be prevented by colonoscopy with polypectomy of premalignant lesions. With respect to the screening age of CRC, since there is a significant increase in the incidence of CRC during the sixth decade of life, most CRC guidelines recommend that screening colonoscopy begin at age 50 for asymptomatic, average-risk individuals [5–7].

Although the frequency of colon cancer over 50 years has decreased in Western countries, the incidence of CRC has increased in 12 per 100,000 in 1987 to 18 per 100,000 in 2006, which is a 50% increase over 20 years among persons aged 40–44 years [8]. Persons younger than 50 years of age account for 7–9% of those diagnosed with CRC, and they tend to present with more advanced disease and have a less favorable prognosis than those older than 50 [9]. These clinical characteristics of younger persons with CRC may be associated with a time delay in diagnosis; hence, current CRC screening guidelines exclude the younger population. To minimize the amount of younger CRC patients who are not captured by the screening program, a tailored approach based on the risk of advanced adenoma that considers cost-effectiveness may be needed because the prevalence of colonic neoplasm in this age group is significantly lower than that in those aged ≥50 years [10, 11].

* Correspondence: JAEJPARK@yuhs.ac
†Equal contributors
[1]Department of Internal Medicine, Gangnam Severance Hospital, Yonsei University College of Medicine, 211 Eonjuro, Gangnam-gu, Seoul 135-720, South Korea
Full list of author information is available at the end of the article

Regarding advanced adenoma, which is the most reliable target lesion for CRC screening, several markers, including the westernization of lifestyles, obesity, and metabolic syndrome, have been reported as risk factors for this neoplasm in the younger population, especially in those aged 40–49 years. Although these risk factors can be tailored in CRC screening for the younger age group, the systematic application of scattered risk factors may be limited in daily clinical practice. Therefore, the aim of this study was to identify risk factors and develop a simple prediction model for advanced colorectal neoplasm in asymptomatic individuals aged 40–49 years.

Methods

This study was conducted in two steps. First, we identified risk factors associated with the occurrence of advanced colorectal neoplasm in the development set, and developed a simple scoring model for the prediction of advanced colorectal neoplasm based on independent risk factors. Subsequently, we evaluated the clinical effectiveness of a prediction model for advanced neoplasm in the validation set. This study was approved by the institutional review board of Gangnam Severance Hospital.

Study population

A cross-sectional study was conducted with 2781 asymptomatic adults aged 40–49 years who underwent screening colonoscopy for the first time from January 2008 to January 2012 at the Health Promotion Center of the Gangnam Severance Hospital in Seoul, South Korea. We excluded the following criteria: 1) previous colorectal examinations, including colonoscopy, sigmoidoscopy, or barium enema; 2) colonoscopies that had inadequate bowel preparation and did not reach the cecum; 3) individuals who had a personal history of colorectal neoplasm and inflammatory bowel disease; 4) a history of colorectal surgery, and 5) any symptoms, weight loss, anemia, or bleeding. Subjects were randomly allocated to a development or validation set in a 2:1 ratio.

Colonoscopy

Bowel preparation was performed using 4 L of polyethylene glycol solution, and subjects underwent a 3-day dietary restriction. The quality of bowel preparation was determined by the physician who used the following descriptors: excellent, good, fair/adequate, inadequate, and poor. Those that were inadequate and poor were labeled as poor preparation and were not included in the final analysis. Colonoscopies were performed by four endoscopists who had performed a minimum of 1000 colonoscopies, and all endoscopists were gastroenterology fellowship-trained and board-certified in their respective field. All examinations were performed using a standard video colonoscope (CF-H260AI; Olympus, Tokyo, Japan). All detected polyps were biopsied or removed. All polyp characteristics such as the size, number, shape, and location were documented. Polyp size was grossly estimated using open-biopsy forceps (Olympus FB-28U-1; Aomori Olympus Co., Ltd., Aomori, Japan). The polyp shape was classified as sessile (Is), semipedunculated (Isp), or pedunculated (Ip) type [12].

Data collection

Subjects' information, including demographics, laboratory tests, colonoscopic findings, and pathology reports, by review of electronic medical records was collected. Age was categorized into two groups: 40–44 years and 45–49 years. Body mass index (BMI) was categorized by the Western Pacific Regional Office of the World Health Organization criteria: normal (<23 kg/m^2), overweight (23–24.9 kg/m^2), or obese (≥25 kg/m^2) [13]. According to the American Joint Committee's (Joint National Committee) seventh report, blood pressure was classified as normal (<120/80 mmHg), prehypertension (120–139/80–89 mmHg), or hypertension (≥140–90 mmHg or taking antihypertensive drugs). Laboratory tests included immunoglobulin G specific for *Helicobacter pylori*, which was screened by an enzyme-linked fluorescence assay in each serum (ELFA, enzyme-linked via Vidas; bioMerieux Vitek, Inc., USA); elevated total cholesterol (≥240 mg/dL); elevated triglycerides (≥200 mg/dL); elevated low-density cholesterol (≥100 mg/dL); and low high-density lipoprotein cholesterol (HDL-c, <40 mg/dL). All lipid and lipoprotein levels were measured using a Hitachi 7600 Modular Dp-110 auto-analyzer, which included enzymatic colorimetric tests. Based on the normal reference range, serum lipid profiles were classified as normal or abnormal results.

We collected polyp data from colonoscopy reports. Advanced colorectal neoplasms were defined as follows: 1) CRC; 2) adenoma with a diameter of ≥10 mm; 3) tubular adenoma with high-grade dysplasia; and 4) tubulovillous or villous adenoma. When two or more adenoma were detected, the most advanced lesion was analyzed based on the largest diameter or advanced histology. All polyps were evaluated histologically by gastroenterology pathologists.

Statistical analysis

Continuous variables were presented as mean ± standard deviation, and categorical variables were expressed as percentages. Continuous variables were compared using Student *t*-test, whereas categorical variables were compared using chi-square or Fisher exact tests. For prediction model development, differences between variables were compared in the training set. Before univariate analysis, continuous variables were converted to categorical variables. Variables with a P-value <0.1 in univariate analysis were included in subsequent multivariate regression analysis in order to select variables to be implemented in the final model. Backward elimination (i.e., removing the covariate with the largest P value, one at a time) was performed until we developed a final model with statistically significant covariates. We established a risk score model by excluding less significant variables in a risk assessment. We intentionally only used categorized variables that captured easy but relevant and validated information in the prediction model to develop an easy to use screening score. We used a weighted scoring system by rounding down odds ratios (ORs) to the nearest integer in the final model. For example, an OR of 1.96 was rounded to 1 and an OR of 2.26 was rounded to 2. Based on this statistical analysis, we developed a formula for predicting asymptomatic subjects aged 40–49 years with advanced neoplasm, and these subjects may be primary candidates for screening colonoscopy. To validate the model, we assessed the diagnostic accuracy of the model in the validation set. The sensitivity, specificity, positive predictive value (PPV), and negative predictive value (NPV) were calculated using the computed area under receiver operating characteristic curve (AUROC). Thereafter, we validated the diagnostic value of the scoring model. $P < 0.05$ was considered to indicate statistical significance. All analyses were performed using SPSS software (version 20.0; SPSS Inc.) and MedCalc software (version 11.1; Mariakerke) for the receiver operating characteristic analysis.

Table 1 Clinical characteristics of subjects aged 40–49 years

Advanced neoplasm	Total subjects (n = 2,781)
Sex	
Male	1,633 (58.7)
Female	1,148 (41.3)
Age	44.8 ± 2.8
Age group	
40–44	1,259 (45.3)
45–49	1,522 (54.7)
Blood pressure (mmHg)	
Systolic blood pressure	120.9 ± 13.9
Diastolic blood pressure	76.3 ± 9.6
Body mass index (kg/m^2)	23.4 ± 3.0
Anti-*H. pylori* IgG (serum)	
Positive	1,623 (58.4)
Negative	1,158 (41.6)
Total cholesterol	198.3 ± 34.1
Triglyceride	124.3 ± 81.5
LDL-cholesterol	124.0 ± 31.0
HDL-cholesterol	
Men	48.4 ± 10.4
Women	58.6 ± 13.0
Advanced neoplasm	70 (2.5)
Overall neoplasm	561 (20.2)

LDL low-density lipoprotein, *HDL* high-density lipoprotein, *H. pylori*, *Helicobacter pylori*

Results

Baseline characteristics of the total subjects

Among 2781 subjects, mean age was 44.8 ± 2.8 years, and 58.7% (1633/2781) were men. Helicobacter serology positivity was observed in 1623 (58.4%) patients. Regarding the prevalence of colorectal neoplasm, advanced neoplasm was detected in 70 (2.5%) of patients, whereas any type of colorectal neoplasm was found in 561 (20.2) of patients. Baseline characteristics of 2781 patients in the training and validation sets are summarized in Table 1. There was no statistically significant difference in patient characteristics between the training and validation sets.

Clinicopathological characteristic of the colorectal neoplasm

Details of the clinicopathological findings of neoplasm are summarized in Table 2. Among 561 neoplasms, 64 (11.4%) were larger than 10 mm, 537 (95.7%) had a low-grade tubular adenoma, and 24 (4.3%) had advanced neoplasm, including 2 patients (0.4%) with cancer.

Factors associated with advanced colorectal neoplasm in the development dataset

Univariate analysis showed that male sex ($P \leq 0.001$), the obese group ($P = 0.016$), positive serology of *H. pylori* ($P = 0.009$), low HDL level ($P \leq 0.001$), and high triglyceride level ($P \leq 0.001$) were significantly associated with the presence of advanced neoplasm. Moreover, the older age group (45–49 years) was marginally associated with the presence of advanced neoplasm ($P = 0.053$). Details of the statistical analysis are summarized in Table 3. In subsequent multivariate analysis, the older age group (OR 1.967, 95% CI 1.191–3.749, $P = 0.040$), male sex (OR 2.763, 95% CI 1.032–6.409, $P = 0.018$), positive serology of *H. pylori* (OR 2.262, 95% CI 1.108–4.621, $P = 0.025$), low HDL level (OR 2.219, 95% CI 1.073–4.308, $P = 0.031$), and high triglyceride level (OR 1.967, 95% CI 1.143–4.252, $P = 0.018$) were identified as independent factors for advanced neoplasm. BMI (body mass index) was not significant in multivariable analysis. Details of these values are depicted in Table 4.

Table 2 Overall colorectal neoplasm in subjects aged 40–49 years

	N = 561	%
Number		
One	312	55.7
Two	152	27.1
Three or more	96	17.2
Size (mm)*		
< 10	496	88.6
≥ 10	64	11.4
Histology*		
Low-grade tubular adenoma	537	95.7
High-grade tubular, villous adenoma	22	3.9
Adenocarcinoma	2	0.4
Shape*		
Sessile	384	66.9
Semipedunculated	158	28.3
Pedunculated	27	4.8
Location*		
Ascending colon	124	22.3
Transverse colon	131	23.4
Descending colon	80	14.3
Rectosigmoid	225	40.0

*Results are summarized according to the most advanced lesion

Table 3 Comparison of variables based on the presence of advanced neoplasm in the training set

Advanced neoplasm	Development set (n = 1,844)		P-value
	No (n = 1,798)	Yes (n = 46)	
Sex			<0.001
Male	1,044 (96.4)	39 (3.6)	
Female	754 (99.1)	7 (0.9)	
Age group			0.053
40–44	805 (98.3)	14 (1.7)	
45–49	993 (96.9)	32 (3.1)	
Blood pressure (mmHg)			0.151
Normal	809 (98.2)	15 (1.8)	
Pre-HTN	741 (97.2)	21 (2.8)	
HTN	248 (96.1)	10 (3.9)	
BMI (kg/m^2)			0.016
< 23.0	845 (98.6)	12 (1.4)	
< 25.0	458 (96.8)	15 (3.2)	
25.0	495 (96.3)	19 (3.7)	
Anti-H. pylori IgG			0.009
Positive	1,062 (96.7)	36 (3.3)	
Negative	736 (98.7)	10 (1.3)	
Total cholesterol			0.755
Normal	1,529 (97.8)	40 (2.2)	
Elevation (≥240 mg/dL)	222 (97.5)	5 (2.5)	
LDL-c			0.237
Normal	140 (100)	0	
Elevation (≥100 mg/dL)	998 (99.0)	10 (1.0)	
HDL-c (<40 mg/dL)			<0.001
Normal	1,554 (98.1)	30 (1.9)	
Low (<40 mg/dL)	244 (93.8)	16 (6.2)	
Triglyceride			<0.001
Normal	1,588 (98.0)	32 (2.0)	
Elevation (≥200 mg/dL)	210 (93.8)	14 (6.3)	

HTN hypertension, *BMI* body mass index, *LDL-c* low-density lipoprotein, *HDL-c* high-density lipoprotein, *H. pylori*, *Helicobacter pylori*

Development of a simple scoring model for predicting advanced neoplasm

A simple scoring model was constructed based on five independently significant variables in multivariate analysis by using rounded down ORs of each variable (Table 4). The final model is as follows:

A simple scoring model for advanced colorectal neoplasm = Age [0: 40–44, 1: 45–49 years] × 1 + Sex [0: female, 1: male] × 2 + Serology of *H. pylori* [0: negative, 1: positive] × 2 + High triglyceride level [0: normal range, 1: high] × 2 + Low HDL level [0: normal range, 1: low] × 2

The range of the total score for this risk model was 0–9. This model yielded an AUROC of 0.74 for predicting advanced neoplasm in the development set (Fig. 1a).

Validation of the scoring model in the validation set

We investigated the predicted value of different total score cut points in the validation sets (Table 5). A cutoff point of 4 was selected because it results in the highest value for the AUROC to indicate an individual at high risk for advanced neoplasm. In the validation set, this cutoff point designated 43.1% of subjects at high risk for advanced colorectal neoplasm, and yielded a sensitivity of 79.2%, specificity of 57.8%, PPV of 4.7%, and NPV of 99.1% with an AUROC of 0.72 (Fig. 1b). The prevalence of advanced neoplasm gradually increased as the total risk score increased, and these findings are depicted in Fig. 2.

Discussion

To the best of our knowledge, our study is the first study to propose a prediction model for advanced neoplasm in the 40–49-year-old population. In the 40–49-year-old group, an increased risk of advanced neoplasm was associated with those aged ≥45 years, male sex, positive serology of *H. pylori*, and high triglyceride and low HDL levels. We developed a simple scoring model for

Table 4 Multivariate regression analysis in the development set

	Odds ratio (95% CI)	*P*-value	Score assigned
Older age (45–49 years)	1.967 (1.191–0.040)	0.040	1
Male sex	2.763 (1.032–0.018)	0.018	2
Positive serology of *H. pylori*	2.262 (1.108–0.025)	0.025	2
High triglyceride level	2.219 (1.073–0.031)	0.031	2
Low HDL-c	2.136 (1.143–4.252)	0.018	2

CI confidence interval, *H. pylori*, *Helicobacter pylori*, *HDL-c* high-density lipoprotein cholesterol
A simple scoring model for advanced colorectal neoplasm = Age [0: 40–44, 1: 45–49 years] × 1 + Sex [0: female, 1: male] × 2 + Serology of *H. pylori* [0: negative, 1: positive] × 2 + Triglyceride level [0: normal range, 1: high] × 2 + High-density lipoprotein level [0: normal range, 1: low] × 2

predicting advanced colorectal neoplasm (range 0–9), and a cutoff point of ≥4 in this model yielded a sensitivity of 78% and specificity of 56% (AUROC = 0.74) (data not shown). Comparable results were obtained in the validation datasets (sensitivity 79%, specificity 58%, and AUROC = 0.72).

It has been reported that the prevalence of advanced colorectal neoplasm in individuals aged 40–49 years is 1.3–3.5% [10, 14–17]. Similar to these results, our study showed a 2.5% prevalence for advanced neoplasm in an asymptomatic population. Currently, advanced adenoma is regarded as the most feasible target for CRC screening [2, 6, 7]. Based on our prediction model, the prevalence of advanced neoplasm gradually increased as the risk score increased. This finding suggests that our prediction model can be a reliable tool for identifying target subjects for CRC screening among persons aged 40–49 years. Our prediction model produced moderate accuracy for predicting advanced neoplasm, producing an AUROC value of 0.72 in the validation cohort.

Regarding age-related risk stratification, our study showed that the risk for advanced neoplasm was approximately two times higher in the 45–49 age group than in the 40–44 age group. This finding suggests that further subgroup classification can be helpful in identifying the population at risk within the 40–49 age group, and it was eventually incorporated into our prediction model. Similar to our results, Hong et al. [10] also reported that the 45–49 age group had a high adjusted OR of 1.68 compared to the 40–44 age group for detecting advanced neoplasm.

Among lipid profile indices, we found that hypertriglyceridemia and low HLD-c were independently associated with advanced neoplasm. In accordance with our findings, a previous study showed that higher levels of serum triglyceride were significantly associated with an increasing prevalence of both non-advanced and advanced colorectal adenoma in a population aged 40–79 years [18]. Concerning the association between hypertriglyceridemia and advanced neoplasm, although the exact mechanism is currently unclear, several mechanisms have been suggested. First, hyperinsulinemia and insulin resistance is affected by apoptosis, thereby a lower rate of apoptosis in normal colonic mucosa is associated with the carcinogenesis process, and they may develop into colorectal adenoma, or even cancer [19–21]. Second, hypertriglyceridemia can also increase proinflammatory cytokine levels, and damage deoxyribonucleic acid. These also affect carcinogenesis through abnormal growth, apoptosis, and the proliferation of colorectal cells [22–24].

Meanwhile, similar to our results of association between a low HDL-c level and the risk of advanced neoplasm, trends for an increased prevalence of advanced adenoma with decreasing levels of HDL cholesterol was also found in previously reported data [18]. Other studies have also shown that a reduction in HDL cholesterol levels slightly increases the risk of adenomatous colon polyps, and consequently colon cancer [25, 26]. Although the underlying mechanism for the relationship

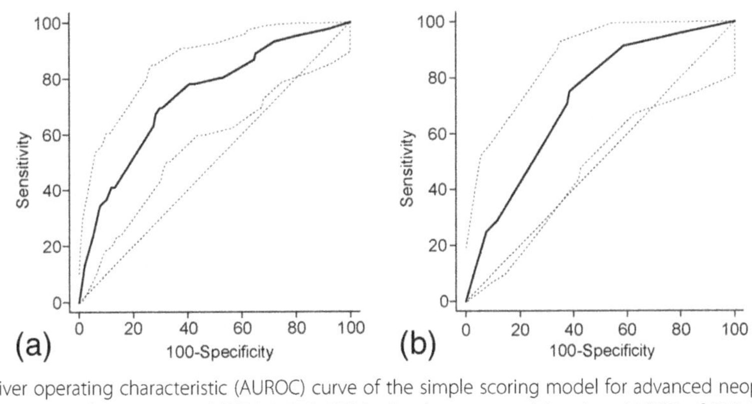

Fig. 1 Area under the receiver operating characteristic (AUROC) curve of the simple scoring model for advanced neoplasm in subjects aged 40–49 years. An AUROC of 0.74 (95% confidence interval [CI] 0.717–0.757) in development set (**a**) and an AUROC of 0.72 (95% CI 0.0695–0.753) in the validation set (**b**)

Table 5 Performance of the simple scoring model in the validation datasets ($n = 937$)

Score	High risk (%)	Sensitivity	Specificity	PPV	NPV	AUROC
≥0	100	100	0	2.8	0	0.50
≥1	90.2	100	10.1	2.8	100	0.55
≥2	81.1	95.8	19.3	3.0	99.4	0.58
≥3	64.2	87.5	36.4	3.5	99.1	0.62
≥4	43.1	79.2	57.8	4.7	99.1	0.72
≥5	30.3	62.5	70.5	5.3	98.6	0.68
≥6	13.6	37.5	87.1	7.1	98.1	0.62
≥7	8.0	25.0	92.4	8.0	97.9	0.59
≥8	3.4	8.3	96.7	6.2	97.6	0.53
≥9	1.5	4.2	98.6	7.1	97.5	0.51

PPV positive predictive value, *NPV* negative predictive value, *AUROC* area under the receiver operating characteristic curve

between a low HLD level and the risk of advanced neoplasm is still elusive, a low HDL level may result from interactions with triglyceride and HDL cholesterol, and the aforementioned possible molecular mechanism associated with hypertriglyceridemia and colonic adenoma may also be involved in these processes. Further extensive molecular biological studies are needed to clarify the association between dyslipidemia and the risk of colonic neoplasm.

An association between colorectal neoplasm and *H. pylori* infection has been steadily suggested, and meta-analysis data also demonstrated that *H. pylori* infection increase the risk of colorectal neoplasm by 1.4–1.6 times [27]. In addition, a recent large cross-sectional study showed that the OR of the group with *H. pylori* gastritis is about 1.24–2.35 [28]. In accordance with these observations, our study also showed that patients with *H. pylori* infection are 2.26 times more likely to have advanced neoplasm compared to patients without *H. pylori* infection in subjects aged 40–49 years. Although the relationship between *H. pylori* infection and increased risk of colorectal adenoma is unclear, several pathogenic mechanisms have been suggested. Increased gastrin induced by *H. pylori* infection may contribute to carcinogenesis by cell proliferation in the colon mucosa, and *H. pylori* itself can act on the colorectal epithelium through inflammatory responses and affect polyp growth or promote mucosal dysplasia [29–31].

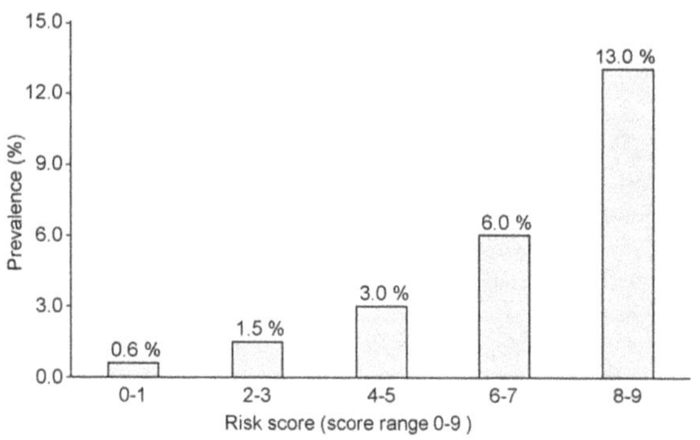

Fig. 2 Estimated prevalence of advanced neoplasm according to the risk score in the validation set. The proportion of subjects with scores of 0–1, 2–3, 4–5, 6–7, and 8–9 correspond to 0.6, 1.5, 3.0, 6.0, and 13.0%, respectively. A cutoff point of ≥4 (sensitivity 79%, specificity 58%) indicates that 43% of subjects are at high risk for advanced colorectal neoplasm

There are several advantages to our study. First, our prediction model was developed based on a large study population that included 1844 and 937 asymptomatic subjects in the training and validation cohort, respectively. Second, our model consisted of basic demographic factors and readily available serologic indices. Moreover, the final score of our model can be calculated in daily practice; thus, it has potential for high clinical utility in selective screening colonoscopy among the 40–49-year-old population. Lastly, our model allows for the adjustment of a cutoff value for subgroup targeting based on population characteristics and endoscopic resources.

Several limitations of our study should be mentioned. First, this study was performed in a health promotion center of a single university hospital in Korea. Therefore, generalizability of our results to the general population and other ethnicities is uncertain. Second, our study did not include lifestyle factors such as drinking, smoking, physical activity, and medication history. It has been reported that these lifestyle factors and some drugs are associated with the development of colorectal neoplasm [32–34]. Nevertheless, previous data have shown that some lifestyle factors, including smoking, alcohol, and medication, use were not significant predictors of advanced neoplasm in average risk screenees aged 40–49 years [10]. Hypertriglyceridemia is associated with alcohol consumption and a degree of smoking. Moreover, low HDL levels are related with a smoking habit, and its value in serum can be increased by regular exercise [35–38]. These observations imply that lipid indices can partly reflect lifestyle characteristics of each single person, and these lipid indices are incorporated in our prediction model. Finally, the retrospective nature of this study poses some limitations. However, our data were gathered prospectively, and our model largely consisted of objective results of serology, which were measured on the same day of colonoscopy. Thus, the influence of this limitation seems to be minimal. Further prospective studies incorporating diverse demographic, clinical, and serological parameters should be conducted.

Conclusions

In conclusion, older age (45–49 years), male sex, positive serology of *H. pylori*, and high triglyceride and low HDL levels were identified as independent risk factors for advanced colorectal neoplasm. A simple scoring model that consists of five parameters may be useful for selecting patients who benefit from screening colonoscopy in asymptomatic persons aged 40–49 year. We hope that researchers will evaluate the performance of our prediction model in an independent population to confirm and validate our results.

Acknowledgements
Not applicable.

Funding
This research received no specific grant.

Authors' contributions
Study concept and design, analysis and interpretation of data, statistical analysis, and drafting of manuscript: YMP, MD. Acquisition of data: YMP, MD and HSK, MD, PhD. Study supervision for important intellectual content: SJB, JHK YHY, and HJP, MD, PhD. Study concept and design, analysis and interpretation of data, and critical revision of the manuscript for important intellectual content: JJP, MD, PhD. All authors read and approved the final manuscript.

Competing interests
The authors declare that they have no competing interests.

Author details
[1]Department of Internal Medicine, Gangnam Severance Hospital, Yonsei University College of Medicine, 211 Eonjuro, Gangnam-gu, Seoul 135-720, South Korea. [2]Health Promotion Center, Gangnam Severance Hospital, Yonsei University College of Medicine, Seoul, South Korea.

References

1. Ferlay J, Soerjomataram I, Dikshit R, Eser S, Mathers C, Rebelo M, Parkin DM, Forman D, Bray F. Cancer incidence and mortality worldwide: sources, methods and major patterns in GLOBOCAN 2012. Int J Cancer. 2015;136(5):E359–86.
2. Sung JJ, Lau JY, Goh KL, Leung WK, Asia Pacific Working Group on Colorectal C. Increasing incidence of colorectal cancer in Asia: implications for screening. Lancet Oncol. 2005;6(11):871–6.
3. Toyoda Y, Nakayama T, Ito Y, Ioka A, Tsukuma H. Trends in colorectal cancer incidence by subsite in Osaka, Japan. Jpn J Clin Oncol. 2009;39(3):189–91.
4. Hill MJ, Morson BC, Bussey HJ. Aetiology of adenoma–carcinoma sequence in large bowel. Lancet. 1978;1(8058):245–7.
5. Winawer S, Fletcher R, Rex D, Bond J, Burt R, Ferrucci J, Ganiats T, Levin T, Woolf S, Johnson D, et al. Colorectal cancer screening and surveillance: clinical guidelines and rationale-Update based on new evidence. Gastroenterology. 2003;124(2):544–60.
6. Davila RE, Rajan E, Baron TH, Adler DG, Egan JV, Faigel DO, Gan SI, Hirota WK, Leighton JA, Lichtenstein D, et al. ASGE guideline: colorectal cancer screening and surveillance. Gastrointest Endosc. 2006;63(4):546–57.
7. Lee BI, Hong SP, Kim SE, Kim SH, Kim HS, Hong SN, Yang DH, Shin SJ, Lee SH, Park DI, et al. Korean guidelines for colorectal cancer screening and polyp detection. Clin Endosc. 2012;45(1):25–43.
8. Wachter K. Colorectal cancer rates up in people aged 40 to 44. GI & Hepatology News. AGA Institute. 2010;4:1–4.
9. Fairley TL, Cardinez CJ, Martin J, Alley L, Friedman C, Edwards B, Jamison P. Colorectal cancer in US adults younger than 50 years of age, 1998–2001. Cancer. 2006;107(5):1153–61.
10. Hong SN, Kim JH, Choe WH, Han HS, Sung IK, Park HS, Shim CS. Prevalence and risk of colorectal neoplasms in asymptomatic, average-risk screenees 40 to 49 years of age. Gastrointest Endosc. 2010;72(3):480–9.
11. Thoma MN, Castro F, Golawala M, Chen R. Detection of colorectal neoplasia by colonoscopy in average-risk patients age 40–49 versus 50–59 years. Dig Dis Sci. 2011;56(5):1503–8.
12. The Paris Workshop. The Paris endoscopic classification of superficial neoplastic lesions: esophagus, stomach, and colon: November 30 to December 1, 2002. Gastrointest Endosc. 2003;58(6 Suppl):S3-43.
13. Anuurad E, Shiwaku K, Nogi A, Kitajima K, Enkhmaa B, Shimono K, Yamane Y. The new BMI criteria for asians by the regional office for the western pacific region of WHO are suitable for screening of overweight to prevent metabolic syndrome in elder Japanese workers. J Occup Health. 2003; 45(6):335–43.
14. Imperiale TF, Wagner DR, Lin CY, Larkin GN, Rogge JD, Ransohoff DF. Results of screening colonoscopy among persons 40 to 49 years of age. N Engl J Med. 2002;346(23):1781–5.
15. Rundle AG, Lebwohl B, Vogel R, Levine S, Neugut AI. Colonoscopic screening in average-risk individuals ages 40 to 49 vs 50 to 59 years. Gastroenterology. 2008;134(5):1311–5.
16. Chung SJ, Kim YS, Yang SY, Song JH, Park MJ, Kim JS, Jung HC, Song IS. Prevalence and risk of colorectal adenoma in asymptomatic Koreans aged 40–49 years undergoing screening colonoscopy. J Gastroenterol Hepatol. 2010;25(3):519–25.
17. Liu HH, Wu MC, Peng Y, Wu MS. Prevalence of advanced colonic polyps in asymptomatic Chinese. World J Gastroenterol. 2005;11(30):4731–4.
18. Yang MH, Rampal S, Sung J, Choi YH, Son HJ, Lee JH, Kim YH, Chang DK, Rhee PL, Kim JJ, et al. The association of serum lipids with colorectal adenomas. Am J Gastroenterol. 2013;108(5):833–41.
19. Burchfiel CM, Abbott RD, Curb JD, Sharp DS, Rodriguez BL, Arakaki R, Yano K. Association of insulin levels with lipids and lipoproteins in elderly Japanese-American men. Ann Epidemiol. 1998;8(2):92–8.
20. Giovannucci E. Insulin, insulin-like growth factors and colon cancer: a review of the evidence. J Nutr. 2001;131(11 Suppl):3109S–20.
21. Martin C, Connelly A, Keku TO, Mountcastle SB, Galanko J, Woosley JT, Schliebe B, Lund PK, Sandler RS. Nonsteroidal anti-inflammatory drugs, apoptosis, and colorectal adenomas. Gastroenterology. 2002;123(6):1770–7.
22. Vogelstein B, Fearon ER, Hamilton SR, Kern SE, Preisinger AC, Leppert M, Nakamura Y, White R, Smits AM, Bos JL. Genetic alterations during colorectal-tumor development. N Engl J Med. 1988;319(9):525–32.
23. Tabuchi M, Kitayama J, Nagawa H. Hypertriglyceridemia is positively correlated with the development of colorectal tubular adenoma in Japanese men. World J Gastroenterol. 2006;12(8):1261–4.
24. Lee HL, Son BK, Lee OY, Jeon YC, Han DS, Sohn JH, Yoon BC, Choi HS, Hahm JS, Lee MH, et al. Abdominal obesity, insulin resistance, and the risk of colonic adenoma. Korean J Gastroenterol = Taehan Sohwagi Hakhoe chi. 2007;49(3):147–51.
25. Bayerdorffer E, Mannes GA, Richter WO, Ochsenkuhn T, Seeholzer G, Kopcke W, Wiebecke B, Paumgartner G. Decreased high-density lipoprotein cholesterol and increased low-density cholesterol levels in patients with colorectal adenomas. Ann Intern Med. 1993;118(7):481–7.
26. Kono S, Honjo S, Todoroki I, Nishiwaki M, Hamada H, Nishikawa H, Koga H, Ogawa S, Nakagawa K. Glucose intolerance and adenomas of the sigmoid colon in Japanese men (Japan). Cancer Causes Control. 1998;9(4):441–6.
27. Zhao YS, Wang F, Chang D, Han B, You DY. Meta-analysis of different test indicators: Helicobacter pylori infection and the risk of colorectal cancer. Int J Color Dis. 2008;23(9):875–82.
28. Sonnenberg A, Genta RM. Helicobacter pylori is a risk factor for colonic neoplasms. Am J Gastroenterol. 2013;108(2):208–15.
29. Ciccotosto GD, McLeish A, Hardy KJ, Shulkes A. Expression, processing, and secretion of gastrin in patients with colorectal carcinoma. Gastroenterology. 1995;109(4):1142–53.
30. Georgopoulos SD, Polymeros D, Triantafyllou K, Spiliadi C, Mentis A, Karamanolis DG, Ladas SD. Hypergastrinemia is associated with increased risk of distal colon adenomas. Digestion. 2006;74(1):42–6.
31. Jones M, Helliwell P, Pritchard C, Tharakan J, Mathew J. Helicobacter pylori in colorectal neoplasms: is there an aetiological relationship? World J Surg Oncol. 2007;5:51.

32. Giovannucci E, Colditz GA, Stampfer MJ, Hunter D, Rosner BA, Willett WC, Speizer FE. A prospective study of cigarette smoking and risk of colorectal adenoma and colorectal cancer in U.S. women. J Natl Cancer Inst. 1994; 86(3):192–9.
33. Cho E, Smith-Warner SA, Ritz J, van den Brandt PA, Colditz GA, Folsom AR, Freudenheim JL, Giovannucci E, Goldbohm RA, Graham S, et al. Alcohol intake and colorectal cancer: a pooled analysis of 8 cohort studies. Ann Intern Med. 2004;140(8):603–13.
34. Chan AT, Giovannucci EL, Meyerhardt JA, Schernhammer ES, Curhan GC, Fuchs CS. Long-term use of aspirin and nonsteroidal anti-inflammatory drugs and risk of colorectal cancer. JAMA. 2005;294(8):914–23.
35. Craig WY, Palomaki GE, Haddow JE. Cigarette smoking and serum lipid and lipoprotein concentrations: an analysis of published data. BMJ. 1989; 298(6676):784–8.
36. Celada MM, Reguero JR, Cubero GI. The interrelationship among tobacco consumption, high-density lipoprotein cholesterol and leukocyte counts. J Cardiovasc Risk. 1997;4(4):279–81.
37. Connelly PW, Petrasovits A, Stachenko S, MacLean DR, Little JA, Chockalingam A. Prevalence of high plasma triglyceride combined with low HDL-C levels and its association with smoking, hypertension, obesity, diabetes, sedentariness and LDL-C levels in the Canadian population. Canadian Heart Health Surveys Research Group. Can J Cardiol. 1999;15(4):428–33.
38. Hata Y, Nakajima K. Life-style and serum lipids and lipoproteins. J Atheroscler Thromb. 2000;7(4):177–97.

6

A potential anatomic subtype of short bowel syndrome

Wencheng Kong[1†], Jian Wang[2†], Rongchao Ying[1†], Yousheng Li[2,4*], Huicheng Jin[1], Qi Mao[2], Danhua Yao[2] and Mingxiao Guo[3]

Abstract

Background: Fundamental researches suggest that ileum presents greater adaptive potential than the jejunum. However, few studies estimate the association between ileum and adaptive potential in human. To discover the association, we conducted this matched case-control study.

Methods: A 1:2 pair-matched, case-control study was conducted from January 1, 2001 to January 1, 2015 in Intestinal Rehabilition and Transplant Center. The case group was ileum predominated (IP) group and the control group was jejunum predominated (JP) group. Demographic data, medical history and progression of each patient were collected.

Results: There were 24 IP cases and 48 JP controls in this study. The cumulative probabilities of parenteral nutrition (PN) weaning in IP group were higher than that in JP group. The Bristol stool scale scores of IP group were lower than that of JP group at third month. The Cox proportional hazards regression model confirmed that IP had a higher odds of PN weaning (OR = 2.69; 95 % CI: 1.27, 5.70, $p = 0.01$) as compared with JP group. The conditional logistic regression with 1:2 matching also confirmed IP group had a higher odds (OR = 4.84; 95 % CI: 2.02, 11.56, $p < 0.01$).

Conclusions: Our results indicated that ileum presents greater adaptive potential than the jejunum in nutrition and fluid absorption. And a potential anatomic subtype of short bowel syndrome was proposed. Further research need to be conducted to more fully understand the adaptive potential of ileum besides nutrition and fluid absorption.

Keywords: Short bowel syndrome, PN weaning, Ileum, Bristol stool scale, Anatomic subtype

Background

Short bowel syndrome (SBS) is a disabling malabsorptive disease usually following massive resection of the small intestine and characterized by the inability to maintain their nutritional status through normal oral intake alone [1]. For those irreversible intestinal failure patients, intestinal transplantation offers the potential to regain intestinal function and clinical nutritional autonomy. Along with improvements in immunosuppression, operative techniques and critical care, the survivals of patient and graft have gradually increased over time [2]. Whereas, it is still low as compared with the survival of patients who receive long-term parenteral nutrition [2, 3]. Recent years, some progress has been achieved in intestinal rehabilitation therapy, especially in the pharmacologic (glucagon-like peptide 2 [GLP-2] analogue and growth hormone) treatment which may augment the adaptive process and help patients wean off parenteral nutrition [4, 5]. Another important factor which effects intestinal adaptation is anatomic feature, including the length, anatomic site and function of residual intestine.

Interestingly, it seems that ileum presents greater adaptive potential than the jejunum [2, 6]. However, as far as we know, this conclusion is mainly concluded from animal study [7, 8]. Therefore, our understanding of intestinal adaptation still requires exploration in

* Correspondence: liys@medmail.com.cn
[†]Equal contributors
[2]Intestinal Rehabilition and Transplant Center, Jinling Hospital, School of Medicine, Nanjing University, Nanjing 210002, China
[4]Department of Surgery, Jinling Hospital, School of Medicine, Nanjing University, 305 East Zhongshan Road, Nanjing 210002, China
Full list of author information is available at the end of the article

humans. And current study can only confirm the ileum decrease diarrhea and steatorrhea because of its absorption of water [9]. The other benefits, such as electrolyte balance and long transit time, are all in theory. Little clinical evidence is found in comparing the intestinal adaptation between ileum and jejunum.

Consequently, to further clarify the difference between ileum and jejunum in intestinal adaptation, we conducted this case-control study in our Intestinal Rehabilition and Transplant Center (IRTC).

Methods

Study design

The study was performed in accordance with the Declaration of Helsinki of the World Medical Association. With the approval of Institutional Review Committee of Jinling Hospital, we retrospectively reviewed all SBS patients between January 1, 2001 and January 1, 2013 in IRTC, China. SBS patients were identified by searching the diagnosis of "Short Bowel Syndrome" in the electronic medical record systems. Individual operative notes were physician-abstracted to obtain additional patient and operation information. A cohort of 356 SBS patients was achieved.

We elected two groups from the cohort and defined them as ileum predominated group (IP group, case group) and jejunum predominated group (JP group, control group). To be eligible as a case or control, the ileocecal valve and the colon were preserved in these patients. No surgery on the stomach, duodenum, or pancreas. The length of the intestine was between 100 and 20 cm. All patients must have longer than 2 years of adaptive phase and be followed. Intestine transplantation, malignancy, irradiation injury and Crohn's disease were excluded. Benign diseases, such as mesenteric vascular disease and volvulus and trauma, were included. IP patients were defined that the ratio of residual ileum/jejunum was larger than 4:1. Inversely, the ratio of JP patients was less than 1:4. IP cases and JP controls were matched 1:2 randomly by sex and length of intestine(±10 cm). Patients who met the inclusion criteria were selected by two independent researchers.

Content and data collection

The primary end-point of this study was development of intestinal adaptation, including weaning from parenteral nutrition (PN) and tolerance of enteral nutrition (EN) or regular diet during our study period (ending at January 1, 2015). The definition of "wean from PN" was absolute enteral independence and intermittent PN or fluid replacement was not included. We used Bristol stool form scale to score the typical stool form [10]. The secondary end-points were the hepatobiliary complications with PN management: steatosis, cholestasis, and gallbladder sludge/stones. We diagnosed "Steatosis" according to physical examination which might notice the liver was enlarged when the abdomen was palpated, blood tests including elevations of the serum alanine aminotransferase (ALT) and aspartate aminotransferase (AST) and ultrasonic diagnosis. Cholestasis was defined by elevation of conjugated bilirubin >2 mg/dL. Gallbladder sludge/stones were detected by ultrasound. Other chronic complications, such as metabolic bone disease and renal insufficiency, were also recorded.

Demographic, anatomic and therapeutic features of both group patients were collected. In our center, we had a procedure in dealing with SBS patients, which was illustrated in Fig. 1. If SBS patients from other medical centers were hospitalized, they would accept bowel rest and PN therapy until nutritional status improved and tissue edema regressed. If patients had undergone massive enterectomy in our center, they required PN for 7–14 days in order to maintain hemodynamic stability and pass the crisis. All patients were provided approximately 25–30 kcal/kg/day and 1.0–1.5 kg/day of protein. Patients would accept EN gradually via mouth, nasogastric tube, nasojejunal tube, percutaneous endoscopic gastrotomy tube or percutaneous endoscopic jejunostomy tube. EN started with amino acid formula (Vivonex, Nestle', Minneapolis, USA) or peptide-based formula (Peptisorb, Nutricia, Wuxi, China), followed by a transition towards whole protein formula (Nutrison or Nutrison Fiber, Nutricia, Wuxi, China). The total calory and protein goal of EN combined PN were consistent with those of PN. If patients developed diarrhea, multiple antidiarrheal drugs includes antimotility agents, antisecretory drugs, antibiotics and probiotics were given to effectively control fecal output. Diarrhea was defined as having three or more loose or liquid stools per day, or as having more stools than is normal for that person. Once patients were EN intolerance mainly including high gastric residuals and vomiting, they would receive PN again. If tolerated, patients would receive home parenteral nutrition (HPN) and EN or intestinal rehabilitation therapy (IRT) according to the intestine function and patients' wills. The IRT program was performed as described by Byrne et al. in 1995 [11]. If patients were EN tolerated but instable in body weight, they also underwent IRT. If patients were stable in body weight and EN tolerated, they were all encouraged to eat small and frequent meals. Some of them received IRT in order to wean EN and have normal diet. We routinely followed these patients through phone calls, and in-person visits with a well-designed questionnaire. This questionnaire main content included Bristol stool scale scores, starting

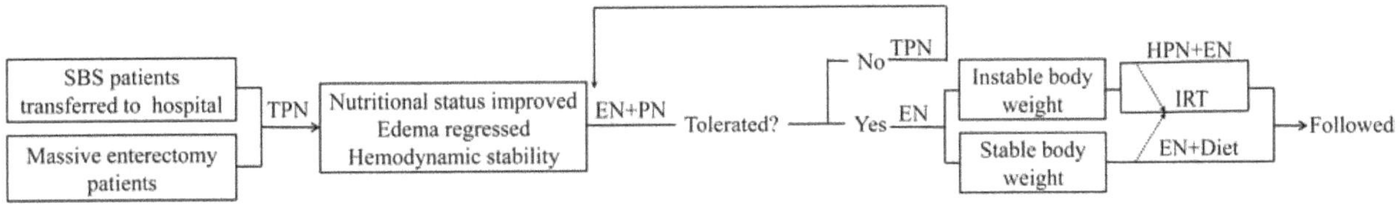

Fig. 1 Schematic illustration of treatment procedure of short bowel syndrome and follow-up

and ending time of new nutrition method, BMI and complications. Each patient was followed at least four times at 1st, 3rd, 6th and 12th month. If patients had not weaned off PN in first year, they would be irregular followed-up.

Statistical analysis

Cox proportional hazards regression and conditional logistic regression were used to estimate the odds of PN dependence stratified by jejunoileostomy types. Univariate analyses of demographic, anatomic and therapeutic features were performed to describe the study population. Missing data ranged from 0 to 5 % for all independent variables studied. Shapiro-Wilk W test for testing normality were conducted on all continuous variables. Normally distributed continuous variables were analyzed using Student's t test and paired t-test. Categorical variables were analyzed using Chi-square test or Fisher's exact test if expected frequency was less than five. The cumulative percentage of patients weaned over time was plotted using the Kaplane-Meier survivorship analysis and log-rank test for statistical comparison. Significance was set as p <0.05.

Results

Figure 2 illustrated the selection of patient. Eventually, 24 IP cases and 48 JP controls were selected. The demographic and clinical characteristics of both groups were summarized in Table 1. The characteristics of JP patients were similar to that of IP patients, but longer jejunum (49.5 ± 26.3 cm) and shorter ileum (8.4 ± 7.1 cm).

Table 2 showed both groups had similar duration of PN or EN support, but the duration of PN+EN was significantly prolonged in JP group than that in IP group. About 1/3 (33 % in IP group, 42 % in JP group) of the patients accepted IRT. Almost all patients (88 % in IP group, 85 % in JP group) presented diarrhea after initiating EN. Steatosis and cholestasis were the other two main complications presented in roughly half of patients. The incidence of gallbladder sludge/stones in IP group was lower than that in JP group, but did not have a statistical significance. The other complications were rare during hospitalization.

The average follow-up time was 968.5 ± 252 days. The cumulative probabilities of PN weaning were shown in Fig. 3. The curves of two groups had statistically significant difference (P = 0.046). The incidence of PN weaning in IP group (83.3 %) is higher than that in JP group (68.8 %). The changes of Bristol stool scale scores of two groups were shown in Fig. 4. The Bristol stool scale scores of both groups decreased to normal levels gradually during 1 year follow-up. However, the score of IP group (median, interquartile range; 4, 4–5) was significantly lower than that of JP group (5, 5–6, p = 0.004) at third month. The complications during follow-up were shown in Table 2. Three patients (1 IP patient, 2 JP patients) were dead during our study period. One IP patient and one JP patient were dead caused by end-stage liver disease and another JP patient were dead caused by infection (suspecting catheter-related infections). There were no statistical significances in complications during follow-up. But the complications of nephrolithiasis, gallbladder sludge/stones, and metabolic bone disease may be underestimated.

Table 3 showed adjusted odds ratio (OR) for PN weaning, calculated by Cox proportional hazards regression. Compared with JP group, IP had a significantly higher odds of PN weaning (OR = 2.69; 95 % CI: 1.27, 5.70, p = 0.01). The younger age (OR = 0.94; 95 % CI: 0.88, 1.00, p = 0.06) or higher BMI (OR = 1.41; 95 % CI: 0.98, 2.03, p = 0.06) might increase the possibility of PN weaning, but the difference was not statistically significant. Table 3 also showed the odds of PN weaning estimated using the 1:2 case (IP patients) to control (JP patients) matched design. And the IP group had a higher odds (OR = 4.84; 95 % CI: 2.02, 11.56, p <0.01).

Discussion

As far as we know, this was the first clinical study to address the question whether the ileum have a better functional adaption than the jejunum. The functional adaption included transporter/cell, crypt cell, transit time, nutrition and fluid absorption [6]. In fact, we had more interest in nutrition and fluid absorption. Our study suggested that the ileum predominated SBS patients were easier to wean PN than jejunum predominated SBS patients within 1.5 years

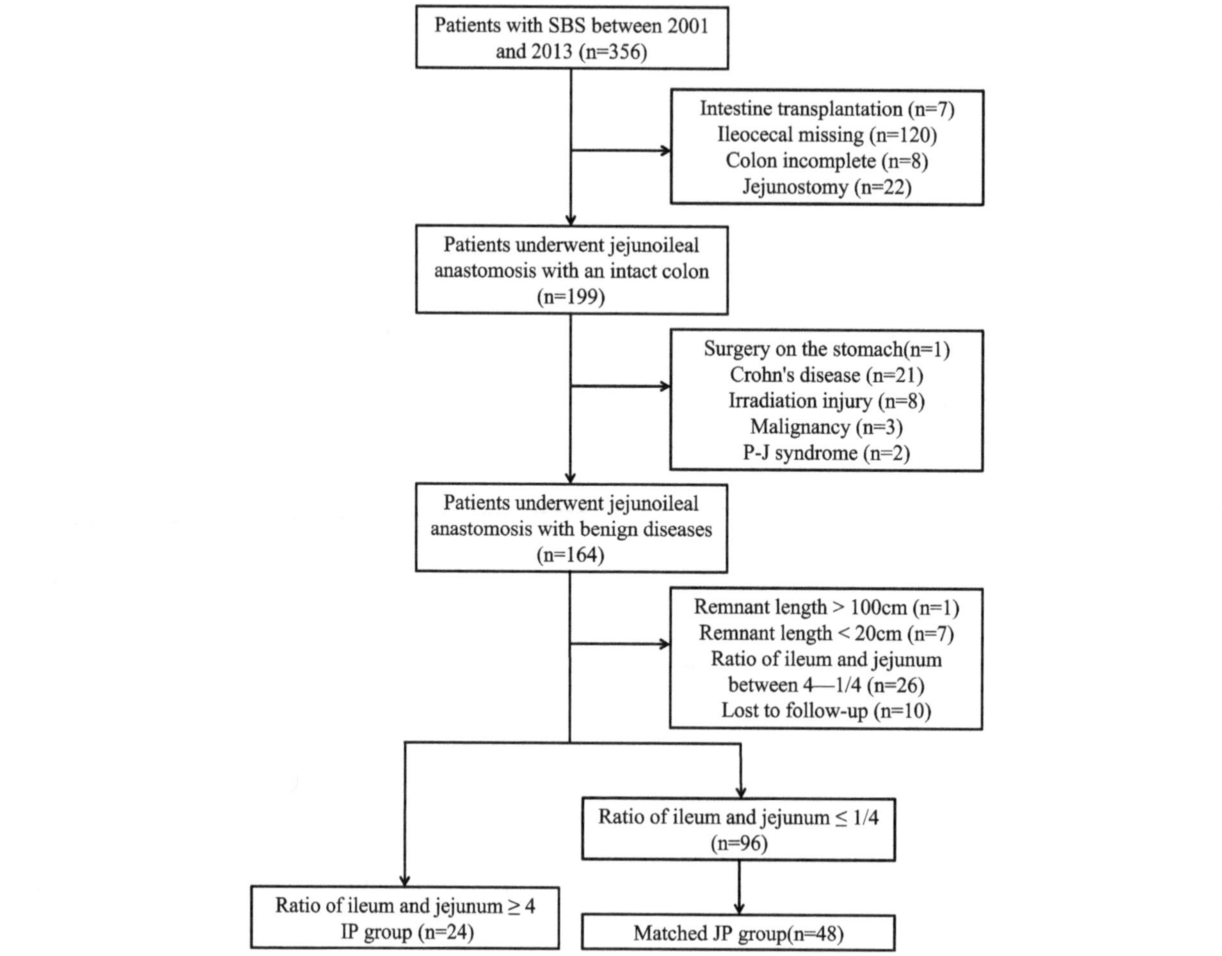

Fig. 2 Flowchart of patient inclusion and exclusion. P-J syndrome, Peutz-Jeghers syndrome

Table 1 Demographic and clinical characteristics of two groups

Characteristic	IP group (n = 24)	JP group (n = 48)	p value
Patient demographics			
Age (years),median (range)	40(26–63)	45(30–65)	0.42
Male gender (%)	67 %	67 %	1.00
BMI, kg/m^2 (Mean ± SD)	17.5 ± 2.6	18.0 ± 2.5	0.35
Transferred patients	3	5	0.29
Etiology for SBS			0.80
Mesenteric vascular disease	13	23	
Small bowel volvulus	7	12	
Intestinal adhesion/obstruction	2	7	
Others	2	6	
Anatomic features			
Remnant intestine length,cm(Mean ± SD)	54.8 ± 28.8	57.9 ± 29.4	0.68
Jejunum, cm	7.3 ± 5.4	49.5 ± 26.3	**<0.01**
Ileum, cm	47.5 ± 25.0	8.4 ± 7.1	**<0.01**

following resection. This result was in agreement with previous animal study but with a shorter duration of intestinal adaptation. It was generally believed that most of intestinal adaptation in adults occurs within 2 years following resection [12]. And some studies suggested the adaptation can occur beyond 2 years especially in adults. A study which followed 124 SBS patients who were weaned off PN showed more than a quarter of them were weaned off PN beyond 2 years following resection [13]. So we inferred this type of SBS defined as type 3 anatomy in some studies had a faster intestinal adaptation because the intact colon had a good adaptation in nutrition and fluid absorption [14].

Diarrhea was another main difficulty affecting SBS patients' quality of life. Massive intestinal resection, gastric hypersecretion, intestinal bacterial overgrowth, bile acids malabsorption and other factors contributed to diarrhea in SBS patients [15]. In this study, the scores of Bristol stool scale of patients were improved continuously to normal value within 1 years following resection. It seemed that

Table 2 Therapic characteristics and complications of two groups

Characteristic	IP group ($n = 24$)	JP group ($n = 48$)	p value
Time of PN (Mean ± SD, d)	10.8 ± 2.8	10.7 ± 2.4	0.87
Time of PN+EN	7.5 ± 3.1	10.3 ± 3.7	**0.002**
Time of EN	4.4 ± 1.7	4.8 ± 2.0	0.42
Intestinal rehabilitation therapy	8(33 %)	20(42 %)	0.49
Complications in hospital [a, b]			
Diarrhea	21(88 %)	41(85 %)	0.71
Catheter-related infections	2(8.3 %)	3(6.3 %)	0.34
Steatosis	11(46 %)	19(40 %)	0.61
Cholestasis	5(21 %)	12(25 %)	0.22
Gallbladder sludge/stones	1(4 %)	5(10 %)	0.26
Metabolic bone disease [c]	2(8 %)	3(6 %)	0.34
Renal insufficiency	1(4 %)	1(2 %)	0.45
Complications during follow-up [a]			
Death	1(4 %)	2(4 %)	0.45
Catheter-related infections	7(29 %)	16(33 %)	0.20
Steatosis	13(54 %)	23(48 %)	0.62
Cholestasis	8(33 %)	17(35 %)	0.86
Renal insufficiency	2(8 %)	5(10 %)	0.32
Nephrolithiasis [d]	1(4 %)	6(13 %)	0.20
Gallbladder sludge/stones [d]	1(4 %)	5(10 %)	0.26
Metabolic bone disease [d]			
All cases	0(0 %)	2(4 %)	0.44
Tested cases	0/5(0 %)	2/8(25 %)	0.43

[a] Some are overlapping
[b] Occurred during hospitalization and diagnosed by the latest test results before discharge
[c] Diagnosed by dual-energy X-ray absorptionmetry measurements of bone mineral density in suspect patients
[d] Only a portion of patients were examined

these patients' diarrhea was improved more quickly as compared to other studies [16, 17]. But as compared between groups, IP patients had better scores of Bristol stool scale than JP patients at the third month. This result implied ileum might adapt faster than jejunum in controlling diarrhea. The ileum's capability of bile acids absorption and potentiality of fluid absorption might be the mechanisms. While, the scores of Bristol stool scale had no significant differences between the two groups after 1 year adaptation. Besides, we found that the improvement of diarrhea always occurs earlier than weaning PN. This was a remarkable phenomenon which researchers should pay more attention to when study the intestinal adaptation.

Hormone therapy became a popular method to help SBS patients accelerate intestinal adaptation with successful application of growth hormone and GLP-2 [18]. Some studies showed intestinal hormones had multiple physiological effects in SBS patients because of lacking intestinal hormones. For instance, secretin and cholecystokinin played regulatory roles in hepatobiliary system which was often disorder in SBS patients [19, 20]. Serotonin and glucose-dependent insulinotropic peptide had a great effect on maintaining bone mass [21, 22]. As is well known, ileum and jejunum have different preferable hormones [18]. So we intended to find the differences of complications between IP group and JP group in this study. But no significant difference was found in duration of hospital stay or follow-up.

In the regression analysis, we found IP group was associated with 2- to 5-fold greater probability of PN weaning than JP group. Remnant intestine length was another significantly associated factor. Besides, BMI and age were two potential factors in borderline. These two factors were supported by previous studies among SBS patients [3, 23]. In this study, we studied the difference between ileum and jejunum in patients' intestinal adaptation. The existing evidence and indications suggested ileum has greater adaptive potential than the jejunum in nutrition and fluid absorption. Whereas, it still need prospective studies to demonstrate ileum's adaptive potential in other aspects

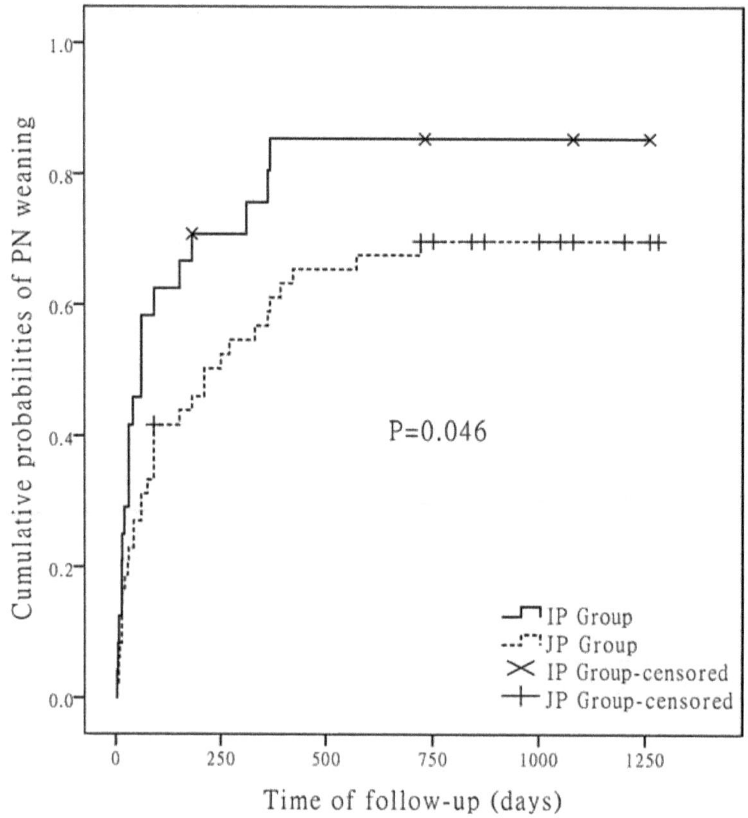

Fig. 3 Cumulative probabilities of PN weaning in IP group and JP group during follow-up

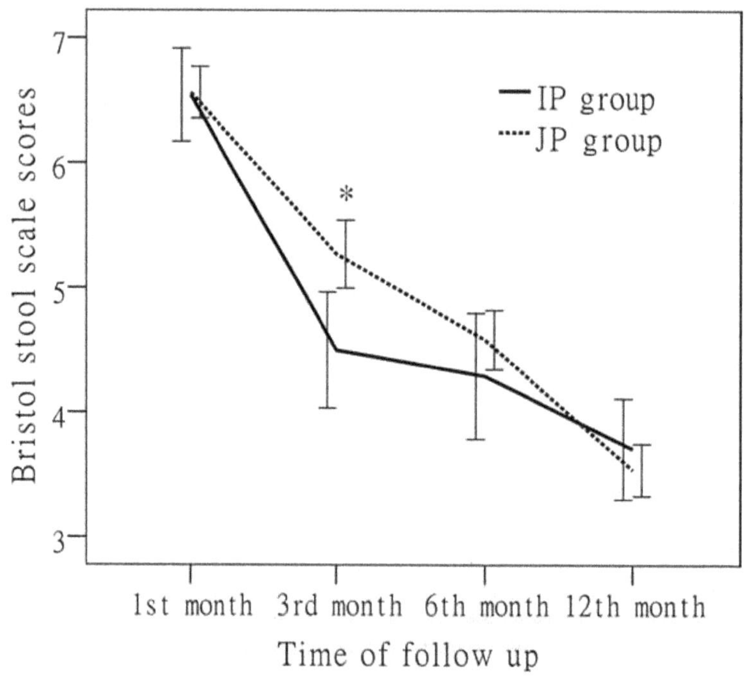

Fig. 4 Bristol stool scale scores of IP group and JP group during follow-up. * $p = 0.003$

Table 3 Estimated risks of PN weaning

	Unadjusted model			Adjusted model		
	Odds ratio	95 % CI	*p*-value	Odds ratio	95 % CI	*p*-value
a) Using Cox proportional hazards regression						
IP group[a]	1.74	[0.99, 3.05]	**0.05**	2.69	[1.27, 5.70]	**0.01**
Age	1.01	[0.99, 1.03]	0.59	0.94	[0.88, 1.00]	0.06
Male	0.84	[0.46, 1.54]	0.57	1.67	[0.68, 4.08]	0.26
BMI	1.06	[0.95, 1.18]	0.32	1.41	[0.98, 2.03]	0.06
Etiology for SBS[b]	1.14	[0.58, 2.42]	0.70	0.60	[0.28, 1.28]	0.18
Remnant intestine length	1.07	[1.05, 1.09]	**<0.01**	1.09	[1.06, 1.12]	**<0.01**
b) Using conditional logistic regression with 1:2 matching[c]						
IP group	4.84	[2.02, 11.56]	**<0.01**			

[a] IP group, ileum predominated group; Jejunum predominated group was reference group
[b] Mesenteric vascular disease was covariates; Small bowel volvulus was reference group
[c] IP cases and JP controls were matched by sex and length of intestine (±10 cm)

such as hormone and transit time. According to this study, we proposed to divide type 3 anatomy SBS into three subtypes: Type 3a, the main remnant intestine was jejunum; Type 3b, the main remnant intestine was ileum (Fig. 5); Type 3c, the mixed type.

There were several limitations of this article. This was a retrospective cohort study with no standardization protocol for patients to decide if and when to accept IRT or wean PN, thus introducing potential bias from unmeasured confounders.

Conclusions

In conclusion, we found that the length and type (ileum or jejunum) were associated with an increased possibility of PN weaning in SBS patients. Our results indicated that ileum presents greater adaptive

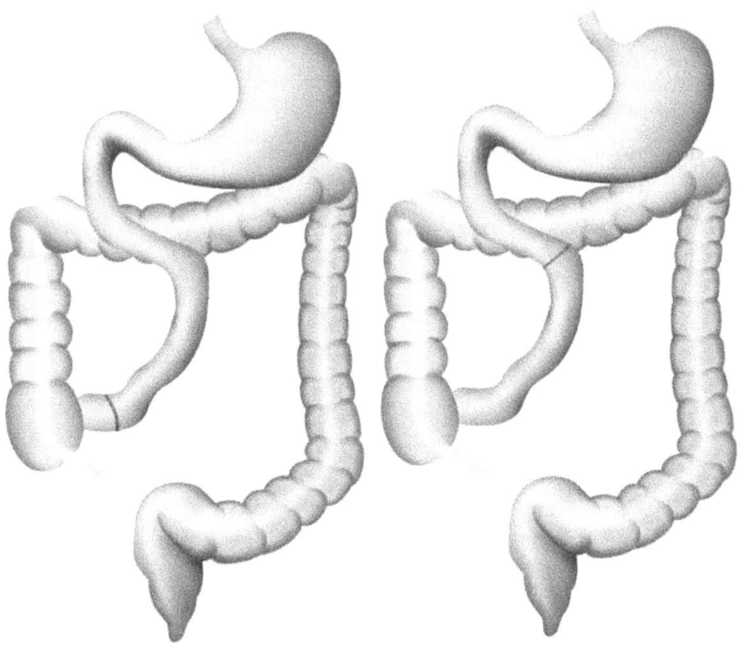

Fig. 5 Intestinal anatomic subtype of short bowel syndrome: *Type 3a*, the main remnant intestine is jejunum; *Type 3b*, the main remnant intestine is ileum. The black line shows the anastomosis

potential than the jejunum in nutrition and fluid absorption. Further research need to be conducted to more fully understand the adaptive potential of ileum besides nutrition and fluid absorption.

Abbreviations

EN: enteral nutrition; IP: ileum predominated; IRT: intestinal rehabilitation therapy; JP: jejunum predominated; PN: parenteral nutrition; SBS: short bowel syndrome.

Competing interests

The authors state that there is no conflict of interests related to this paper.

Authors' contributions

WK, JW and RY are co-first authors, and they contributed equally to the work; WK, JW and RY designed the research; QM, DY, MG collected cases and data; YL, HJ analysed the data; WK, JW and RY follow up all cases and wrote the paper. All authors read and approved the final manuscript.

Acknowledgments

This work was financially supported by National Natural Science Foundation of China (Grant No. 81270945, No.81200327 and No.81500688).

Author details

[1]Department of Gastroenterological Surgery, Hangzhou First People's Hospital, School of Clinical Medicine, Nanjing Medical University, Hangzhou 310006, China. [2]Intestinal Rehabilition and Transplant Center, Jinling Hospital, School of Medicine, Nanjing University, Nanjing 210002, China. [3]Department of Gastroenterological Surgery, Linyi People's Hospital, Shandong 276000, China. [4]Department of Surgery, Jinling Hospital, School of Medicine, Nanjing University, 305 East Zhongshan Road, Nanjing 210002, China.

References

1. O'Keefe SJ, Buchman AL, Fishbein TM, Jeejeebhoy KN, Jeppesen PB, Shaffer J. Short bowel syndrome and intestinal failure: consensus definitions and overview. Clin Gastroenterol Hepatol. 2006;4:6–10.
2. Thompson JS, Rochling FA, Weseman RA, Mercer DF. Current management of short bowel syndrome. Curr Probl Surg. 2012;49:52–115.
3. Vantini I, Benini L, Bonfante F, Talamini G, Sembenini C, Chiarioni G, et al. Survival rate and prognostic factors in patients with intestinal failure. Dig Liver Dis. 2004;36:46–55.
4. Matarese LE. Nutrition and fluid optimization for patients with short bowel syndrome. JPEN J Parenter Enteral Nutr. 2013;37:161–70.
5. Jeppesen PB, Pertkiewicz M, Messing B, Iyer K, Seidner DL, O'Keefe SJ, et al. Teduglutide reduces need for parenteral support among patients with short bowel syndrome with intestinal failure. Gastroenterology. 2012;143:1473–81.
6. Tappenden KA. Intestinal adaptation following resection. JPEN J Parenter Enteral Nutr. 2014;38:23S–31S.
7. Appleton GV, Bristol JB, Williamson RC. Proximal enterectomy provides a stronger systemic stimulus to intestinal adaptation than distal enterectomy. Gut. 1987;28(Suppl):165–8.
8. Thompson JS, Quigley EM, Adrian TE. Factors affecting outcome following proximal and distal intestinal resection in the dog: an examination of the relative roles of mucosal adaptation, motility, luminal factors, and enteric peptides. Dig Dis Sci. 1999;44:63–74.
9. Cosnes J, Gendre JP, Le Quintrec Y. Role of the ileocecal valve and site of intestinal resection in malabsorption after extensive small bowel resection. Digestion. 1978;18:329–36.
10. Lewis SJ, Heaton KW. Stool form scale as a useful guide to intestinal transit time. Scand J Gastroenterol. 1997;32:920–4.
11. Byrne TA, Persinger RL, Young LS, Ziegler TR, Wilmore DW. A new treatment for patients with short-bowel syndrome. Growth hormone, glutamine, and a modified diet. Ann Surg. 1995;222:243–55.
12. Buchman AL, Scolapio J, Fryer J. AGA technical review on short bowel syndrome and intestinal transplantation. Gastroenterology. 2003;124:1111–34.
13. Amiot A, Messing B, Corcos O, Panis Y, Joly F. Determinants of home parenteral nutrition dependence and survival of 268 patients with non-malignant short bowel syndrome. Clin Nutr. 2013;32:368–74.
14. Carbonnel F, Cosnes J, Chevret S, Beaugerie L, Ngo Y, Malafosse M, et al. The role of anatomic factors in nutritional autonomy after extensive small bowel resection. JPEN J Parenter Enteral Nutr. 1996;20:275–80.
15. Kumpf VJ. Pharmacologic management of diarrhea in patients with short bowel syndrome. JPEN J Parenter Enteral Nutr. 2014;38:38S–44S.
16. Cosnes J, Carbonnel F, Beaugerie L. Functional adaptation after extensive small bowel resection in humans. Eur J Gastroenterol Hepatol. 1994;6:197–202.
17. Mitchell JE, Breuer RI, Zuckerman L, Berlin J, Schilli R, Dunn JK. The colon influences ileal resection diarrhea. Dig Dis Sci. 1980;25:33–41.
18. Tappenden KA. Pathophysiology of short bowel syndrome: considerations of resected and residual anatomy. JPEN J Parenter Enteral Nutr. 2014;38:14S–22S.
19. Kanno N, LeSage G, Glaser S, Alpini G. Regulation of cholangiocyte bicarbonate secretion. Am J Physiol Gastrointest Liver Physiol. 2001;281:G612–25.
20. Chandra R, Liddle RA. Cholecystokinin. Curr Opin Endocrinol Diabetes Obes. 2007;14:63–7.
21. Cui Y, Niziolek PJ, MacDonald BT, Zylstra CR, Alenina N, Robinson DR, et al. Lrp5 functions in bone to regulate bone mass. Nat Med. 2011;17:684–91.
22. Mieczkowska A, Irwin N, Flatt PR, Chappard D, Mabilleau G. Glucose-dependent insulinotropic polypeptide (GIP) receptor deletion leads to reduced bone strength and quality. Bone. 2013;56:337–42.
23. Thompson JS, Weseman RA, Rochling FA, Grant WJ, Botha JF, Langnas AN, et al. Pre-resection gastric bypass reduces post-resection body mass index but not liver disease in short bowel syndrome. Am J Surg. 2014;207:942–8.

7

Diagnosis of celiac disease and applicability of ESPGHAN guidelines in Mediterranean countries

Andrea Smarrazzo[1,2], Zrinjka Misak[3], Stefano Costa[4], Dušanka Mičetić-Turk[5], Mona Abu-Zekry[6], Aydan Kansu[7], Abdelhak Abkari[8], Karim Bouziane-Nedjadi[9], Mongi Ben Hariz[10], Eleftheria Roma[11], Virtut Velmishi[12], Maria Legarda Tamara[13], Thomas Attard[14], Veselinka Djurisic[15], Luigi Greco[1,2] and Giuseppe Magazzù[4*]

Abstract

Background: We assessed how the diagnosis of Celiac Disease (CD) is made and how the new ESPGHAN guidelines can be applied in children from countries with different resources.

Methods: A *real life* prospective study was performed in 14 centres of 13 different Mediterranean countries. Participants were asked to apply the usual diagnostic work-up for CD according to their diagnostic facilities.

Results: There were 1974 patients enrolled in the study, mean age 4 years, 10 months; 865 male, 1109 female. CD was confirmed in 511 (25.9%) and was unconfirmed in 1391 (70.5%) patients; 14 patients were diagnosed as having CD according to the new ESPGHAN guidelines, 43 patients were classified as having potential CD. In all participating countries the diagnosis of CD relied on histology of duodenal biopsy; in 5 countries, HLA, and in one country endomysial antibodies (EMA) were not available. Symptoms did not add a significant increase to the pre-test probability of serological tests. The positive predictive value of tissue transglutaminase type 2 (tTG) antibodies performed with different kits but all corresponding to those recommended by ESPGHAN was 96.1% (95% CI 94–97.9%) in presence of tTG > 10xULN. In 135 patients with tTG >10xULN, HLA genotyping was performed and in all it was compatible with CD.

Conclusions: The results of our study show that CD diagnosis still relies on intestinal biopsy in the Mediterranean area. New ESPGHAN criteria are not applicable in 5 countries due to lack of resources needed to perform HLA genotyping and, in one country, EMA assay. Further simplification of the new ESPGHAN guidelines might be made according to what preliminarily the present results suggest if confirmed by new prospective studies.

Keywords: Celiac disease, Diagnosis, Mediterranean area, ESPGHAN

Background

Prevalence of celiac disease (CD) has been estimated at around 1% in Western populations [1] but most patients remain undiagnosed. The burden of unrecognized CD in countries with poor resources and facilities for diagnosis is very heavy [2]. Factors influencing the onset of this non communicable epidemics have been taken into consideration also recently [3–8]. New ESPGHAN guidelines [9] state that the protocol for the diagnosis of CD changed as a result of the availability of CD-specific tissue transglutaminase type 2 antibodies (tTG). As in children and adolescents with signs or symptoms suggestive of CD and high tTG titers with levels >10 times Upper Limits of Normal (ULN), the likelihood of villous atrophy (Marsh type 3) is very high, it has been suggested [9] that histological assessment may be omitted in symptomatic patients in whom these high tTG levels are verified by endomysial antibodies (EMA) positivity and are HLA-DQ2 and/or HLA-DQ8 heterodimer positive.

However ESPGHAN states that it is necessary to perform prospective research studies.

* Correspondence: magazzug@unime.it
[4]Celiac Regional Centre, Pediatric Gastroenterology and Cystic Fibrosis Unit, University of Messina, Via Consolare Valeria 1, 98125, Messina, Italy
Full list of author information is available at the end of the article

After the publication of the new ESPGHAN criteria, apart from a large study investigating antibody diagnostics in paediatric CD [10], 2 prospective studies [11, 12] have been performed to our knowledge. One other prospective study adopted criteria other than those suggested by the guidelines [13].

Two main problems should be highlighted:

- there are many different tTG antibody tests;
- new ESPGHAN criteria were applied in some studies, but these studies have been performed, with only one exception [12], in tertiary centres of affluent countries in subjects with classical gastrointestinal disease.

Therefore, the conclusions of a recent commentary on the applicability of the new ESPGHAN Guidelines for diagnosing CD in children from resource limited countries [14] rely on a single centre prospective study comprising only 142 children.

The Mediterranean Network for the Management of Food-Induced Diseases (MEDICEL) is a EUROMED-based action in which Mediterranean countries with different resources and diagnostic facilities participate. It, therefore, represents the *real life* ideal setting in which the new ESPGHAN guidelines can be prospectively applied.

The objectives of this prospective study were to assess how the diagnosis of CD is made in different countries and how the new ESPGHAN guidelines can be applied in different Mediterranean countries.

Methods

Study design

A *real life* prospective study was performed in 14 centres of 13 different Mediterranean countries participating to the MEDICEL network; all unselected new cases referred to these Centres for suspected CD and asymptomatic subjects with autoimmune CD-associated diseases or familiarity for CD were enrolled, from April 2013 to July 2014.

Participants were asked to apply the usual diagnostic work-up for CD according to their diagnostic facilities and to classify enrolled subjects as confirmed or unconfirmed CD according to shared criteria, as done in their usual clinical practice. Two sessions of shared agreement on diagnostic criteria were run through the MEDICEL network before starting the study.

Criteria for admission were: age below 18 years, clinical signs and symptoms of CD (systemic, gastrointestinal, extraintestinal) and/or associated autoimmune diseases (type 1 diabetes mellitus, thyroiditis, other autoimmune diseases) and/or no symptoms but familiarity for CD (1st and 2nd degree).

Criteria for exclusion were: already known diagnoses of CD only.

Familiarity, associated diseases, clinical symptoms, tTG as N x Upper Limit Normal (ULN), EMA, histology (Marsh-Oberhuber classification) [15], were collected into the database.

HLA-DQ2/DQ8 and follow-up were performed to confirm uncertain cases.

Diagnostic procedures

The tTG, EMA and HLA typing methods utilized by the Centres participating in the study, if available, are shown in Table 1.

tTG were determined with a kit of the 14 most frequently applied serum anti-TG2 IgA antibody assays taken in consideration in the new ESPGHAN guidelines (9).

Table 1 tTG, EMA and HLA typing methods utilized by the Centres participating in the study

Country	tTG kit	EMA substrate	HLA typing kit
Albania	Orgentec	Monkey esophagus	NA
Algeria	Phadia - EliA Celikey	Monkey esophagus	NA
Croatia	Phadia - EliA Celikey	Monkey esophagus	Tepnel LIfecodes Corporation
Egypt	Euroimmun	NA	NA
Greece	Inova	Monkey esophagus	Olerup, HLA typing kits
Italy (ME)	Euroimmun	Umbilical cord	BioDiagene - DQ-CD Typing Plus kit
Italy (NA)	Eurospital	Monkey esophagus	BioDiagene - DQ-CD Typing Plus kit
Malta	Orgentec	Monkey esophagus	Invitrogen / Life technologies
Montenegro	Aesku	Monkey esophagus	Olerup, HLA typing kits
Morocco	Orgentec	Monkey esophagus	NA
Slovenia	Eurospital	Monkey esophagus	Olerup, HLA typing kits
Spain	Celikey; Pharmacia & Upjohn	Monkey esophagus	Tepnel LIfecodes Corporation
Tunisia	Inova	Monkey esophagus	NA
Turkey	Orgentec	Monkey esophagus	Olerup, HLA typing kits

With the exception of 1 centre, that utilized umbilical cord as substrate, all Centres assayed EMA on monkey esophagus as substrate.

In each Centre at least 4 endoscopic biopsy samples from duodenum, including one from bulbus, were taken.

Data provided by participants to the study were re-evaluated by A.S., L.G. and G.M, and classified as shown in Table 2.

Crosstabs and stepwise statistics were generated by SPSS and t-Test, Relative Risk (RR) and Positive Predictive Value (PPV) were estimated for each variable assuming histology as the gold standard.

Results

Population

Demographic data of all the patients, and according to the final diagnosis, are shown in Table 3.

There were 1974 patients enrolled in the study, mean age 4 years, 10 months; 865 male, 1109 female. A global view of the classification and investigations performed by each Centre can be seen in the Flow Chart (Fig. 1) and in Table 4. CD was confirmed (CCD) in 511 (25.9%) and was unconfirmed (UCD) in 1391 (70.5%) patients. Apart from 14 patients diagnosed as having CD according to the new ESPGHAN guidelines (NCCD: New Criteria Celiac Disease), 2.47% of the final amount of diagnoses of CD, 43 patients were classified as having Potential Celiac Disease (PCD), 7.4% of the CD population, and 16 defined as having "high probability" of CD, as EMA or HLA were positive, but not both were done.

Symptoms

The proportion of asymptomatic cases enrolled for familiarity and of symptoms in CCD and UCD are shown in Table 5. A higher prevalence of asymptomatic cases, food refusal, globose abdomen and paleness was found in CCD, whereas abdominal pain and constipation were more common in the UCD. No difference was found for diarrhoea and failure to thrive between the two groups.

Diagnostic tools

Table 4 shows the frequency of various investigations performed in different countries: in 5 countries, HLA, and in one EMA assays were not available. HLA was not performed in Malta because it was not considered necessary.

Serology

In 91 patients, tTG antibodies were not performed; out of these, 7 patients showed positivity for EMA and histology, allowing to classify them as CCD, while in the other 84 cases CD was excluded (thus, they were classified as UCD, see Fig. 1). Of 1883 patients evaluated for tTG: 1219 were negative, while 664 were positive.

Among the 1307 UCD patients in whom tTG were performed, 1215 resulted negative, while 92 resulted positive: 70/1307 (5.4%) had tTG titre higher than 2 x ULN, and 22/1307 (1.7%) had tTG titre higher than 10 x ULN.

Four patients received diagnosis of CD despite having negative titre of tTG in presence of EMA positve: one was classified as PCD because of Marsh type 0, while the other 3 presented a Marsh type equal to or higher than 2. tTG sensitivity and specificity were 99.3% (95% CI 98.6-99.9%) and 93% (95% CI 91.6-94.3%) respectively, with a RR 1888.53 (95% CI 690.61-5164.35) of being celiac.

Results of EMA assay are shown in Fig. 2. EMA sensitivity and specificity were 99.5% (95% CI 98.8-100%) and 90.1% (95% CI 87.5-92.7%) respectively.

Both EMA and tTG were performed in 464 patients who underwent intestinal biopsy as well: 66 were EMA negative and 398 EMA positive. The reliability of tTG versus EMA is defined by its sensitivity 95.7% (95% CI 93.86-97.54%) and specificity 95.8% (95% CI 93.91-97.69%). High titers of tTG > 10 x ULN were found in 427 patients, out of whom EMA were performed in 289 and were found absent in only 3 patients (1.04%). Intestinal biopsy was performed in 2 of these latter patients and in both, histology showed a Marsh type 3c confirming CD diagnosis. The third was classified as UCD because of having done neither HLA nor intestinal biopsy.

Table 2 Classification of the patients' diagnoses

Classification	Histology	tTG	EMA	HLA
CCD[a]	≥ Marsh type 2	Positive or not done	Positive or not done	Positive or not done
NCCD	Not done	>10 x ULN	Positive	Positive
UCD	Not done or Marsh type 0-1	<5 x ULN	Negative	Not done
PCD	Marsh 0-1	Positive	Positive	Positive
High probability CD[b]	Not done	>10 x ULN	Positive or not done	Positive or not done

CD Celiac Disease, *CCD* Confirmed Celiac Disease, *NCCD* New Criteria Celiac Disease, *UCD* Unconfirmed Celiac Disease, *PCD* Potential Celiac Disease, *tTg* tissue transglutaminase type 2 antibodies, *EMA* endomysial antibodies, *ULN* Upper Limit of Normal

[a]at least tTG or EMA positive or both positive; [b]EMA or HLA positive but not both done. This category was not taken into account for comparison of the variables considered in the study

Table 3 Demographic data according to the final diagnosis

	No. (%)	Gender (F/M)	Age (M ± SD)
PATIENTS	1974	1109/865	4.83 ± 4.72
Confirmed	511 (25.9%)	320/191	4.1 ± 4.11
Unconfirmed	1391 (70.5%)	739/652	5.11 ± 4.89
Potential	42 (2.1%)	28/14	4.25 ± 4.51
Diagnosed according new ESPGHAN guidelines	14 (0.7%)	10/4	3.97 ± 3.59
High probability	16 (0.8%)	12/4	2.98 ± 2.93

In 135 patients with tTG > 10 x ULN, HLA genotyping was performed and in all of them it was compatible with CD.

Out of the 413 patients with tTG > 10 x ULN (excluding 14 patients diagnosed according to the new ESPGHAN criteria) both EMA and HLA were performed in 88. In all these patients a duodenal biopsy was performed, and in 85/88 the diagnosis would have been correctly made according to the new criteria; in 3 (3.41%) the diagnosis of PCD would have been missed in absence of the biopsy.

Biopsy was performed in 382 out of the 427 patients with high titre tTG, and histology showed at least a Marsh type 2 in 367 patients (96.1%). Thus, in this subgroup of patients, the positive predictive value of tTG > 10 x ULN was 96.1% (95% CI 94-97.9%).

Biopsy

Of 1974 cases included in this study, 1002 underwent an intestinal biopsy and in 542 at least Marsh type 2 mucosal damage was found: 511 (94%) were classified as CCD, because of positivity of tTG or EMA, 31 (6%) were classified as UCD because of negativity of both tTG and EMA.

Out of 460 patients with Marsh type 0-1, 42 (9%) were classified as PCD in light of the positivity of EMA or tTG antibodies. In particular, 8 of them had tTG > 10 x ULN, 6 between 5 and 10 x ULN, 27 between 1 and 5 x ULN. One patient had a negative titre of tTG (0.9 x ULN), but he was symptomatic (abdominal pain) and had positive EMA with compatible HLA.

In 364/460 with a Marsh type 0-1 at biopsy, no antibodies were produced and they were classified as UCD.

Overall, 568 patients were diagnosed as having CD (including CCD, NCCD and PCD), 2.47% of whom according to the new guidelines.

The presence of high titre of tTG correlates with villous atrophy (Fig. 3).

HLA

Less than 20% (382) of the total number of enrolled patients underwent a HLA analysis: in 63, that were both DQ2 and DQ8 negative, CD was finally excluded they were classified as UCD.

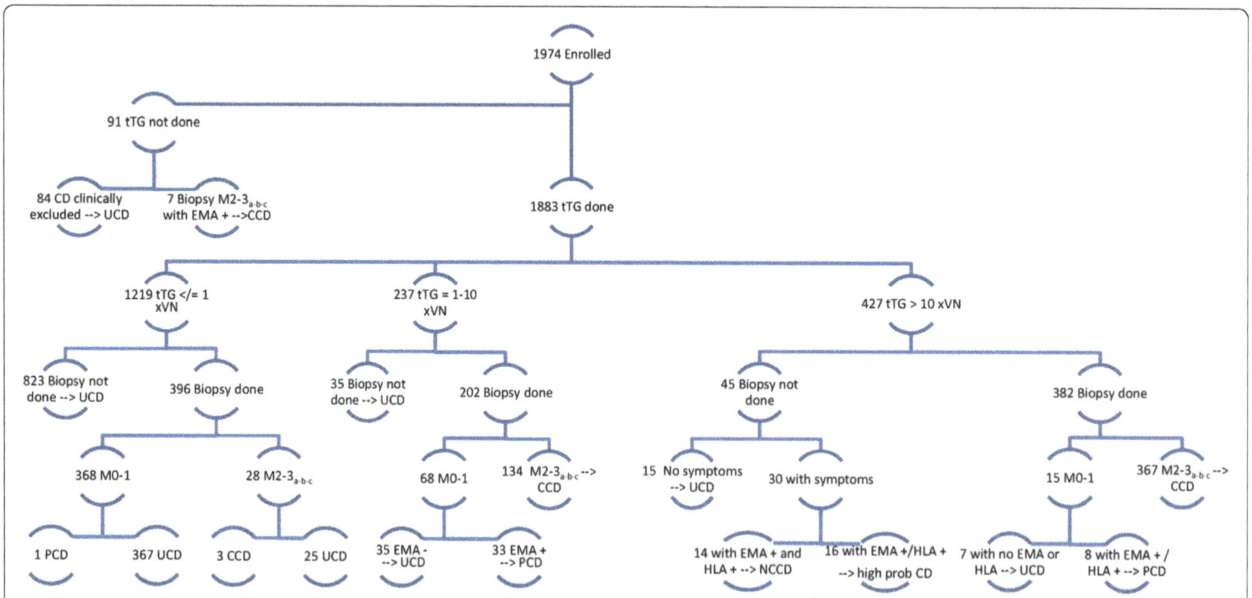

Fig. 1 Prospective study design. Detailed legend: tTG: tissue transglutaminase; CD: celiac disease; CCD: confirmed celiac disease; UCD: unconfirmed celiac disease; PCD: potential celiac disease; NCCD: celiac disease diagnosed according to new EPSGHAN criteria; M: Marsh degree

Table 4 Distribution of patients by study centers and according to the final diagnosis and performed diagnostic investigations

Country	N. Pts.	N. CCD + NCCD[a]	N. UCD	N. PCD	N. tTG	N. EMA (in CCD)	N. Intestinal biopsy (in CCD)	N. HLA
Albania	45	25	20	0	45	7 (1)	32 (25)	0
Algeria	71	17	54	0	70	6 (2)	54 (17)	0
Croatia	310	12 + 1	293	3	304	25 (6)	202 (12)	14
Egypt	200	5	195	0	159	0	21 (5)	0
Greece	46	35	10	1	46	40 (31)	46 (35)	27
Italy (ME)	332	111	199	15	307	273 (108)	142 (111)	13
Italy (NA)	339	152 + 9	153	17	330	281 (151)	202 (152)	109
Malta	27	14	13	0	26	16 (14)	27 (14)	0
Montenegro	18	11	4	2	17	5 (3)	16 (11)	11
Morocco	106	45	61	0	100	1 (1)	90 (45)	0
Slovenia	234	29 + 1	203	1	234	234 (29)	34 (29)	66
Spain	40	4 + 3	32	1	40	10 (4)	8 (4)	9
Tunisia	67	22	44	1	66	23 (11)	43 (22)	0
Turkey	139	29	109	1	139	5 (1)	85 (29)	133
TOTAL	1974	511 + 14	1391	42	1883	926 (362)	1002 (511)	382

N. Pts Number of Patients, *N. CCD* Number of Patients with Confirmed Celiac Disease, *N. UCD* Number of Patients with Unconfirmed Celiac Disease, *N. PCD* N. of Patients with potential celiac disease, *N. tTG* Number of tissue TransGlutaminase antibody assays, *N. EMA* Number of EndoMysial Antibody assays
[a]diagnosed according to new ESPGHAN criteria omitting biopsy

Associated diseases

About 80% of the total study population had no other disease. The significant differences in prevalence of associated diseases in UCD and CCD are shown in Table 6. The frequency of thyroiditis, type 1 diabetes mellitus and dermatitis herpetiformis was higher in CCD, whereas IgA deficiency and hypertransaminasemia were higher in UCD.

Discussion

Our study, for the first time, provides a wide picture of CD diagnosis feasibility in 13 Mediterranean countries with different health resources and facilities. It is also the largest one investigating antibody diagnostics in paediatric CD that prospectively evaluates the new ESPGHAN guidelines in different countries including those with poor resources.

Table 5 Distribution of symptoms in UCD and CCD patients

Symptoms	UCD (%)	CCD (%)	χ^2	*p*
No symptoms	93 (6.7%)	120 (20.6%)	82.4	<0.0001
Abdominal pain	402 (28.9%)	69 (11.8%)	65.9	<0.0001
Constipation	89 (6.4%)	17 (2.9%)	9.8	0.002
Diarrhea	297 (21.4%)	145 (24.9%)	2.93	0.087
Failure to thrive	266 (19.1%)	98 (16.8%)	1.46	0.227
Food refusal	16 (1.2%)	14 (2.4%)	4.3	0.038
Globose abdomen	29 (2.1%)	22 (3.8%)	4.66	0.031
Mood changes	5 (0.4%)	6 (1%)	3.33	0.068
Paleness	46 (3.3%)	31 (5.3%)	4.43	0.035
Vomiting	103 (7.4%)	30 (5.1%)	3.34	0.068
Others	45 (3.2%)	31 (5.3%)	4.81	0.028

UCD Unconfirmed Celiac Disease, *CCD* Confirmed Celiac Disease

In all participating countries, the diagnosis of CD relied on histology of duodenal biopsy, but other diagnostic procedures were not always available. In particular, in 5 countries, HLA, and in 1, EMA were not performed. Even though HLA was not required when the diagnosis was not in doubt, in some countries the limitation of performing it derives from its cost. The same is true for EMA assay.

On the other hand, in order to apply what is suggested by the new ESPGHAN guidelines, apart from the presence of symptoms and high antibody levels, HLA has to be compatible and EMA have to be present if the diagnosis of CD is to be made without a biopsy. In 4 centres, the diagnosis of CD was made for a total of 14 patients according to these new guidelines, omitting a duodenal biopsy.

Even though CD can be reliably diagnosed following the latest ESPGHAN and BSPGHAN guidelines [16], as not all diagnostic procedures required by the new guidelines are available in all countries, our results may suggest to further simplify the new ESPGHAN guidelines. As a matter of fact, it is not useful nor necessary to perform an expensive determination, such as HLA, as in all patients with tTG higher than 10 x ULN who had HLA heterodimer determined it was compatible with CD. Moreover EMA, which is not easily performed in all countries, does not add diagnostic accuracy to tTG, as

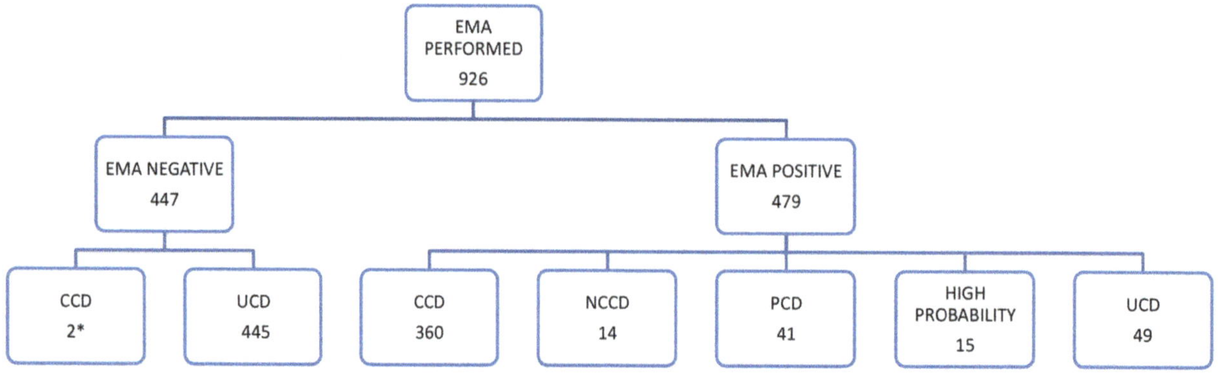

Fig. 2 Role of EMA assay in the diagnosis. Detailed legend: *tTg and Histology positive

suggested by the cases in which both tests were performed and tTG was > 10 x ULN. In 3 cases of our study, in whom EMA were negative, histology showed a picture that allowed us to make the diagnosis of CD. Rather than determining EMA, in the presence of such a high titre tTG, it is better to repeat a second test for tTG according also to what is suggested by the Joint BSPGHAN and Coeliac UK guidelines for diagnosis and management of CD in children [17]. In a commentary regarding applicability of the new ESPGHAN guidelines for diagnosing celiac disease in children from resource limited countries [14], it has been suggested that positive HLA-DQ2/DQ8 serotype and EMA are necessary in order to apply the ESPGHAN guidelines for serological diagnosis of CD, and that CD should not be diagnosed on the basis of a single high tTG-titre. Our study comprising many countries with limited resources suggests that both HLA and EMA may be omitted and CD may be diagnosed on the basis of repeated high tTG titres. Altogether, the diagnosis would have been correctly made according to the new criteria in 85 out 88 patients with tTG > 10 x ULN who underwent tTG and EMA determination, together with intestinal biopsy. In 3 patients (3.41%), the diagnosis of PCD would have been missed in absence of the biopsy.

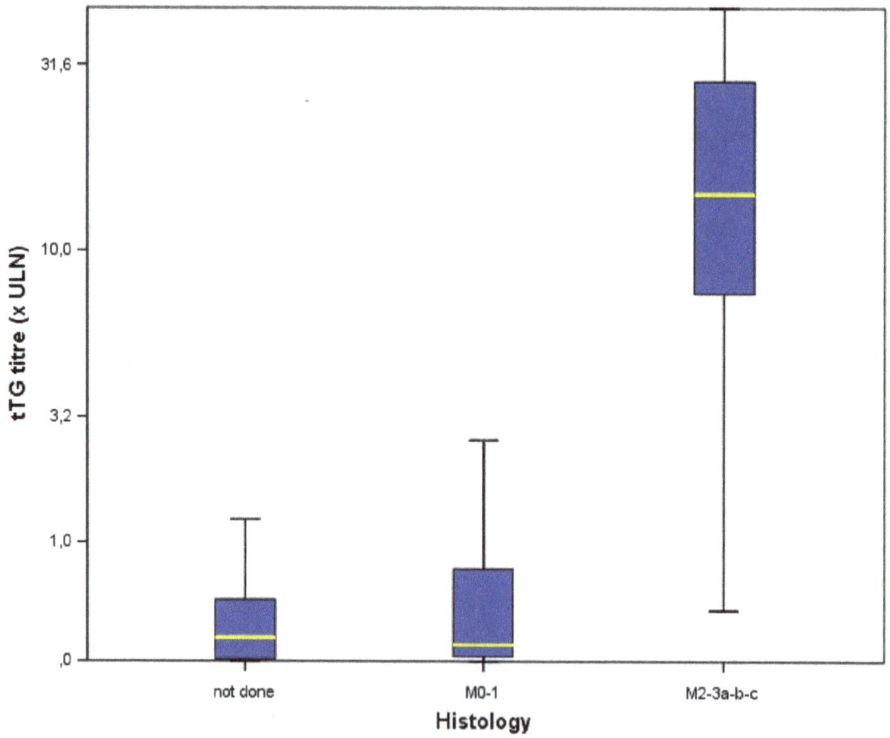

Fig. 3 Correlation among tTG titre and villous atrophy

Table 6 Significant differences in prevalence of associated diseases in unconfirmed celiac disease (UCD) and confirmed celiac disease (CCD)

Associated diseases	UCD (%)	CCD (%)	χ^2	*p*
Thyroiditis	1	5.7	38.7	0.0001
Type 1 Diabetes Mellitus	7	3	16	0.0001
Dermatitis herpetiformis	0.1	1.5	17.1	0.0001
IgA deficiency	1.8	0.3	6.3	0.012
Hypertransaminasemia	2.7	0.7	7.87	0.005

Thus, some practical issues need to be addressed. In adopting the new ESPGHAN criteria, it has to be kept in mind that there is a chance that patients might have a potential CD. In a prospective cohort study [18], which describes the long term natural history of potential CD by a 9 years follow-up, the risk of becoming atrophic was estimated at 18% especially in subjects with persistent positive serology, while serology became negative in 20% of potential patients on follow up. Even if rarely, potential celiac patients showed a TTG value >10 x ULN: hence this limit does not exclude the chance of finding potential celiac cases. Starting from this point, the decision to omit biopsy and the chance of being a potential CD should be thoroughly discussed with families considering the life-long diagnosis of CD. The new ESPGHAN guidelines also state that it is important to be precise in the clinical evaluation of patients and to perform prospective research studies. To the best of our knowledge, our prospective study is the largest one including 511 (+14) CD patients and 1391 controls and it shows that symptoms are not able to assign a pre-test probability to serological tests. On the other hand, Webb et al. [11] found no difference in terms of diagnostic accuracy of tTG in asymptomatic children diagnosed as having CD detected by screening.

We are aware of the limitations of our study, mostly due to the unequal distribution of enrolled patients across participating countries, although the total number is the largest one reported.

Therefore, further prospective multicentre studies with an homogeneous enrolment of patients should be planned also in order to try a further simplification of ESPGHAN guidelines.

Moreover, due to different test kinetics the 10 x UNL is not the same with all tTG tests. However, all the centres participating in the study utilized one of the 14 most frequently applied serum tTG assays in Europe taken in consideration in the new ESPGHAN guidelines Appendix. All these assays underwent United Kingdom National External Quality Assessment according to which the 10 x ULN was suggested by the new guidelines in order to omit intestinal biopsy. Considering that all the centres took at least 4 duodenal biopsy samples always including a sample from the bulbus we are confident that histology is the right gold standard chosen in this study.

Conclusions

This is the largest prospective study providing a wide picture of CD diagnosis feasibility in Mediterranean countries with different health resources and facilities. The results of our study show that CD diagnosis still relies on intestinal biopsy in the Mediterranean area. New ESPGHAN criteria are not applicable in 5 countries due to lack of resources needed to perform HLA genotyping and, in one country, EMA assay. Further simplification of the new ESPGHAN guidelines might be made according to what preliminarily the present results suggest if confirmed by new prospective studies. This would be a result of great value especially for countries with limited resources, even though the chance of a potential CD has to be taken into account and discussed with the families when intestinal biopsy is omitted.

Abbreviations

BSPGHAN: British society for pediatric gastroenterology, hepatology and nutrition; CCD: Confirmed celiac disease; CD: Celiac disease; ESPGHAN: European society for pediatric gastroenterology, hepatology and nutrition; NCCD: New criteria celiac disease; PCD: Potential celiac disease; PPV: Positive predictive value; RR: Relative risk; tTG: tissue transglutaminase type 2 antibodies; UCD: Unconfirmed celiac disease; ULN: Upper limit of normal

Acknowledgement

We thank Trays MacDonnell for revising the English of the article.

Funding

Italian Department of Health, Direction of International Affairs; Euromed action. Project: MEDICEL-Mediterranean Network for Celiac Disease–Phase II" (CUP n° E61J11000450001); ELFID – European Laboratory for Food Induced Disease

Authors' contributions

AS, LG and GM conceptualized and designed the study, carried out the initial analyses, drafted the initial manuscript, and approved the final manuscript as submitted. ZM drafted the initial manuscript, reviewed and revised the manuscript and approved the final manuscript as submitted. SC, DM-T, MA-Z, AK, AA, KB-N, MBH, ER, VV, MLT, TA and VD reviewed and revised the manuscript, and approved the final manuscript as submitted. All authors approved the final manuscript as submitted.

Competing interests

The authors declare that they have no competing interests.

Authors' information

Not applicable.

Author details

[1]Department of Translational Medical Sciences, School of Medicine, University "Federico II", Naples, Italy. [2]European Laboratory for Food Induced Diseases, Naples, Italy. [3]Children's Hospital Zagreb, Zagreb, Croatia. [4]Celiac Regional Centre, Pediatric Gastroenterology and Cystic Fibrosis Unit, University of Messina, Via Consolare Valeria 1, 98125, Messina, Italy. [5]Paediatric Department, University Medical Centre, Maribor, Slovenia. [6]Cairo University Children Hospital, El Cairo, Egypt. [7]Department of Pediatric

Gastroenterology, School of Medicine, Ankara University, Ankara, Turkey. [8]Centre Hospitalier Universitaire Ibnou Rochd, Casablanca, Morocco. [9]Faculté de Médecine d'Oran, Oran, Algeria. [10]Pediatric Unit, Mongi SLIM's Hospital of Tunis, Marsa, Tunisia. [11]First Department of Pediatrics, University of Athens, Athens, Greece. [12]Service of Pediatric Gastroenterology "Mother Teresa" Hospital, Tirana, Albania. [13]Paediatric Gastroenterology Unit, Cruces University Hospital, Bilbao, Spain. [14]University of Malta, Msida, Malta. [15]Clinical Center of Montenegro, Podgorica, Montenegro.

References

1. Green PH, Cellier C. Celiac disease. N Engl J Med. 2007;357:1731–43.
2. Greco L, Timpone L, Abkari A, Abu-Zekry M, Attard T, Bouguerrà F, Cullufi P, Kansu A, Micetic-Turk D, Mišak Z, Roma E, Shamir R, Terzic S. Burden of celiac disease in the Mediterranean area. World J Gastroenterol. 2011;17: 4971–8.
3. Emilsson L, Magnus MC, Størdal K. Perinatal risk factors for development of celiac disease in children, based on the prospective Norwegian Mother and Child Cohort Study. Clin Gastroenterol Hepatol. 2015;13:921–7.
4. Mårild K, Stephansson O, Montgomery S, Murray JA, Ludvigsson JF. Pregnancy outcome and risk of celiac disease in offspring: a nationwide case-control study. Gastroenterology. 2012;142:39–45.
5. Lionetti E, Castellaneta S, Francavilla R, Pulvirenti A, Tonutti E, Amarri S, Barbato M, Barbera C, Barera G, Bellantoni A, Castellano E, Guariso G, Limongelli MG, Pellegrino S, Polloni C, Ughi C, Zuin G, Fasano A, Catassi C, SIGENP (Italian Society of Pediatric Gastroenterology, Hepatology, and Nutrition) Working Group on Weaning and CD Risk. Introduction of gluten, HLA status, and the risk of celiac disease in children. N Engl J Med. 2014; 371:1295–303.
6. Vriezinga SL, Auricchio R, Bravi E, Castillejo G, Chmielewska A, Crespo Escobar P, Kolaček S, Koletzko S, Korponay-Szabo IR, Mummert E, Polanco I, Putter H, Ribes-Koninckx C, Shamir R, Szajewska H, Werkstetter K, Greco L, Gyimesi J, Hartman C, Hogen Esch C, Hopman E, Ivarsson A, Koltai T, Koning F, Martinez-Ojinaga E, te Marvelde C, Pavic A, Romanos J, Stoopman E, Villanacci V, Wijmenga C, Troncone R, Mearin ML. Randomized feeding intervention in infants at high risk for celiac disease. N Engl J Med. 2014;371: 1304–15.
7. Andrén Aronsson C, Lee HS, Koletzko S, Uusitalo U, Yang J, Virtanen SM, Liu E, Lernmark Å, Norris JM, Agardh D, TEDDY Study Group. Effects of Gluten Intake on Risk of Celiac Disease: A Case-Control Study on a Swedish Birth Cohort. Clin Gastroenterol Hepatol. 2016;14:403–9.
8. Mårild K, Kahrs CR, Tapia G, Stene LC, Størdal K. Infections and risk of celiac disease in childhood: a prospective nationwide cohort study. Am J Gastroenterol. 2015;110:1475–84.
9. Husby S, Koletzko S, Korponay-Szabó IR, Mearin ML, Phillips A, Shamir R, Troncone R, Giersiepen K, Branski D, Catassi C, Lelgeman M, Mäki M, Ribes-Koninckx C, Ventura A, Zimmer KP, ESPGHAN Working Group on Coeliac Disease Diagnosis; ESPGHAN Gastroenterology Committee; European Society for Pediatric Gastroenterology, Hepatology, and Nutrition. European Society for Pediatric Gastroenterology, Hepatology, and Nutrition guidelines for the diagnosis of coeliac disease. J Pediatr Gastroenterol Nutr. 2012;54: 136–60.
10. Wolf J, Hasenclever D, Petroff D, Richter T, Uhlig HH, Laaß MW, Hauer A, Stern M, Bossuyt X, de Laffolie J, Flemming G, Villalta D, Schlumberger W, Mothes T. Antibodies in the diagnosis of coeliac disease: a biopsy-controlled, international, multicentre study of 376 children with coeliac disease and 695 controls. PLoS ONE. 2014;9:e97853.
11. Webb C, Norström F, Myléus A, Ivarsson A, Halvarsson B, Högberg L, Lagerqvist C, Rosén A, Sandström O, Stenhammar L, Carlsson A. Celiac disease can be predicted by high levels of anti-tissue transglutaminase antibodies in population-based screening. J Pediatr Gastroenterol Nutr. 2015;60:787–91.
12. Bhattacharya M, Lomash A, Sakhuja P, Dubey AP, Kapoor S. Clinical and histopathological correlation of duodenal biopsy with IgA anti-tissue transglutaminase titers in children with celiac disease. Indian J Gastroenterol. 2014;33:350–4.
13. Kurppa K, Salminiemi J, Ukkola A, Saavalainen P, Löytynoja K, Laurila K, Collin P, Mäki M, Kaukinen K. Utility of the new ESPGHAN criteria for the diagnosis of celiac disease in at-risk groups. J Pediatr Gastroenterol Nutr. 2012;54:387–91.
14. Paul SP, Mazhar H, Spray CH. Applicability of the New ESPGHAN Guidelines for Diagnosing Coeliac Disease in Children from Resource Limited Countries. J Coll Physicians Surg Pak. 2015;25:455–7.
15. Oberhuber G, Granditsch G, Vogelsang H. The histopathology of coeliac disease: time for a standardized report scheme for pathologists. Eur J Gastroenterol Hepatol. 1999;11:1185–94.
16. Benelli E, Carrato V, Martelossi S, Ronfani L, Not T, Ventura A. Coeliac disease in the ERA of the new ESPGHAN and BSPGHAN guidelines: a prospective cohort study. Arch Dis Child. 2016;101:172–6.
17. Murch S, Jenkins H, Auth M, Bremner R, Butt A, France S, Furman M, Gillett P, Kiparissi F, Lawson M, McLain B, Morris MA, Sleet S, Thorpe M, BSPGHAN. Joint BSPGHAN and Coeliac UK guidelines for the diagnosis and management of celiac disease in children. Arch Dis Child. 2013;98:806–11.
18. Auricchio R, Tosco A, Piccolo E, Galatola M, Izzo V, Maglio M, Paparo F, Troncone R, Greco L. Potential celiac children: 9-year follow-up on a gluten-containing diet. Am J Gastroenterol. 2014;109:913–21.

8

Chronic constipation diagnosis and treatment evaluation: the "CHRO.CO.DI.T.E." study

Massimo Bellini[1*], Paolo Usai-Satta[2], Antonio Bove[3], Renato Bocchini[4], Francesca Galeazzi[5], Edda Battaglia[6], Pietro Alduini[7], Elisabetta Buscarini[8], Gabrio Bassotti[9] and ChroCoDiTE Study Group, AIGO

Abstract

Background: According to Rome criteria, chronic constipation (CC) includes functional constipation (FC) and irritable bowel syndrome with constipation (IBS-C). Some patients do not meet these criteria (No Rome Constipation, NRC). The aim of the study was is to evaluate the various clinical presentation and management of FC, IBS-C and NRC in Italy.

Methods: During a 2-month period, 52 Italian gastroenterologists recorded clinical data of FC, IBS-C and NRC patients, using Bristol scale, PAC-SYM and PAC-QoL questionnaires. In addition, gastroenterologists were also asked to record whether the patients were clinically assessed for CC for the first time or were in follow up. Diagnostic tests and prescribed therapies were also recorded.

Results: Eight hundred seventy-eight consecutive CC patients (706 F) were enrolled (FC 62.5%, IBS-C 31.3%, NRC 6.2%). PAC-SYM and PAC-QoL scores were higher in IBS-C than in FC and NRC. 49.5% were at their first gastroenterological evaluation for CC. In 48.5% CC duration was longer than 10 years. A specialist consultation was requested in 31.6%, more frequently in IBS-C than in NRC. Digital rectal examination was performed in only 56.4%. Diagnostic tests were prescribed to 80.0%. Faecal calprotectin, thyroid tests, celiac serology, breath tests were more frequently suggested in IBS-C and anorectal manometry in FC. More than 90% had at least one treatment suggested on chronic constipation, most frequently dietary changes, macrogol and fibers. Antispasmodics and psychotherapy were more frequently prescribed in IBS-C, prucalopride and pelvic floor rehabilitation in FC.

Conclusions: Patients with IBS-C reported more severe symptoms and worse quality of life than FC and NRC. Digital rectal examination was often not performed but at least one diagnostic test was prescribed to most patients. Colonoscopy and blood tests were the "first line" diagnostic tools. Macrogol was the most prescribed laxative, and prucalopride and pelvic floor rehabilitation represented a "second line" approach. Diagnostic tests and prescribed therapies increased by increasing CC severity.

Keywords: Functional constipation, Irritable bowel syndrome, Diagnosis, Treatment

* Correspondence: mbellini@med.unipi.it
[1]Gastrointestinal Unit, Department of Gastroenterology, University of Pisa, Via Paradisa, 2, 56127 Pisa, Italy
Full list of author information is available at the end of the article

Background

Chronic constipation (CC) is a common and extremely troublesome disorder that has a negative impact on social and professional life, reduces the quality of life (QoL) and represents a heavy economic burden [1–5]. CC affects about 12–17% of the world population, with a higher prevalence among females and elderly people [6–9].

A considerable amount (16 to 40%) of CC patients in different countries use laxatives, and their use is related to increasing age, symptom frequency and duration of constipation; in the USA more than $800 million are spent on laxatives each year [10, 11].

The most widely used criteria to assess CC are the Rome Criteria [12] (Table 1) which separate constipation in functional constipation (FC) and irritable bowel syndrome with constipation (IBS-C). The presence of abdominal pain relieved by defecation characterizes IBS-C. Moreover, some patients consider themselves constipated even when not showing signs or symptoms consistent with Rome criteria (here defined as "No-Rome Constipation", NRC) [13].

Table 1 Rome III criteria for functional constipation and irritable bowel syndrome

Functional Constipation
Diagnostic criteria[a]
1. Must include two or more of the following:
α. Straining during at least 25% of defecations
β. Lumpy or hard stools in at least 25% of defecations
γ. Sensation of incomplete evacuation for at least 25% of defecations
δ. Sensation of anorectal obstruction/blockage for at least 25% of defecations
ε. Manual manoeuvres to facilitate at least 25% of defecations (e.g. digital evacuation, support of the pelvic floor)
η. Fewer than three defecations per week
2. Loose stools are rarely present without the use of laxatives
3. Insufficient criteria for irritable bowel syndrome
[a]Criteria fulfilled for the last 3 months with symptoms onset at least 6 months prior to diagnosis
Irritable Bowel Syndrome with Constipation
Diagnostic criteria[a]
Recurrent abdominal pain or discomfort [b] at least 3 days/month in the last 3 months associated with two or more of the following:
-Improvement with defecation
-Onset associated with a change in frequency of stool
-Onset associated with a change in form (appearance) of stool (hard or lumpy stools ≥25% and loose or watery stools <25% of bowel movements)

[a]Criteria fulfilled for the last 3 months with symptoms onset at least 6 months prior to diagnosis

[b] "Discomfort" means an uncomfortable sensation not described as pain

At present it is unclear whether gastroenterologists use the same diagnostic and therapeutic approach in these different groups of patients.

Objective of the study

Primary endpoints

- To describe the diagnostic tools used and the treatments suggested by Italian gastroenterologists for CC patients.

Secondary endpoints

- To assess, among CC patients, the distribution of FC, IBS-C and NRC and the severity of symptoms and QoL.
- To evaluate whether the diagnosis of FC, IBS-C and NRC could affect the use of the diagnostic tools and the choice of the therapy.
- To evaluate other possible potential factors affecting the use of the diagnostic tools and the therapeutic choices in CC patients.

Methods

Study population and questionnaires

Fifty two gastroenterologists belonging to different gastroenterological units in Italy on behalf of the Italian Association of Hospital Gastroenterologists and Endoscopists (AIGO), recorded clinical and demographic data of all patients consecutively referred for CC in a two month period (September-October 2013).

Bristol scale [14] was used to assess the stool consistency in the previous three months, while symptoms were classified according to Rome III criteria in order to verify whether the patients could be diagnosed as FC, IBS-C, or NRC. In addition, gastroenterologists were also asked to record whether the patients were clinically assessed for CC for the first time or were in follow up. Diagnostic tests, recommended specialist consultations and prescribed therapies were also recorded.

Furthermore, patients were required to fill the Patient Assessment of Constipation-Symptoms (PAC-SYM) and the Patient Assessment of Constipation-Quality of Life (PAC-QoL) questionnaires.

PAC-SYM is a 12-item self-reported questionnaire developed to assess the frequency and severity of CC symptoms. It is divided into three symptom subscales: abdominal (items 1–4), rectal (items 5–7), and stool (items 8–12) [15].

PAC-QoL is a 28 item self-reported questionnaire used to measure the patient's QoL. It is divided into four subscales: physical discomfort (items 1–4), psychosocial discomfort (items 5–12), worries and concerns (items 12–23), and satisfaction (items 24–28) [16].

For both questionnaires, items are scored on a five-point Likert scale (0–4), with 4 indicating the worst symptom severity.

Inclusion criteria

-Patients aged over 18 years evaluated for CC.

Exclusion criteria

-Presence of known or suspected severe organic disease potentially causing constipation and/or psychiatric disease potentially interfering with questionnaires compilation.

-Patients assuming potentially constipating drugs or the onset of constipation after starting any kind of drug.

Statistical analysis

Data were analyzed by means of the SAS® System for Windows, version 9.2.

A prevalence approach was adopted and no imputation was performed for any missing data.

The association between categorical variables was analyzed using Chi-Square test or Fisher's exact test (for cell frequencies < 5). In order to correct for multiple comparisons, pairwise tests were adjusted using the Bonferroni method.

The association between a continuous and a categorical variable (with two categories) was analyzed by the Wilcoxon-Mann–Whitney test. Finally, the association between a continuous and a categorical variable was analyzed by the Kruskal-Wallis test (or by the ANOVA in case of normal distribution). In case of pairwise comparisons, the Dunn's test was performed. The correlation between two continuous variables was summarized by the Pearson's correlation coefficient in case of normal data distribution, or by the Spearman's correlation coefficient otherwise.

All statistical tests were performed with a two-sided significance level $\alpha = 0.05$, therefore p-values lower than 0.05 were considered statistically significant.

The PAC-SYM and PAC-QoL total and domain scores were calculated as detailed in Additional file 1, respectively.

PAC-SYM total score and PAC-QoL total score were also analyzed through multivariate regression models, adjusting for the following independent variables: age, sex, diagnosis, duration of CC.

Results

Data from 878 CC patients (33.9% in Northern Italy, 32.4% in Center Italy and 33.7% in Southern Italy), 706 women (80.4%) and 172 men (19.6%), mean age: 51.0 ± 16.8 years (F 49.6 ± 16.6 years; M 56.9 ± 16.5 years) were obtained. Their body mass index (BMI) was 23.7 ± 4.0 kg/m^2. Four hundred thirty-five out of 878 patients (49.5%) were at their first gastroenterological evaluation for CC. According to Rome III criteria the patients were classified as FC: 549 (62.5%); IBS-C: 275 (31.3%); NRC: 54 (6.2%).

IBS-C patients were younger (46.9 ± 16.2 years) than FC (52.8 ± 16.6) and NRC (53.1 ± 18.6) ($p < 0.0001$). The gender distribution was significantly different between the three groups (IBS-C: women 234/275 (85.1%); FC: women 433/549 (78.9%); NRC: women 39/54 (72.2%) ($p < 0.05$) .

The duration of CC was ">1–4 years" in 23.1% (IBS-C: 33.0%; FC: 59.1%; NRC: 7.9%), "≥5years" in 21.1% (IBS-C: 27.0%; FC: 65.4%; NRC: 7.6%) and ">10 years" in 48.5% of the patients (IBS-C: 32.2%; FC: 63.9%; NRC: 4.0%). No significant difference was observed between groups but only a trend toward a shorter duration in NRC could be detected.

Bristol 1–2 was reported in 628/878 (71.5%) patients (IBS-C: 208/275, 75.6%; FC:394/549, 71.8%; NRC: 26/54, 48.2%) (IBS-C vs FC: ns; IBS-C vs. NRC: $p < 0.001$; FC vs NRC: $p < 0.005$).

As shown in Table 2, 73.2% of patients reported at least one comorbidity in the previous year: depression and anxiety were more frequent in IBS-C compared to FC ($p < 0.01$) and NRC ($p < 0.005$), as well as dyspepsia ($p < 0.05$ vs. FC and NRC). Gastroesophageal reflux disease was more frequent in IBS-C compared to NRC ($p < 0.01$) and in FC compared to NRC ($p < 0.05$). Hypertension was found more frequently in FC than in IBS-C ($p < 0.05$).

The results of PAC-SYM are shown in Table 3: IBS-C mean total score was higher than FC and NRC ($p < 0.0001$) ones. The multivariate regression model suggested that the total score of PAC-SYM (mean: 1.6 ± 0.7) was directly related to the duration of constipation ($p < 0.01$), and to younger age ($p < 0.0001$). Abdominal symptoms subscale was significantly higher in IBS-C than in FC ($p < 0.05$) and in NRC ($p < 0.0001$). In particular, a positive association was detected between each of the first four items (discomfort, pain, bloating and stomach cramps) which constitutes the abdominal subscale and IBS-C ($p < 0.0001$). Fecal symptoms subscale was significantly higher in FC and IBS-C than NRC ($p < 0.01$). Furthermore, there was a positive correlation of the total PAC-SYM score with the number of diagnostic tests ($p < 0.0005$) and of suggested therapies ($p < 0.05$).

In Table 4 the results of PAC-QoL are shown: IBS–C mean total score was higher than FC and NRC ($p < 0.001$); all the subscales, excluding the satisfaction subscale, were significantly higher in IBS-C and in FC than in NRC. Moreover, the multivariate regression model for the total score of PAC-QoL (mean: 1.8 ± 0.7) shows that this was neither related to

Table 2 Prevalence of comorbidities

	IBS-C: 275	FC: 549	NRC: 54	*p*-value[1]
Dyspepsia	128 (46.5%)	200 (36.4%)	14 (25.9%)[#]	<0.005
Depression/anxiety	111 (40.4%)	164 (29.9%)*	9 (16.7%)**	<0.0005
GERD	98 (35.6%)	167 (30.4%)	8 (14.8%)[## ###]	<0.01
Sleep disturbances	87 (31.6%)	141 (25.7%)	13 (24.1%)	ns
Hypertension	45 (16.4%)	135 (24.6%)[§]	11 (20.4%)	<0.05
Urinary disturbances	52 (18.9%)	115 (20.9%)	8 (14.8%)	ns
Thyroid disease	26 (9.4%)	65 (11.8%)	6 (11.1%)	ns
Vaginitis	29 (10.5%)	46 (8.4%)	4 (7.4%)	ns
Dyspareunia	30 (10.9%)	38 (6.9%)	4 (7.4%)	ns
Diabetes	7 (2.5%)	29 (5.3%)	3 (5.6%)	ns
Fibromyalgia	16 (5.8%)	18 (3.3%)	-	ns
Other	36 (13.1)	56 (10.2%)	7 (13%)	ns

IBS-C irritable bowel syndrome with constipation, *FC* functional constipation, *NRC* patients do not accomplish Rome III criteria, *GERD* gastroesophageal reflux disease
[1]*p* values are referred to the differences between IBS-C, FC and NRC groups, in particular
$*p < 0.01$ vs IBS-C; $**p < 0.005$ vs IBS-C; $\#p < 0.05$ vs IBS-C and FC; $\#\#p < 0.01$ vs IBS-C
$\#\#\#p < 0.05$ vs FC; $§p < 0.05$ vs IBS-C; ns: not statistically significant

gender, nor to age or duration of constipation. There was a statistically significant positive correlation with the number of diagnostic tests ($p < 0.05$), the number of suggested therapies ($p < 0.0001$) and the number of specialist consultations ($p < 0.005$).

Digital rectal examination (DRE) was performed in 495/878 (56.4%), independently from the patients being at their first evaluation (54.7%) or at a follow up visit (56.6%). No relationship with gender was found (104 M: 61.3%; F 391: 55.2%). Patients in whom a DRE was performed were older (52.6 ± 16.6 years vs. 49.4 ± 16.7; $p < 0.01$), and DRE was more often performed by gastroenterologists aged over 40 years than by younger ones (60.1% vs. 44.6%; $p < 0.0001$).

At least a specialist consultation was requested in 277/878 (31.6%) patients, mostly psychiatric/psychological (11.5%), urological (8.1%) and gynecological (12.3% of the women) (Table 5). In IBS-C psychiatric/psychological and gynaecological consultations were more frequently requested than in NRC ($p < 0.05$).

Diagnostic tests were requested in 702/878 (80.0%) of the patients. Table 6 shows the different tests requested in the whole sample and in the different diagnosis subgroups (IBS-C, FC and NRC). Fecal calprotectin was more frequently prescribed in IBS-C than in FC and NRC ($p < 0.0001$ and $p < 0.05$, respectively). Thyroid function tests ($p < 0.05$), serology for celiac disease ($p < 0.005$), lactose breath test ($p < 0.01$) and glucose breath test ($p < 0.05$) were more frequently suggested in IBS-C than in FC, whereas in FC anorectal manometry was more frequently prescribed than in IBS-C ($p < 0.05$) and defecography more frequently than in NRC ($p < 0.05$). Abdominal ultrasonography was suggested in 22% of the patients without significant differences among groups.

Colonoscopy was suggested more in patients ≥50 years than in those <50 years (52.3% vs. 22.5%; $p < 0.0001$), more in males than in females (51.2% vs. 35.6%; $p < 0.001$) and more often at first evaluation than at follow-up (43.2% vs. 32.8%; $p < 0.005$). Also, routine blood tests

Table 3 PAC-SYM total score and abdominal, rectal and faecal symptoms subscales: mean values ± SD in all patients and in IBS-C, FC and NRC subgroups

	ALL PATIENTS	IBS-C	FC	NRC	*p*-value[1]
Total score	1.6 ± 0.70	1.75 ± 0.70*	1.56 ± 0.68	1.31 ± 0.70	$p < 0.0001$
Abdominal symptoms	1.53 ± 0.88	1.91 ± 0.74#§	1.37 ± 0.88	1.19 ± 0.86	$p < 0.0001$
Rectal symptoms	0.88 ± 0.86	0.98 ± 0.92	0.85 ± 0.83	0.70 ± 0.78	ns
Faecal symptoms	2.09 ± 0.91	2.09 ± 0.88	2.13 ± 0.92	1.74 ± 0.88^	$p < 0.01$

IBS-C irritable bowel syndrome with constipation, *FC* functional constipation, *NRC* patients do not accomplish Rome III criteria
[1]*p* values are referred to the differences between IBS-C, FC and NRC groups, in particular * $p < 0.0001$ vs FC and NRC; # $p < 0.0001$ vs NRC; § $p < 0.05$ vs FC;
^ $p < 0.01$ vs IBS-C and FC; ns: not statistically significant

Table 4 PAC-QoL total score and subscales (mean values ± SD) in all patients and in IBS-C, FC and NRC subgroups

	ALL PATIENTS	IBS-C	FC	NRC	*p*-value[1]
Total score	1.77 ± 0.69	1.97 ± 0.70	1.71 ± 0.68	1.44 ± 0.62*	$p < 0.001$
Physical discomfort	1.85 ± 0.88	2.13 ± 0.82	1.75 ± 0.88	1.42 ± 0.82*	$p < 0.001$
Psychosocial discomfort	1.12 ± 0.83	1.38 ± 0.83	1.02 ± 0.80	0.77 ± 0.73*	$p < 0.001$
Worries and concerns	1.72 ± 0.92	1.92 ± 0.93	1.65 ± 0.90	1.36 ± 0.80*	$p < 0.001$
Satisfaction	2.90 ± 0.71	2.89 ± 0.72	2.92 ± 0.69	2.74 ± 0.81	ns

IBS-C irritable bowel syndrome with constipation, *FC* functional constipation, *NRC* patients do not accomplish Rome III criteria
[1]*p* values are referred to the differences between IBS-C, FC and NRC groups, in particular
* $p < 0.001$ vs IBS-C and FC; ns: not statistically significant

(61.2% vs. 46.6%; $p < 0.0001$), thyroid function tests (52.0% vs. 40.2%,; $p < 0.001$), carcinoembryonic antigen (11.3% vs. 6.4%; $p < 0.05$), serology for celiac disease (19.1% vs. 13.2%; $p < 0.05$); and stool culture and test for ova and parasites (9.7% vs. 4.2%; $p < 0.005$) were requested more often at first evaluation than at follow-up. On the contrary defecography (2.5% vs. 5.6%; $p < 0.05$) was suggested less frequently at first visit than at follow-up. Serology for celiac disease was suggested more frequently in patients <50 years old than in patients ≥50 years old (22.0% vs. 11.3%; $p < 0.0001$).

Table 7 shows the suggested therapies, overall and by diagnosis. In 863/878 patients (98.3%) at least one treatment was given. Lifestyle and dietary changes were the most frequent suggestions, whereas macrogol and fiber supplements were largely the most frequently prescribed substances.

Macrogol was suggested more frequently in FC (71.6%) and IBS-C (70.9%) than in NRC (42.6%; $p < 0.0001$). A fiber supplements prescription was slightly more frequent in IBS-C, but no significant difference was detected among IBS-C, FC and NRC. In IBS-C antispasmodics were used more frequently compared to FC and NRC (27.6% vs. 11.7% vs. 11.1%; $p < 0.0001$ and $p > 0.05$, respectively). Antibloating agents (29.1% vs. 18.6%; $p < 0.005$) and psychotherapy (6.9% vs. 2.7%; $p < 0.05$) were most frequently prescribed in IBS-C than in FC, whereas pelvic floor rehabilitation was more frequently suggested in FC than in IBS-C (22.2% vs. 14.6%; $p < 0.05$).

Lactulose/lactitole (8.6% vs. 4.3%; $p < 0.05$), suppositories/micro-enemas (26.4% vs. 18.2%; $p < 0.005$), intestinal antibiotics (9.0% vs. 3.0%; $p < 0.0005$), antidepressants (10.0% vs. 3.0%; $p < 0.0001$), anxiolytics (15.9% vs. 8.1; $p < 0.001$) and pelvic floor rehabilitation (22.0% vs. 15.7%; $p < 0.05$) were more frequently suggested in patients ≥50 years than in patients <50 years, whereas antispasmodics were more frequently prescribed in patients <50 years than in patients ≥50 years (20.0% vs. 13.8%; $p < 0.05$).

Enemas and micro-enemas/suppositories were mainly prescribed not on a daily basis but usually every other day or on demand (24.2% and 19.7%, respectively). Lifestyle changes (87.5% vs. 80.9%; $p < 0.05$) and dietary suggestions (91.1% vs. 83.9%; $p < 0.05$) were more frequently prescribed in males than in females, but anorectal surgery only in females (2.8%).

Table 5 Specialist consultations requested by the gastroenterologists after their visit

CONSULTATION	878 pts. (%)	IBS-C (%)	FC (%)	NRC (%)	*p*-value[1]
Psychiatrist/psychologist	101 (11.5)	16.0	10.0	3.7*	<0.01
Gynaecologist[a]	87(12.3)	15.4	11.6	2.6*	<0.05
Urologist	71 (8.1)	8.0	8.4	5.6	ns
Surgeon	66 (7.5)	6.6	7.8	9.3	ns
Physiatrist/Physiotherapist	49 (5.6)	6.2	5.8	-	ns
Dietician	46 (5.2)	4.0	5.8	5.6	ns
Rheumatologist	15 (1.7)	2.6	1.3	1.9	ns
Neurological	15 (1.7)	1.8	1.6	1.9	ns
Other	17 (1.9)	2.6	1.8	-	ns

IBS-C irritable bowel syndrome with constipation, *FC* functional constipation, *NRC* patients do not accomplish Rome III criteria
[a]calculated on the women sample visited
[1]*p* values are referred to the differences between IBS-C, FC and NRC groups, in particular; *vs IBS-C and FC; ns: not statistically significant

Table 6 Diagnostic test requested by the gastroenterologist after their visit

DIAGNOSTIC TEST	878 pts.(%)	IBS-C (%)	FC (%)	NRC (%)	*p*-value[1]
Routine blood tests	472 (53.8)	58.9	51.6	50.0	ns
Thyroid function tests	400 (45.6)	52.4 #	43.2	35.2	<0.05
Colonoscopy	339 (38.6)	34.6	40.6	38.9	ns
Anorectal manometry	306 (34.9)	29.8 #	38.6	22.2	<0.01
Colonic transit time	228 (26.0)	30.6	24.6	16.7	ns
Abdominal ultrasonography	193 (22.0)	22.6	22.2	16.7	ns
RX Defecography	167 (19.0)	16.4	21.5 °	7.4	<0.05
Faecal blood test	153 (17.4)	14.9	18.8	16.7	ns
Coeliac serology	142 (16.2)	22.6^	13.1	14.8	<0.005
Carcinoembryonic antigen assay	78 (8.9)	6.6	9.8	11.1	ns
Faecal calprotectin	64 (7.3)	15.3 * **	3.8	1.9	<0.0001
Stool culture, test for ova and parasites	62 (7.1)	6.6	8.0	-	ns
Lactose Breath Test	35 (4.0)	7.3 §	2.7	-	<0.005
MR Defecography	33 (3.8)	2.6	4.2	5.6	ns
Trans-anal ultrasound	30 (3.4)	4.7	2.9	1.9	ns
Rectosigmoidoscopy	22 (2.5)	2.9	2.6	-	ns
Virtual colonoscopy	19 (2.2)	1.8	2.4	1.9	ns
Barium Enema	14 (1.6)	1.1	1.8	1.9	ns
Glucose Breath test	12 (1.4)	2.9 #	0.7	-	<0.05
Colonic manometry	12 (1.4)	1.8	1.1	1.9	ns
Anal Sphincter Electromyography	5 (0.6%)	0.7	0.6	-	ns
Other	34 (3.9)	4.7	3.6	1.9	ns

IBS-C irritable bowel syndrome with constipation, *FC* functional constipation, *NRC* patients do not accomplish Rome III criteria
[1]*p* values are referred to the differences between IBS-C, FC and NRC groups, in particular
# $p < 0.05$ vs FC; * $p < 0.0001$ vs FC; ** $p < 0.05$ vs NRC; ^ $p < 0.005$ vs FC; § $p < 0.01$ vs FC; ° $p < 0.05$ vs NRC; ns: not statistically significant

Probiotics were most frequently prescribed at first visit than at follow-up (40.9% vs. 31.5%; $p < 0.01$), whereas prucalopride and pelvic floor rehabilitation were more often prescribed during a follow-up visit than at first evaluation (20.1% vs. 10.6%, $p < 0.0001$; 23.8% vs. 15.4%, $p < 0.005$, respectively).

A mix of suggestions and drugs was used in many patients: in 59.5% lifestyle suggestions, changes in diet and macrogol; in 50.8% lifestyle suggestions, changes in diet and fiber supplementation; in 37.2% changes in diet, fiber supplementation and macrogol; in 37.1% lifestyle suggestions, fiber supplementation and macrogol; in 33.3% lifestyle suggestions, changes in diet and probiotics.

Discussion

The present study conveys an important educational message for general practitioners, who see the majority of constipated patients, and for other specialists who could visit patients for possible comorbidities: when collecting the patient's history, the presence of constipation should be accurately searched and treated (if possible). Waiting so many years before sending constipated patients to a gastroenterologist simply means worsening a patient's symptoms and his/her QoL [4] and increasing the risk to develop important anatomical alterations such as perineal descent, rectocele, rectal intussusceptions, prolapse, enterocele or sigmoidocele, or increase his/her cardiovascular mortality [17].

Rome criteria seemed accurate to identify constipated patients, since only 6.2% showed NRC.

NRC patients were usually older and often male than IBS-C, and reported fewer and less severe symptoms, softer stools and a better QoL than FC and IBS-C. On the other hand, IBS-C patients were younger and more often female, reported more severe symptoms, harder stools and a worse QoL than NRC

Table 7 Suggested therapies requested by the gastroenterologist after their visit

THERAPIES	878 pts.(%)	IBS-C (%)	FC (%)	NRC (%)	p-value[1]
Life style recommendations	722 (82.2)	84.7	81.8	74.1	ns
Dietary suggestions	749 (85.3)	85.5	85.8	79.6	ns
Fibre supplements	489 (55.7)	60.7	53.2	55.6	ns
Herbal remedies	46 (5.2)	6.2	4.9	3.7	ns
Probiotics	318 (36.2)	40.4	33.5	42.6	ns
Lactulose/lactitole	58 (6.6)	4.7	7.8	3.7	ns
Macrogol	609 (69.4)	71.6	70.9	42.6 #	<0.0001
Saline laxatives	31 (3.5)	4.0	3.5	1.9	ns
Stimulant laxatives	55 (6.3)	6.2	6.7	1.9	ns
Softening laxatives	46 (5.2)	5.1	5.7	1.9	ns
Prucalopride	126 (14.4)	13.1	15.7	7.4	ns
Suppositories/micro-enemas	198 (22.6)	23.6	21.3	29.6	ns
Enemas	238 (27.1)	29.5	26.6	20.4	ns
Antispasmodics	146 (16.6)	27.6 * **	11.7	11.1	<0.0001
Anti-bloating agents	191 (21.8)	29.1 ^	18.6	16.7	<0.005
Intestinal antibiotics	55 (6.3)	7.3	5.5	9.3	ns
Anxiolytics	108 (12.3)	14.6	11.5	9.3	ns
Antidepressants	60 (6.8)	8.0	6.0	9.3	ns
Psychotherapy	35 (4.0)	6.9 §	2.7	1.9	<0.05
Pelvic floor rehabilitation	169 (19.3)	14.6	22.2 °	13.0	<0.05
Sacral neurostimulation	3 (0.3)	//	0.4	1.9	ns
Anorectal surgery	20 (2.3)	1.5	2.7	1.9	ns
Colectomy	1 (0.1)	//	//	1.9	ns
Other	18 (2.1)	2.2	2.2	//	ns

IBS-C irritable bowel syndrome with constipation, *FC* functional constipation, *NRC* patients do not accomplish Rome III criteria
[1]*p* values are referred to the differences between IBS-C, FC and NRC groups, in particular
# $p < 0.0001$ vs IBS-C and NRC; * $p < 0.0001$ vs FC; ** $p < 0.05$ vs NRC; ^ $p < 0.005$ vs FC; § $p < 0.05$ vs FC; ° $p < 0.05$ vs IBS-C; ns: not statistically significant

and FC. Our results show that Rome III criteria identify patients with more severe constipation.

Recently the new Rome IV criteria have been published [18]. No substantial differences have been introduced regarding definition and classification of functional constipation: simply they state that "abdominal pain and/or bloating may be present but are not predominant symptoms (ie, the patient does not meet criteria for IBS)". Regarding IBS the term discomfort was eliminated and the frequency of abdominal pain became at least 1 day per week instead of 3 days per month. However we think that these changes would not have a significant impact on the results of our study.

PAC-SYM and PAC-QoL questionnaires showed higher scores in IBS-C group than in FC and NRC: PAC-SYM abdominal symptom subscale, PAC-QoL mean total score, physical discomfort, psychosocial discomfort and worries and concerns subscales were found to be higher in IBS-C. This reflects the close association between the first four items of PAC-SYM (abdominal discomfort, abdominal pain, bloating, stomach cramps) and the typical symptoms of IBS. These symptoms are likely responsible for the lower QoL in IBS-C. Thus, the increase in perception of constipation severity increases impairment of the QoL, also increasing request of diagnostic tests and therapies.

Different clinical characteristics, such as type of constipation and comorbidities, may influence the clinical approach of the gastroenterologists; thus, our primary endpoint was to assess the diagnostic tools and treatment suggested by Italian gastroenterologists to their constipated patients, and the impact on the clinical subgroups.

A surprising result, deserving discussion, is that DRE was not performed in more than 40% of the patients, independently from being at first visit or at follow-up. DRE is the simplest and the most immediate method to assess anal tone and to collect information about the pelvic floor conditions and to detect early forms of rectal cancer or benign diseases [19–22]. These data should be carefully taken into account when carrying out educational campaigns on the diagnosis and treatment of CC.

The presence of comorbidities was likely the main reason for the more frequent requested consultations (psychiatric/psychological, urological, gynecological) underlining the need for a stronger collaboration among different specialists for the correct management of CC, possibly creating multidisciplinary teams.

Regarding the attitude towards diagnostic tests, we want to stress that in about four out of five patients gastroenterologists were not so confident on Rome III criteria, and prescribed at least one diagnostic test, more often in patients at first evaluation, mainly blood tests, but also colonoscopy (requested more frequently in patients older than 50 years), anorectal manometry and measurement of colonic transit time. As already shown in previous studies in a general practitioner setting, abdominal ultrasound, although not recommended by current guidelines, was quite frequently requested, especially when abdominal pain is present [23–26].

To exclude conditions potentially mimicking IBS, laboratory and breath tests were more frequently requested in these patients, whereas in FC, defecography and anorectal manometry were more frequently requested to evaluate the presence of dyssynergic defecation. In NRC patients fewer diagnostic tests were overall required, probably due to less severe symptoms and lesser impairment of the QoL.

Overall, dietetic and lifestyle suggestions were the most frequently suggested therapeutic options (>90% of the patients) (Table 7). However, in the present study, the gastroenterologists were often not confident that these could be sufficient to solve the problem and used macrogol as the first line laxative, both in association with dietetic and lifestyle suggestion and fibers.

Macrogol is effective and safe, and new liquid formulations make it easier to dose; because taste is an important factor for patients' adherence, particularly for long-time treatment, the formulations without aroma made it more acceptable to patients [27]. On the other hand further increasing fibers intake could induce bloating and abdominal discomfort without improving colonic transit time [28]. To control the different symptoms of IBS (mainly abdominal pain and bloating) gastroenterologists also used antispasmodic drugs, psychotherapy and anti-bloating agents, whereas pelvic floor rehabilitation was suggested more often in FC patients, in whom functional defecation disorders should be more frequent.

Surgery procedures (and sacral neurostimulation) were infrequently suggested by gastroenterologists.

The gastroenterologists involved in this study rarely prescribed laxatives such as lactulose/lactitole, and stimulant, emollient or saline laxatives which still represent the most used laxatives in Italy. These drugs, which cover about 40% of the Italian market [29], are more often prescribed by general practitioners [23] and other specialists than gastroenterologists.

Prucalopride, recently available on the Italian market, was prescribed in about 13% of patients although it was considered, probably because expensive, a second/third line treatment, and prescribed more frequently at a follow-up. At the time of the study, linaclotide was not yet available on the Italian market.

As previously reported for diagnostic tools, the amount of therapy prescribed also increased by increasing PAC-SYM and PAC-QoL scores; in NRC patients, who displayed lighter symptoms, fewer therapies were suggested. In conclusion, in our country a gastroenterological evaluation of CC is often delayed in patients with long lasting symptoms, colonoscopy and blood tests are considered a "first line" diagnostic tool, and DRE is insufficiently performed. Furthermore, constipation is associated with several comorbidities in most patients. Among Italian gastroenterologists macrogol is the most frequently used laxative, while in IBS-C patients a larger amount of drugs is prescribed than in FC and NRC patients.

The study also provides several educational ideas to improve the diagnostic and therapeutic approach to CC: general practitioners and other specialists should be suggested to address earlier such patients to a gastroenterologist before long-term complications occur. DRE should be performed in all patients, while echography usefulness should be resized.

Conclusions

Chronic constipation is a common disorder that has a remarkable impact on the quality of life. We report on diagnostic and therapeutical experiences of Italian gastroenterologists.

Patients with irritable bowel syndrome with constipation reported more severe symptoms and worsened quality of life than functional constipation. Colonoscopy and blood tests were the most prescribed tests and Macrogol was the most prescribed laxative.

This study can provide several educational ideas to improve the diagnostic and therapeutic approach to Chronic Constipation.

Appendix
ChroCoDiTE Study Group Members - Collaborators

Last Name, First Name, Degree	Affiliation
Bellini Massimo, MD	U.O. Gastroenterologia Universitaria – AOU Pisana, Pisa
Usai Satta Paolo, MD	S.C. Gastroenterologia - Azienda Ospedaliera G. Brotzu - Cagliari
Bove Antonio, MD	U.O. Gastroenterologia ed Endoscopia Digestiva, Dipartimento di Gastroenterologia - AORN "A. Cardarelli", Napoli
Bocchini Renato, MD	Fisiopatologia ed Endoscopia Digestiva. Gastroenterologia ed Endoscopia Digestiva, Casa di Cura Malatesta Novello, Cesena
Battaglia Edda, MD	S.O.C Gastroenterologia, Ospedale Cardinal Massaja, Asti
Alduini Pietro, MD	U.O. Gastroenterologia; Ospedale di Lucca
Galeazzi Francesca, MD	U.O. Gastroenterologia Universitaria - Azienda Ospedaliero Universitaria Padova
Bassotti Gabrio, MD	Sezione di Gastroenterologia ed Epatologia, Dipartimento di Medicina Interna, Università di Perugia
Balzano Antonio, MD	Azienda Ospedaliera di Rilevanza Nazionale "A. Cardarelli", Napoli
Portincasa Piero, MD	Clinica Medica "A. Murri", Dipartimento di Scienze Biomediche e Oncologia Umana, Università di Bari
Bonfrate Leonilde, MD	Clinica Medica "A. Murri", Dipartimento di Scienze Biomediche e Oncologia Umana, Università di Bari
D'Alba Lucia; MD	U.O.C. Gastroenterologia ed Endoscopia Digestiva, Az. Ospedaliera San Giovanni Addolorata - Roma
Badiali Danilo, MD	Dip. Medicina Interna e Specialità Mediche, La Sapienza, Roma
Marchi Santino, MD	U.O. Gastroenterologia Universitaria – AOU Pisana, Pisa
Gambaccini Dario, MD	U.O. Gastroenterologia Universitaria – AOU Pisana, Pisa
Neri Maria Cristina, MD	Ambulatorio Gastroenterologia ed Endoscopia digestiva – Pio Albergo Trivulzio, Milano,
Muscatiello Nicola, MD	U.O. Gastroenterologia Universitaria, Foggia
Di Stefano Michele, MD	U.O. Medicina Interna I, Fondazione IRCCS Policlinico "S.Matteo", Pavia.
Giannelli Claudio, MD	U.O.C. di Gastroenterologia Riabilitativa – Az. Ospedaliera San Camillo – Forlanini, ROMA
Goffredo Fabio, MD	U.O.C di Gastroenterologia Riabilitativa – Az. Ospedaliera San Camillo – Forlanini, ROMA
Turco Luigi, MD	S. S. Endoscopia Digestiva; U. O. C. Chirurgia Generale; P. O. Copertino, Lecce
Camilleri Salvatore, MD	U.O.C. di gastroenterologia, Ospedale M. Raimondi San Cataldo, Caltanissetta
Ceccarelli Giovanni, MD	U.O.C. di Gastroenterologia ed Endoscopia Digestiva, Ospedale della Versilia - Viareggio
Iovino Paola, MD	Dipartimento di Medicina e Chirurgia-Università di Salerno
Montalbano Luigi Maria, MD	U.O.C. di Gastroenterologia, Ospedali Riuniti Villa Sofia-Cervello Palermo
Morreale Gaetano Cristian, MD	Gastroenterologia ed Epatologia; Policlinico Palermo
Rentini Silvia, MD	U.O.C. Gastroenterologia ed Endoscopia Operativa, Dipartimento Oncologico; Azienda Ospedaliera Universitaria Senese - Siena
Savarino Vincenzo, MD	U.O. Clinica Gastroenterologia con Endoscopia - IRCCS AO Universitaria San Martino - IST - Genova
Segato Sergio, MD	UO Gastroenterologia ed Endoscopia Digestiva. AOU Macchi, Varese
Buscarini Elisabetta, MD	U.O. Gastroenterologia ed Endoscopia Digestiva, Ospedale Maggiore- Crema
Manfredi Guido, MD	U.O. Gastroenterologia ed Endoscopia Digestiva, Ospedale Maggiore- Crema
Cannizzaro Renato, MD	SOC. Gastroenterologia Oncologica, Centro di Riferimento Oncologico - Istituto Nazionale Tumori IRCCS, Aviano
Passaretti Sandro, MD	U.O. Gastroenterologia Ospedale Universitario San Raffaele, Milano, Italy
Alessandri Matteo, MD	U.O. Gastroenterologia Ospedale Universitario San Raffaele, Milano, Italy
Corti Federico, MD	U.O.C. di Gastroenterologia ed Endoscopia Digestiva, Ospedale della Versilia - Viareggio
Cuomo, Rosario, MD	Dipartimento di Medicina Clinica e Sperimentale, Università Federico II, Napoli
Zito Francesco Paolo, MD	Dipartimento di Medicina Clinica e Sperimentale, Università Federico II, Napoli
Mellone Carmine, MD	UOS di Endoscopia Digestiva. Ospedali della Valdichiana, Montepulciano
Barbera Roberta, MD	Ospedale San Giuseppe Multimedica - Milano

(Continued)

Milazzo Giuseppe, MD	UOC Medicina e Lungodegenza, Ospedale Vittorio Emanuele III, Salemi
Pucciani Filippo, MD	Dipartimento di Chirurgia e Medicina Traslazionale - Università di Firenze.
Soncini Marco, MD	UOC Gastroenterologia, Ospedale San Carlo - Milano
Lai Maria Antonia, MD	Dipartimento di Medicina Interna A.O.U. Policlinico di Monserrato, Università di Cagliari
Ruggeri Maurizio, MD	U.O. Gastroenterologia, Ospedale Sant'Andrea - Roma
Savarese Maria Flavia, MD	U.O.C. Endoscopia Digestiva e Gastroenterologia – A.O. Istituti Ospitalieri di Cremona
De Bona Manuela, MD	U.O.C. Gastroenterologia, Ospedale S. Maria Del Prato, Feltre
Surrenti Elisabetta, MD	SOS Fisiopatologia dell'apparato digerente e motilità, AOU Careggi - Firenze
Arini Andrea, MD	U.O. Gastroenterologia ed Epatologia; Policlinico Paolo Giaccone - Palermo
Dinelli Marco, MD	U.O. Endoscopia Digestiva, Azienda Ospedaliera San Gerardo, Monza
Leandro Gioacchino, MD	Dipartimento di gastroenterologia, IRCCS De Bellis – Castellana Grotte
Peralta Sergio, MD	U.O.C di Gastroenterologia ed Epatologia, A.O.U. Policlinico Paolo Giaccone - Palermo
Manta Raffaele, MD	U.O.C. Endoscopia Digestiva ed Interventistica Ospedale Niguarda Ca' Granda , Milano
Quartini Mariano, MD	S.C. Epatologia e Gastroenterologia, A.O. S. Maria, Terni
Torresan Francesco, MD	Dipartimento di Medicina Interna e Gastroenterologia , Policlinico S.Orsola-Malpighi - Università di Bologna,
Vilardo Luigi, MD	U.O.S. Gastroenterologia Ospedale Generale Ferrari, Castrovillari
Pulvirenti D'Urso Antonino, MD	U.O. Chirurgia, Ospedale Nuovo Garibaldi - Catania
Tarantino Ottaviano, MD	U.O. Gastroenterologia, Ospedale S. Giuseppe, Empoli
Noris Roberto Antonio, MD	U.O.C. di Gastroenterologia ed Endoscopia Digestiva - A.O. Bolognini - Seriate
Monica Fabio, MD	S.C. Gastroenterologia ed Endoscopia Digestiva – AOU - Ospedale di Cattinara - Trieste
Carrara Maurizio, MD	U.O.S.D. di Gastroenterologia Ospedale Orlandi, Bussolengo
Losco Alessandra, MD	Gastroenterologia Ospedale San Paolo - MILANO
Lauri Adriano, MD	U.O.C. Gastroenterologia ed Endoscopia Digestiva, Ospedale Civile Spirito Santo, Pescara
Neri Matteo, MD	Dipartimento di Medicina e Scienze dell'Invecchiamento & Ce.S.I., Università G. D'Annunzio, Chieti.
Grassini Mario, MD	S.O.C. Gastroenterologia, Ospedale Cardinal Massaja, Asti

Abbreviations

AIGO: Italian association of hospital gastroenterologists and endoscopists; BMI: Body mass index; CC: Chronic constipation; DRE: Digital rectal examination; FC: Functional constipation; IBS-C: Irritable bowel syndrome with constipation; NRC: No Rome constipation; PAC-QoL: The patient assessment of constipation-quality of life; PAC-SYM: Patient assessment of constipation-symptoms; QoL: Quality of life.

Acknowledgments

The authors are grateful to Dr. Elena Pasquali for her valuable help in carrying out the statistical analysis.
The members of the ChroCoDiTE StudyGroup are listed in Appendix and searchable through their individual PubMed records.

Authors' contributions

MB, PUS, GB, participated in study concept and design, data analysis, interpretation of results, manuscript drafting and approved the final version of the manuscript. AB, RB and FG contributed to the interpretation of results, provided critical revisions to manuscript drafts and approved the final version of the manuscript. EB and PA participated in study concept and design, data collection, interpretation of results, provided critical revisions to manuscript drafts and approved the final version of the manuscript. All members of the ChroCoDiTE study group participated in data collection, provided critical revisions to manuscript drafts and approved the final version of the manuscript.

Competing interests

The authors declare that they have no competing interests.

Author details

[1]Gastrointestinal Unit, Department of Gastroenterology, University of Pisa, Via Paradisa, 2, 56127 Pisa, Italy. [2]Brotzu Hospital, Gastroenterology Unit, Cagliari, Italy. [3]AORN "A. Cardarelli", Naples, Italy. [4]Malatesta Novello, Private Hospital, Cesena, Italy. [5]Division of Gastroenterology, Department of Surgery, Oncology and Gastroenterology, University of Padua, Padua, Italy. [6]Cardinal Massaia Hospital, Gastroenterology Unit, Asti, Italy. [7]San Luca Hospital, Digestive Endoscopy Unit, Lucca, Italy. [8]Gastroenterology and Digestive Endoscopy Unit, Maggiore Hospital, Crema, Italy. [9]Gastrointestinal and Hepatology Section, Clinical & Experimental Medicine, Perugia, Italy.

References

1. Lacy BE, Brunton SA. Partnering with gastroenterologists to evaluate patients with chronic constipation. Med Gen Med. 2005;7:19. PMID: 16369398.
2. Lindberg G, Hamid SS, Malfertheiner P, Thomsen OO, Fernandez LB, Garisch J, Thomson A, Goh KL, et al. World Gastroenterology Organisation global guideline: Constipation–a global perspective. J Clin Gastroenterol. 2011;45: 483–7. doi:10.1097/MCG.0b013e31820fb914. PMID: 21666546.
3. Nellesen D, Yee K, Chawla A, Lewis BE, Carson RT. A systematic review of the economic and humanistic burden of illness in irritable bowel syndrome and chronic constipation. J Manag Care Pharm. 2013;19:755–64. PMID: 24156644.

4. Neri L, Basilisco G, Corazziari E, Stanghellini V, Bassotti G, Bellini M, Perelli I, Cuomo R, LIRS study group. Constipation severity is associated with productivity losses and healthcare utilization in patients with chronic constipation. United European Gastroenterol J. 2014;2:138–47. doi:10.1177/2050640614528175. PMID: 24953097.
5. Nyrop KA, Palsson OS, Levy RL, Von Korff M, Feld AD, Turner MJ, Whitehead WE. Costs of health care for irritable bowel syndrome, chronic constipation, functional diarrhoea and functional abdominal pain. Aliment Pharmacol Ther. 2007;26:237–48. doi:10.1111/j.1365-2036.2007.03370.x. PMID: 17593069.
6. Bharucha AE, Pemberton JH, Locke 3rd GR. American Gastroenterological Association technical review on constipation. Gastroenterology. 2013;144: 218–38. doi:10.1053/j.gastro.2012.10.028. PMID: 23261065.
7. McCrea GL, Miaskowski C, Stotts NA, Macera L, Varma MG. A review of the literature on gender and age differences in the prevalence and characteristics of constipation in North America. J Pain Symptom Manage. 2009;37:737–45. doi:10.1016/j.jpainsymman.2008.04.016. PMID: 18789639.
8. Peppas G, Alexiou VG, Mourtzoukou E, Falagas ME. Epidemiology of constipation in Europe and Oceania: a systematic review. BMC Gastroenterol. 2008;8:5. doi:10.1186/1471-230X-8-5. PMID: 18269746.
9. Suares NC, Ford AC. Prevalence of, and risk factors for, chronic idiopathic constipation in the community: systematic review and meta-analysis. Am J Gastroenterol. 2011;106:1582–91. doi:10.1038/ajg.2011.164. quiz 1, 92. PMID: 21606976.
10. Higgins PD, Johanson JF. Epidemiology of constipation in North America: a systematic review. Am J Gastroenterol. 2004;99:750–9. PMID: 15089911.
11. Wald A, Scarpignato C, Mueller-Lissner S, Kamm MA, Hinkel U, Helfrich I, Schuijt C, Mandel KG. A multinational survey of prevalence and patterns of laxative use among adults with self-defined constipation. Aliment Pharmacol Ther. 2008;28:917–30. doi:10.1111/j.1365-2036.2008.03806.x. [PMID: 18644012.
12. Longstreth GF, Thompson WG, Chey WD, Houghton LA, Mearin F, Spiller RC. Functional bowel disorders. Gastroenterology. 2006;130:1480–91. PMID: 16678561.
13. Gambaccini D, Racale C, Salvadori S, Bassotti G, Pucciani F, Battaglia E, Bocchini R, Bove A, Alduini P, Marchi S, Bellini M. Sa2033 Chronic Constipation: ROME III Criteria and What Patients Think. Are We Talking the Same Language? Gastroenterology. 2014;146:S-360.
14. Lewis SJ, Heaton KW. Stool form scale as a useful guide to intestinal transit time. Scand J Gastroenterol. 1997;32:920–4. PMID: 9299672.
15. Frank L, Kleinman L, Farup C, Taylor L, Miner Jr P. Psychometric validation of a constipation symptom assessment questionnaire. Scand J Gastroenterol. 1999;34:870–7. PMID: 10522604.
16. Marquis P, De La Loge C, Dubois D, McDermott A, Chassany O. Development and validation of the Patient Assessment of Constipation Quality of Life questionnaire. Scand J Gastroenterol. 2005;40:540–51. PMID: 16036506.
17. Bassotti G. Being constipated: a bad omen for your cardiovascular system? Atherosclerosis. 2016;245:240–1. doi:10.1016/j.atherosclerosis.2015.10.001. PMID: 26684285.
18. Lacy BE, Mearin F, Chang L, Chey WD, Lembo AJ, Simren M, Spiller R. Gastroenterology. 2016;150:1393–407. doi:10.1053/j.gastro.2016.02.031.
19. Eckardt VF, Kanzler G. Prevention and early recognition of colorectal carcinoma. Dtsch Med Wochenschr. 1995;120:417–22. PMID: 7705204.
20. Talley NJ. How to do and interpret a rectal examination in gastroenterology. Am J Gastroenterol. 2008;103:820–2. doi:10.1111/j.1572-0241.2008.01832.x. [PMID: 18397419.
21. Gupta PJ. A review of ano-rectal disorders and their treatment. Bratisl Lek Listy. 2006;107:323–31. PMID: 17125068.
22. Wong RK, Drossman DA, Bharucha AE, Rao SS, Wald A, Morris CB, Oxentenko AS, Ravi K, Van Handel DM, Edwards H, Hu Y, Bangdiwala S. The digital rectal examination: a multicenter survey of physicians' and students' perceptions and practice patterns. Am J Gastroenterol. 2012;107:1157–63. doi:10.1038/ajg.2012.23. PMID: 22858996.
23. Bellini M, Gambaccini D, Salvadori S, Tosetti C, Urbano MT, Costa F, Monicelli P, Mumolo MG, Ricchiuti A, De Bortoli N, Marchi S. Management of chronic constipation in general practice. Tech Coloproctol. 2014;18:543–9. doi:10.1007/s10151-013-1093-9. PMID: 24272606.
24. Bellini M, Tosetti C, Costa F, Tosetti C, Urbano MT, Costa F, Monicelli P, Mumolo MG, Ricchiuti A, Bruzzi P, Marchi S. The general practitioner's approach to irritable bowel syndrome: from intention to practice. Dig Liv Dis. 2005;37:934–9. PMID: 16243592.
25. Bove A, Bellini M, Battaglia E, Bocchini R, Gambaccini D, Bove V, Pucciani F, Altomare DF, Dodi G, Sciaudone G, Falletto E, Piloni V. Consensus statement AIGO/SICCR diagnosis and treatment of chronic constipation and obstructed defecation (part II: treatment). World J Gastroenterol. 2012;18: 4994–5013. doi:10.3748/wjg.v18.i36.4994. PMID: 23049207.
26. Tack J, Muller-Lissner S, Stanghellini V, Boeckxstaens G, Kamm MA, Simren M, Galmiche JP, Fried M. Diagnosis and treatment of chronic constipation–a European perspective. Neurogastroenterology Motil. 2011;23:697–710. doi:10.1111/j.1365-2982.2011.01709.x. PMID: 21605282.
27. Lam TJ, Mulder CJ, Felt-Bersma RJ. Differences in taste between three polyethylene glycol preparations: a randomized double-blind study. Patient Prefer Adherence. 2011;5:423–6. doi:10.2147/PPA.S22780. PMID: 21949605.
28. McRorie Jr JW. Evidence-Based Approach to Fiber Supplements and Clinically Meaningful Health Benefits, Part 2: What to Look for and How to Recommend an Effective Fiber Therapy. Nutr Today. 2015;50:90–7. doi:10.1097/NT.0000000000000089. PMID: 25972619.
29. IMS Health. Intercontinental Marketing Services. Available at: http://www.imshealth.com.

9

Life-threatening bleeding from gastric dieulafoy's lesion in a pregnant woman with hellp syndrome

Chen Si[1*], Zhu Xiuli[1], Xie Li[1], Jia Yong[1], Zhou Ying[2] and Zhang Kaiguang[1]

Abstract

Background: Dieulafoy's lesion (DL) is one of the rare causes of upper gastrointestional bleeding. This disease is characterized by small sub-mucosal arteriole that eroded the stomach mucosa and cause severe upper GI bleeding without obvious ulceration. The most common location is fundus area of stomach and usually affects patients over 50 years of age with multiple comorbidities.

Case presentation: We report a case of life-threatening bleeding from DL during late pregnancy 31 weeks. Hemoclips were used twice through upper endoscopy with successful hemostasis. Unfortunately, she developed HELLP syndrome diagnosed 5 days after the GI bleeding was stopped. Her pregnancy had to be terminated with delivery of a premature infant. She recovered from her illness and discharged from hospital uneventfully. There is no current report in literature of DL in pregnant woman subsequently suffered HELLP syndrome.

Conclusion: Endoscopic hemoclip application is an effective technique in the treatment of upper GI bleeding from DL. For this patient, laparoscopic surgery or combination therapy before pregnancy may have been a suitable treatment on preventing rebleeding.

Keywords: Dieulafoy's lesion, Pregnancy, HELLP syndrome

Background

Dieulafoy's lesion (DL) is one of the rare, but potentially life-threatening causes of massive upper gastrointestinal (GI) bleeding. It accounts for about 1–2% of acute upper GI bleeding and occur more common in gastric fundic area at all age [1]. The diagnosis in pregnant women has not been reported. Due to the hemodynamic changes during pregnancy, DL is likely increase the morbidities and mortalities of pregnant women. Here we report a case that a pregnant woman who had massive upper GI hemorrhage from Dieulafoy's lesion of stomach. She was treated successfully with hemoclips endoscopically with supportive care including fluid resuscitation, blood transfusion. Unfortunately, the patient eventually developed HELLP (hemolysis, elevated liver enzymes, and low platelets) syndrome. Termination of pregnancy prematurely to save the mother and baby's life was the only option.

In 1982, Weinstein firstly described the HELLP syndrome which including hemolysis, elevated liver enzymes and low platelets [2]. The incidence of this syndrome is only 0.2%–0.6% in pregnant women and the exact etiology has not been clearly defined. There were case reports about Dieulafoy's disease and HELLP syndrome occurred in women. To our knowledge, sequential occurrence of DL and HELLP syndrome were not reported so far.

Case presentation

A 27-year-old female patient was admitted to the gastroenterology department of our hospital due to hematemesis and melena. She was at 31 weeks and

* Correspondence: css81729@163.com
[1]Department of Gastroenterology, Affiliated Provincial Hospital of Anhui Medical University, Hefei, China
Full list of author information is available at the end of the article

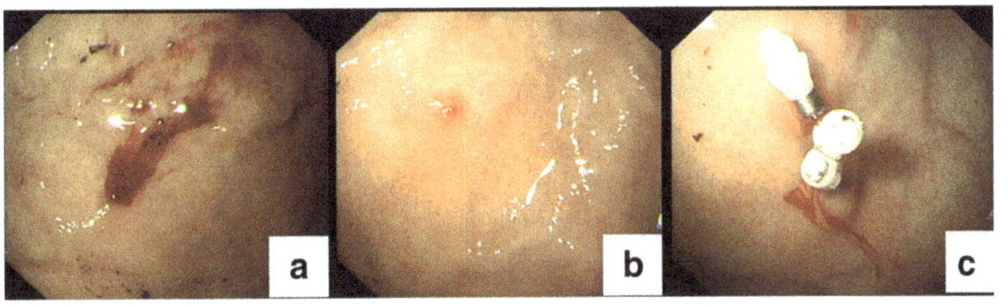

Fig. 1 a, b GI endoscopy revealed active bleeding from gastric fundus and an exposed vessel protruded from a slight defect. **c** The lesion was treated with three hemoclips

4 days gestation. The patient had gastric DL diagnosed by esophagogastroduodenoscopy (EGD) 8 years ago when she presented with frequent hematemesis and black stools. EGD showed an blood vessel with bleeding over her gastric fundus about 6 cm from the gastro-esophageal junction (Fig. 1). She had three episodes of upper GI bleeding from the same lesion without no overt symptoms.

In this case, emergency EGD (GIF Q260, Olympus Optical Co., Japan) revealed no active hemorrhage detected in upper digestive tract, other than the DL. The DL lesion in the fundus of stomach was treated with hemoclips for recurrent bleeding prophylaxis since she is having upper GI bleeding (Fig. 2). Unfortunately, massive hematemesis occurred again 2 days later and a second emergency gastroscopy was performed, which showed a spurting arterial bleeding without underlying ulceration close to the previous hemoclips. Hemoclips were applied again (Fig. 3). Finally, hemostasis based on endoscopic examination was achieved. However, even with blood transfusion support, the patient developed progressively anemia and thrombocytopenia without evidence of GI bleeding such as guaiac negative stools. Because of paroxysmal mild chest tightness and abdominal pains, Dexamethasone and magnesium sulfatate were administered intravenously to prevent eclampsia. Her laboratory examination showed: hemoglobin (HB), 62 g/L, platelet count, 19 × 10^9/L, aspartate aminotransferase (AST) level and glutamic-pyruvic transaminase (ALT) were 136 IU/L and 252 IU/L respectively, serum total bilirubin, 55.7 μmol/L, lactate dehydrogenase (LDH), 1740 IU/L. Peripheral blood smear and elevated indirect bilirubin (38.5 μmol/L) revealed presence of schistocytes. Her blood pressure also increased to 155/91 mmHg. Meanwhile, there was signs of fetal distress and patient presented with acute abdominal pain. With evidence of acute hemolysis, thrombocytopenia and liver dysfunction, the pregnant woman was diagnosed with HELLP syndrome.

To prevent the further deterioration of mother and fatal condition, immediate delivery of the preterm baby by cesarean was recommended by hematology and gynecology consultation. She had uneventful surgery and discharged from hospital a week later. Her laboratory studies prior to discharge showed HB of 80 g/L and platelet count of 88 × 10^9/L. Serum bilirubin, AST and ALT were all within normal limits. No recurrence of GI bleeding was noted within 1-month of outpatient follow-up. Premature baby was also discharged from hospital after delivery within 30 days showing no complications.

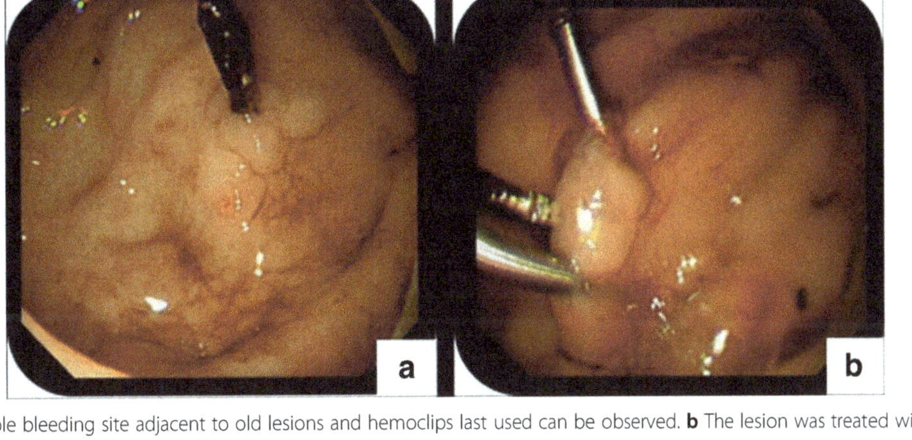

Fig. 2 a The possible bleeding site adjacent to old lesions and hemoclips last used can be observed. **b** The lesion was treated with titanium clamhemoclips for prevention of recurrent bleeding

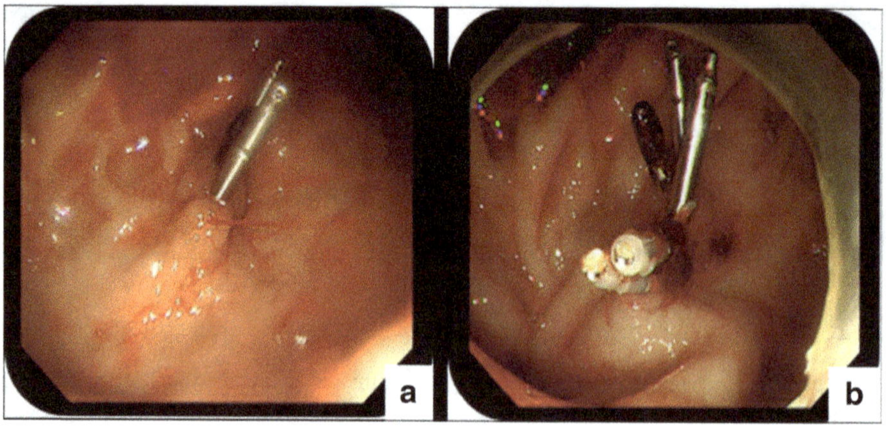

Fig. 3 a A pulsatile bleeding in the upper stomach without underlying ulceration. **b** Resolution of hemorrhage following placement of hemoclips

Discussion and conclusion

DL is one of the rare causes of GI bleeding. It accounts for about 1.5% of all GI hemorrhages [3, 4]. Due to the subtlety of the lesion, endoscopic visual criteria have been established for diagnosis of DL [5]. In this case we observed active arterial spurting from a small (<3 mm) defect in the gastric mucosa. DL associated upper GI bleeding during late pregnancy is extraordinarily rare in clinical practice. There was only one case report of duodenal DL associated bleeding in the first trimester of pregnancy in literature (Table 1) [6]. It can occur anywhere in the gastrointestinal tract. Some lesions are extragastric including duodenum and esophageal [5, 6].

Although there is no consensus on the best techniques to treat DL, GI endoscopy is a vital tool [7, 8]. The common endoscopic treatment for DL associated GI bleeding include thermal probe, regional injection of epinephrine and mechanical methods [9–11]. The use of hemoclips proves to be easy and safe technique in treating DL GI bleeding and preventing rebleeding [11]. In our case, the pregnant woman suffered from pulsatile bleeding has been multiple hospitalizations for hemostasis which was controlled with emergency endoscopy two times. During late pregnancy, enlarged uterus can cause gastrointestinal compression leading to delayed gastric emptying. Retention of gastric juice and food may result in damage to the mucous membranes; thus, the risk of DL rebleeding may be higher in the third trimester.

Surgery is needed in about 3% to 16% of cases in patients with DL bleeding due to rebleeding after endoscopic therapies [12–14]. Laparoscopic surgery has been reported to treat patient with DL bleeding with advantages of minimally invasive intervention, but accurate localization of the bleeding site can be challenged [15]. For this patient rebleeding of DL occurred at the same site of stomach, so wide wedge resection of laparoscopic surgery with intraoperative endoscopy before pregnancy could have been a preferable treatment for patient with frequent recurrence of DL bleeding. Combined modality such as epinephrine injection and application of hemoclips therapy can achieve higher rate of initial hemostasis and lower rate of rebleeding when compared with monotherapy [12, 14]. It also may be a better option for our current case.

Even with the success of endoscopic therapy, massive hemorrhage has led to the progressive decline of PLT and eventually the HELLP syndrome occurred. It may be associated with massive hemorrhage and repeatedly erythrocyte transfusion. Moreover, hypoxia and heterologous related antigen during transfusion triggered immune reaction and inflammatory response that are both included in the etiology and pathogenesis of HELLP [16]. Damage to the vascular endothelial cell by activated platelets and other factors may cause thrombotic microangiopathy. This is considered to be the main pathogenetic mechanism of HELLP [16, 17].

The syndrome is typically observed in patients with severe preeclampsia. Although there was no severe preeclampsia in our case, laboratory results were consistent with the diagnosis of HELLP syndrome. The diagnostic criteria of the HELLP syndrome was initially proposed by Tennessee Classification System [18]. It includes

Table 1 Bleeding DL in pregnant woman: literature review

Author	GA at diagnosis (weeks)	Treatment	Complications	Follow-up (months)	Outcome
Benedetto et al.	9	Endoscopy with HCPs	no	1	Normal
Chen et al.	31	Endoscopy with HCPs	HELLP syndrome	2	Normal

GA gestational age, *HCPs* hemoclips

presence of hemolysis, thrombocytopenia and hepatic changes with increased levels of enzymes. Pregnancy termination is still considered to be the best HELLP treatment method ensuring safety of the mother and infant [17, 18]. Current case presents nonspecific symptoms and stable delivery of the fetus by cesarean section. The mother and infant recovered uneventfully following effective treatment.

The patient with DL followed by HELLP syndrome is rare. Koji et al. have reported a case of HELLP syndrome with pituitary apoplexy [19]. Endoscopic therapy, especially hemoclips, is an initial and main treatment of bleeding caused by DL. However, both combined endoscopic therapies and surgery might be needed in some patients who are in a high risk of life-threatening rebleeding. Pathogenesis of HELLP syndrome in patient with DL is unclear. Massive GI hemorrhage and inflammatory response may be the triggering factors that lead to HELLP syndrome.

Abbreviations

DL: Dieulafoy's lesion; GI: Gastrointestinal; HELLP: H (hemolysis) EL (elevated liver enzymes) LP (low platelet count); PLT: Platelet; EGD: Esophagogastroduodenoscopy

Funding

This report received no specific grant from any funding agency or institution.

Authors' contributions

XL, JY, ZX and CS managed the patient; XL, ZK and CS worked on endoscopic therapy; ZY performed caesarian section; CS and ZX wrote the manuscript and ZY supervised it. All authors approved the final manuscript.

Competing interests

The authors declare that they have no competing interests.

Author details

[1]Department of Gastroenterology, Affiliated Provincial Hospital of Anhui Medical University, Hefei, China. [2]Department of Obstetrics, Affiliated Provincial Hospital of Anhui Medical University, Hefei, China.

References

1. Baxter M, Aly EH. Dieulafoy's lesion: current trends in diagnosis and management. Ann R Coll Surg Engl. 2010;92:548–54.
2. Benedetto C, Marozio L, Tancredi A. Biochemistry of HELLP syndrome. Adv Clin Chem. 2011;53:85–104.
3. Chaer R, Helton WS. Dieulafoy's disease. Am Coll Surg. 2003;196:290–6.
4. Veldhuyzen van Zanten SJ, Bartelsman JF, Schipper ME, et al. Recurrent massive haematemesis from Dieulafoy vascular malformations–a review of 101 cases. Gut. 1986;27:213–22.
5. Malliaras GP, Carollo A, Bogen G. Esophageal Dieulafoy's lesion: an exceedingly rare cause of massive upper GI bleeding. J Surg Case Rep. 2016;6:1–2.
6. Mangiavillano B, Luigiano C, Basile S, et al. Is pregnancy a predisposing factor for Dieulafoy's duodenal lesion or only a coincidence? Clin Res Hepatol Gastroenterol. 2013;37(5):e119–20.
7. Nguyen DC, Jackson CS. The Dieulafoy's lesion: an update on evaluation, diagnosis, and management. J Clin Gastroenterol. 2015;49(7):541–9.
8. Alis H, Oner OZ, Kalayci MU, et al. Is endoscopic band ligation superior to injection therapy for Dieulafoy lesion? Surg Endosc. 2009;23(7):1465–9.
9. Schmulewitz N, Baillie J. Dieulafoy lesions: a review of 6 years of experience at a tertiary referral center. Am J Gastroenterol. 2001;96:1688–94.
10. Iacopini F, Petruzziello L, Marchese M, et al. Haemostasis of Dieulafoy's lesion by argon plasma coagulation. Gastrointest Endosc. 2007;66:20–6.
11. Yamaguchi Y, Yamato T, Katsumi N, et al. Short-term and long-term benefits of endoscopic hemoclip application for Dieulafoy's lesion in the upper GI tract. Gastrointest Endosc. 2003;57:653–6.
12. Eisenberg D, Bell R. Intraoperative endoscopy: a requisite tool for laparoscopic resection of unusual gastrointestinal lesions–a case series. J Surg Res. 2009;155:318–20.
13. Norton ID, Petersen BT, Sorbi D, et al. Management and long-term prognosis of Dieulafoy lesion. Gastrointest Endosc. 1999;50:762–7.
14. Chung IK, Kim EJ, Lee MS, et al. Bleeding Dieulafoy's lesions and the choice of endoscopic method: comparing the hemostatic efficacy of mechanical and injection methods. Gastrointest Endosc. 2000;52(6):721–4.
15. Alva S, Abir F, Tran D. Laparoscopic gastric wedge resection for Dieulafoy's disease following pre-operative endoscopic localisation with India ink and endoscopic clips. J Soc Laparoendosc Surg. 2006;10:244–6.
16. Abildgaard U, Heimdal K. Pathogenesis of the syndrome of hemolysis, elevated liver enzymes, and low platelet count (HELLP): a review. Eur J Obstet Gynecol Reprod Biol. 2013;166(2):117–23.
17. Dusse LM, Alpoim PN, Silv JT, et al. Revisiting HELLP syndrome. Clin Chim Acta. 2015;45 (Pt B):117–20.
18. Barton JR, Sibai BM. Diagnosis and management of hemolysis, elevated liver enzymes, and low platelets syndrome. Clin Perinatol. 2004;31:807–33.
19. Murao K, Imachi H, Muraoka T, et al. Hemolysis, elevated liver enzymes, and low platelet count (HELLP) syndrome with pituitary apoplexy. Fertil Steril. 2011;96(1):260–1.

10

Soluble ST2 is a sensitive clinical marker of ulcerative colitis evolution

David Díaz-Jiménez[1], Marjorie De la Fuente[1,2], Karen Dubois-Camacho[1], Glauben Landskron[1], Janitza Fuentes[3], Tamara Pérez[3], María Julieta González[4], Daniela Simian[2], Marcela A. Hermoso[1*†] and Rodrigo Quera[5*†]

Abstract

Background: The ST2/IL-33 pathway has been related to ulcerative colitis (UC), and soluble ST2 (sST2), to disease severity. We tested the potential usefulness of sST2 as a predictive marker of treatment response and patients' outcome.

Methods: Twenty-six patients with active UC were prospectively recruited and grouped according to an endoscopic score and therapy response. Colonoscopic biopsies were collected at baseline and 6 months or when patients showed clinical activity. The protocol was reinitiated in patients requiring rescue therapy. Blood and stool were collected at baseline, 1, 3, 6 and 12 months. Serum and mucosal ST2, and fecal calprotectin (FC) content were determined by ELISA and correlated to Mayo clinical and endoscopic subscore. Intestinal ST2 was evaluated by immunofluorescence. Wilcoxon signed rank test and Spearman correlations (Rs) were applied (p <0.05).

Results: Follow-up was completed in 24 patients. sST2 levels (median and range) varied from 173.5 [136.6–274.0] to 86.5 [54.6–133.2] in responders ($p < 0.05$), and 336.3 [211.0–403.2] to 385.3 pg/mL [283.4–517.3] in non-responders at baseline and 6 months, respectively. sST2 levels correlated with Mayo clinical and endoscopic subscore, mucosal ST2 and FC (Rs = 0.57, 0.66, 0.74 and 0.42, respectively; $p < 0.0001$) and showed a trend similar to that of FC in responders. Non-responders revealed an increased ST2 content, restricted to the lamina propria's cellular infiltrate.

Conclusions: Consecutive sST2 measurement to follow changes in inflammatory activity of UC patients who respond or not to treatment identifies sST2, like FC, as a useful biomarker in predicting clinical outcome of UC patients.

Keywords: Soluble ST2, Ulcerative colitis, Biomarker, Fecal calprotectin

Abbreviations: 5-ASA, 5-aminosalicylate derivatives; CD, Crohn's disease; ELISA, Enzyme-linked immunosorbent assay; FC, Fecal calprotectin; IBD, Inflammatory bowel diseases; sST2, Soluble ST2; UC, Ulcerative colitis

Background

The two main subtypes of inflammatory bowel diseases (IBD), Crohn's disease (CD) and ulcerative colitis (UC), are characterized by episodes of inflammatory activity and remission. To explain the multifactorial and polygenic nature of IBD, a scenario of chronic and uncontrolled activation of the mucosal immune response in genetically susceptible individuals, exacerbated by environmental factors, has been proposed [1].

Treatment of IBD seeks to induce and maintain remission, as well as reduce inflammation, promote mucosal healing and prevent complications [2], such that the choice of optimal therapy is crucial for patient recovery. In most cases, the disease can be controlled with conventional treatment, such as 5-aminosalicylate (5-ASA) derivatives, corticosteroids and immunosuppressants. However, patients who do not respond to these treatments eventually require biological therapy and, as a final alternative, colectomy. While clinical tools, such as assessment of symptoms/signs, performance of laboratory markers [3], colonoscopy/sigmoidoscopy and imaging modalities may allow monitoring the response to a selected therapy, only endoscopic studies definitively diagnose IBD and evaluate its activity through detection

* Correspondence: mhermoso@med.uchile.cl; rquera@clc.cl
†Equal contributors
[1]Programa Disciplinario de Inmunología, Instituto de Ciencias Biomédicas, Facultad de Medicina, Universidad de Chile, Santiago, CL 8380453, Chile
[5]Servicio de Gastroenterología, Clínica Las Condes, Santiago, CL 7591018, Chile
Full list of author information is available at the end of the article

of intestinal lesions [4]; unfortunately this procedure is invasive and costly. Determination of disease activity remains challenging, with most clinical scores correlating poorly with the inflammatory state [4, 5]. Treatment of IBD patients has recently shifted from controlling symptoms to promoting endoscopic mucosal healing or deep remission [6], features that are now major endpoints in clinical trials and are highly efficient in predicting long-term remission and preventing hospitalization and surgery.

Treatment promoting mucosal healing can slow the progression of the disease [6]. In this context, laboratory biomarkers have gained importance in evaluating and predicting the response to therapy [7, 8]. Recently, key molecules that regulate mucosal immunity and IBD pathogenesis, including those in the IL-33/ST2 signaling pathway, have emerged as suitable biomarkers in inflammatory conditions such as IBD [9, 10]. In humans, *IL1RL1* expression is regulated by distal and proximal promoters that govern expression of the ST2 membrane-anchored receptor (ST2L) and a soluble isoform (sST2) generated by alternative splicing. sST2 is identical to the ST2L extracellular domain and is a decoy receptor for IL33 [11]. The IL-33/ST2 axis has been implicated in numerous other diseases, such as asthma, rheumatoid arthritis, cancer and Alzheimer's disease [9, 12–14].

We previously proposed the sST2 variant as a potential severity biomarker, mainly in UC patients, that might allow differentiation between active and inactive disease [15]. However, sST2 behavior during the clinical course and response to therapy has not been explored. Here, we examined whether changes in serum ST2 levels can predict response to treatment, clinical activity and disease outcome when compared with other biomarkers, such as FC.

Methods

Patients

In this observational study, we prospectively included patients with relapsed IBD from Clínica Las Condes. The diagnosis of UC was established according to international guidelines including clinical, endoscopic, histologic and radiologic criteria [16, 17]. Patients were assessed at a minimum of 3-month intervals or upon relapse. The follow-up period was 12 months in patients showing no relapse and in patients showing activity flares and requiring rescue therapy (Fig. 1a). All relapses were sufficiently severe to warrant a change in treatment.

Patients were excluded from the study based on the following criteria: incomplete ileo-colonoscopy (ileum not intubated), non-classifiable IBD or coexisting cardiopulmonary, renal, hepatic, celiac disease, neurologic, psychiatric, severe allergy and rheumatologic disease, a history of HIV, previous ileostomy or colostomy, and conditions associated with elevated FC levels [18, 19], i.e., non-steroidal anti-inflammatory or anti-coagulant drug use in the 6 months preceding enrollment, a history of erosive/ulcerative upper gastrointestinal disease within 2 months prior to the study or gastrointestinal infection within 4 weeks prior to the study and those patients treated with biological therapy. The source data was encrypted and the data extracted were anonymous. This study was performed in accordance with the Declaration of Helsinki and the protocol was approved by Clinica Las Condes Review Board of the Universidad de Chile, Chile. All patients gave written informed consent.

Clinical activity index

During clinic visits, general well-being, stool frequency, stool consistency and presence or absence of abdominal pain, tenderness, tenesmus, rectal bleeding, and mucus in stool were recorded. Clinical activity indices were scored according to data available in patient records using the Mayo clinical subscore at baseline and at 1, 3, 6 and 12 months or, in the case of flare, during the follow-up period. Three clinical variables were graded: frequency of evacuation, amount of blood in stool, and the physician's global assessment. A Mayo clinical subscore of 0 was defined as remission, 1–3 as mildly active disease, 4–6 as moderately active disease, and ≥7 as severely active disease [20].

All clinical decisions were made independently of ST2 protein level measurements, since detections were performed only after follow-up was completed.

Endoscopic assessment of disease activity

Endoscopic findings were scored according to the Mayo endoscopic subscore, graded as normal (0), mild (1), moderate (2), or severe (3) disease activity. Subscore 0–1 was defined as remission and subscore ≥2 as active disease [21]. Colonoscopic biopsies were collected at baseline (colonoscopy 1) and at 6 months or if patients showed clinical signs of activity (colonoscopy 2). Patients who required rescue therapy reinitiated the protocol. Endoscopic re-evaluation in patients receiving conventional or biological therapy was conducted at 6 months or 14 weeks, respectively, or when flares were evident.

Disease activity was assessed based on the results of clinical activity scoring but blinded to quantitative FC values. Clinical response was defined as a decrease from baseline in the total Mayo score by at least three points and at least 30 %, with an accompanying decrease in the subscore for rectal bleeding of at least one point or an absolute subscore for rectal bleeding of 0 or 1. Mucosal healing was defined as an absolute subscore for endoscopy of 0 or 1. Patients who had a clinical response at

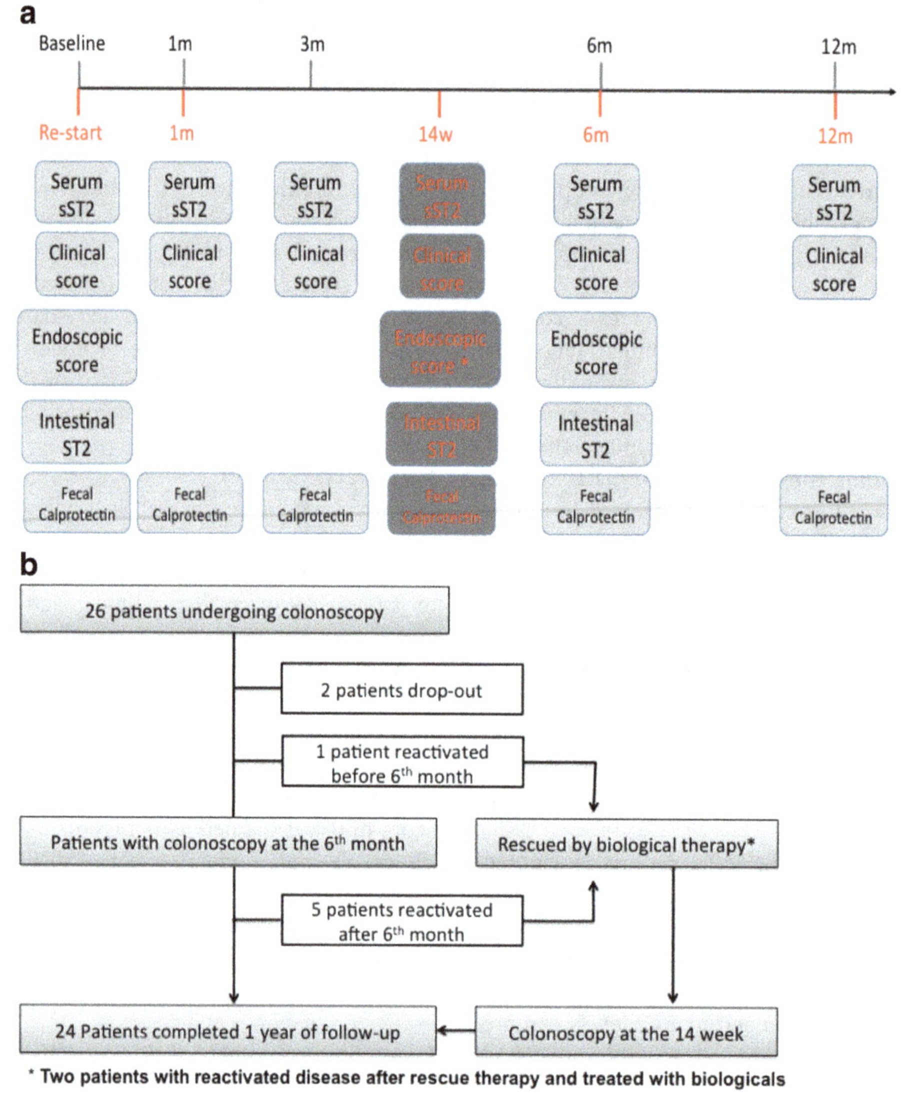

Fig. 1 Study selection and flow-chart of UC patients' 1-year follow-up. **a** Follow-up scheme protocol performed in active UC patients receiving conventional therapy (baseline). Responder UC patients completed the entire follow-up period. Non-responder patients re-started the follow-up with biological therapy and were examined at 1 month, 14 weeks, 6 and 12 months. Clinical subscore, FC and serum sST2 were evaluated at 1, 3, 6 and 12 months. Endoscopic subscore and intestinal ST2 were determined at baseline, 14 weeks (w) and 6 months. **b** Flow-chart of patients enrolled in the follow-up

each time during the follow-up were considered to have a sustained clinical response [22].

Medical treatment

Patients enrolled in the study were treated with conventional therapy, such as 5-ASA derivatives, corticosteroids or immunomodulators (azathioprine/6-mercaptopurine), depending on disease severity. The decision to change medical treatment was based on clinical and/or endoscopic evaluation. Physicians were blinded to results of individual quantitative FC values at the time of the patient's visit. Rescue therapy was defined as: (a) an increased dose of any previously administered medication; or (b) a change in medication to corticosteroids, immunosuppressants (azathioprine/6-mercaptopurine) or anti-TNF (infliximab/adalimumab). Information about the drug, dose and duration of treatment was obtained from the medical history.

Measurement of ST2 and IL-33

A blood sample was collected at baseline and at 1, 3, 6 and 12 months of follow-up on the day of colonoscopy or physical examination (Fig. 1a). Serum and intestinal ST2 concentrations, as well as serum IL-33 content, were measured using an enzyme-linked immunosorbent assay (ELISA) kit for human ST2 or IL-33 (DuoSet,

R&D Systems, Minneapolis, MN, USA) according to the manufacturer's instructions and expressed as pg/mL. Blood samples were centrifuged and serum was stored at −80 °C. For ST2 and IL-33 detection, serum samples were thawed and treated with protein A/G PLUS-agarose (Santa Cruz Biotechnology, Santa Cruz, CA, USA). Protein extracts of colonic mucosa were obtained from each biopsy by homogenization using a lysis buffer supplemented with a protease inhibitor cocktail (Complete Mini, Roche Diagnostics, Basel, Switzerland) and subsequently disrupted by sonication. Levels of total intestinal ST2 were adjusted to total protein concentration determined by Bradford protein assay (Bio-Rad). The ST2 detection assay is stable over time, with a detection limit of 20 pg/mL, while the IL-33 detection assay is less stable over time, with a detection limit of 23.40 pg/mL, according to the manufacturer's information. All samples were analyzed in duplicate; within-run and total coefficients of variation were ≤2.5 and ≤4.0 %, respectively.

Using the cut-off for sST2 previously estimated at <74.87 pg/mL [15], we determined the specificity, sensitivity, positive predictive value and negative predictive value for our patient cohort.

Fecal calprotectin measurement

A fecal sample was collected at baseline and at, 1, 3, 6 and 12 months of follow-up (Fig. 1a) 24 h before colonoscopy or physical examination. Feces (50 mg) was resuspended in 500 μL of extraction buffer, spun for 10 min and centrifuged for 10 min at 10,000 rpm. The supernatant was immediately processed for rapid semi-quantitative test (Calprotectin 50 + 200, CerTest Biotec S.L. Spain) or stored at −80 °C for subsequent quantification using a standard ELISA with a solid bound specific antibody and biotinylated tracer antibody according to the manufacturer's instructions (Hycult Biotech, HK325-02, The Netherlands). Detection levels were 1.6–100 ng/mL, corresponding to 40–2500 μg calprotectin/g of feces, adjusted for the dilution factor.

Clinical decisions to change therapy were based on semi-quantitative analysis of calprotectin and independent of quantitative ELISA after completed follow-up.

Endpoints

The correlation of ST2 and FC measurements with clinical and endoscopic activity scoring was the primary endpoint of the study. Complete response (remission) was defined as the absence of symptoms, normal stool frequency, absence of rectal bleeding, general wellness based on the patient's functional assessment score and endoscopy findings of subscore 0–1 [21]. Biological remission also implies healing of mucosa and normalization of inflammation biomarkers, such as serum sST2 (<74.87 pg/mL) [15] and FC, according to the cut-off obtained from our patient cohort.

Mucosal ST2 detection by immunofluorescence

Intestinal mucosa biopsies were reviewed by a pathologist experienced in IBD who was blinded to any clinical information about the patients. Mucosal tissue sections comprised the most inflamed segment according to chronic inflammatory infiltrate.

Biopsies were obtained at baseline and at 6 months or at baseline and 14 weeks in patients treated with conventional treatment and those rescued with biological therapy, respectively. Total ST2 content was detected in 2 % PFA-fixed, paraffin-embedded UC patient biopsies cut into 4-μm sections and subjected to immunofluorescence analysis. Non-specific binding was blocked and samples were incubated with a mouse monoclonal antibody against human ST2 (MAB523, R&D Systems) followed by an Alexa 546-tagged secondary goat antibody against mouse IgG (Invitrogen/Life Technologies, Carlsbad, CA, USA) to detect ST2. Cell nuclei were stained using Hoechst 33342 (Thermo/Life Technologies, Carlsbad, CA, USA). Images were captured using an Olympus confocal laser scanning biological microscope FV10i (Olympus America Inc., Melville, NY, USA) and processed using ImageJ (NIH, Bethesda, MD USA). Negative controls were prepared under conditions identical to those described above using an isotype control.

Statistical analyses

Data were analyzed using GraphPad Prism5 (La Jolla, CA USA). Results of parametric numerical data are given as mean ± standard deviation (SD) and, in non-parametric distributions, as median and interquartile range (IQR). Serial assessments of change from baseline in serum ST2 and FC levels were compared using the Wilcoxon signed rank test. Differences and significance during follow-up times were analyzed by multiple comparisons using the non-parametric Kruskal-Wallis test with Dunn's multiple comparison post-test. Correlations between sST2 levels and total intestinal ST2, FC, and clinical and activity score were analyzed using Spearman's rank correlation coefficient (r). For each test, differences were considered significant at $p \le 0.05$.

Results

Serum ST2 and clinical characteristics of patients

Table 1 summarizes the clinical characteristics of 26 patients included in the protocol, while Fig. 1a shows the flow-chart of the 1-year follow-up enrollment and sampling overview at each stage of the patient's monitoring.

Baseline ileo-colonoscopy data were available for 26 UC patients. During the study, 24 patients finished the protocol, six of whom showed disease reactivation, once

Table 1 Clinical and demographic data of ulcerative colitis patients

	Number
Number of patients	26
Number of patients dropped out	2
Female/male	16/10
Median [range] age at entry	34.5 [30.0–52.5]
Duration of UC, years (median, range)	4.0 [1.3–11.8]
Age at diagnosis, years (median, range)	32.0 [22.5–44.0]
Location	
Proctitis	6
Left-sided	5
Extensive	15
Clinical disease activity	
Mild/ Moderate/ Severe	0/14/12
Endoscopic severity	
Moderate (score 2) / Severe (score 3)	22/4
Medication used	
No medication	3
5-ASA	11
Corticosteroids and 5-ASA	3
Corticosteroids, 5-asa and azathioprine	5
Corticosteroids and azathioprine	1
5-ASA and azathioprine	3
Response to therapy	21
Reactivation (after/before 6 months)	6 (1/5)
Rescued by anti-TNF-α	6

in four patients after 6 months and twice in two patients before and after 6 months, for a total of eight reactivation episodes in six presumed non-responder patients. Overall, 18 patients responded to treatment and six patients did not (Fig. 1b). Baseline sST2 levels were 189.5 pg/mL [154.1–286.9]; at 1, 3, 6 and 12 months, with levels of 87.3 [70.1–142.2], 73.25 [55.1–145.1], 95.8 [55.7–134.9] and 78.0 [59.9–99.8] pg/mL, respectively (Fig. 2a). When patients were grouped according to treatment response, baseline levels were 173.5 [136.6–274.0], whereas sST2 levels at 6 months decreased to 86.5 [54.6–133.2] pg/mL in responders and increased in the eight reactivation episodes from 336.3 [211.0–403.2] to 385.3 [283.4–517.3] pg/mL in the six non-responders (Fig. 2b). No significant differences between therapy responder and non-responder patients were found in baseline sST2 values ($p = 0.1057$). Quantitation of FC at baseline, at 1, 3, 6 and 12 months revealed levels of 147.0 [102.1–210.2], 107.1 [54.2–161.3], 119.5 [57.7–144.5], 85.4 [63.0–96.7] and 74.7 [48.9–1076.0] μg/g feces, respectively (Fig. 2c). According to treatment, baseline FC levels of 141.4 [92.9–204.6] decreased to 82.8 [59.2–97.8] μg/g feces in responders and from 243.9 [175.1–297.9] to 152.0 [100.1–200.8] μg/g feces in non-responders at 6 months (Fig. 2d). sST2 levels in all follow-up times correlated with the Mayo clinical subscore (Rs = 0.57, $p < 0.0001$); at baseline and 6 months, levels correlated with Mayo endoscopic subscores (Rs = 0.66, $p < 0.0001$) and total ST2 content in mucosa (Rs = 0.74, $p < 0.0001$) (Fig. 2e). Patients in biological remission showed normalization of the inflammation biomarker sST2, with values below the cut-off of 74.87 pg/mL [15]. Considering this cut-off value of sST2, the specificity, sensitivity, PPV and NPV were 0.44, 0.95, 0.62, and 0.90, respectively.

When patients were grouped according to treatment response, IL-33 baseline levels were 199.8 [51.92–372.20], decreasing at 6 months to 141.2 [44.00–352.90] pg/mL in responders, and decreasing from 629.0 [49.56–716.8] to 217.9 [50.39–647.5] pg/mL in the reactivation episodes, both without significant differences ($p > 0.05$) (Additional file 1: Figure S1).

Relationship of ST2 to the FC biomarker

Analysis showed that sST2-circulating levels directly correlated with those of FC (Rs = 0.42, $p < 0.0001$) in all patients (Fig. 3a). Intestinal total ST2 levels in mucosa also correlated with those of FC, although the association was less significant statistically (Rs = 0.35, $p = 0.044$) (Fig. 3b).

sST2 response to biological therapy

In our cohort, six patients were rescued with biological therapy. Immediately after infliximab infusions, sST2 levels were markedly increased, but protein content during the induction period gradually declined between weeks 3 and 24 of monitoring, reaching levels similar to those in patients responding to treatment ($p < 0.01$, Fig. 4a). A similar trend was observed for FC levels, indicating that fecal biomarker content also decreases gradually as a function of type and response to therapy ($p < 0.05$; Fig. 4b).

Intestinal total ST2 immunoreactivity

Because intestinal ST2 levels were highly correlated with sST2 concentrations (Fig. 2e), we tested whether the total mucosal ST2 content, as the source of ST2 in the periphery, might be related to healing and deep remission in responder patients. Mucosal ST2 immunoreactivity detected by immunofluorescence may allow identification of membrane-anchored ST2 and the soluble variant restricted to the intracellular compartment. In responder patients, total ST2 immunoreactivity was maintained in the cellular infiltrate of the lamina propria at 6 months of follow-up, whereas patients showing reactivation revealed increased total ST2 in inflamed mucosa but also confined to the cellular infiltrate (Fig. 5a,b). No immunoreactivity

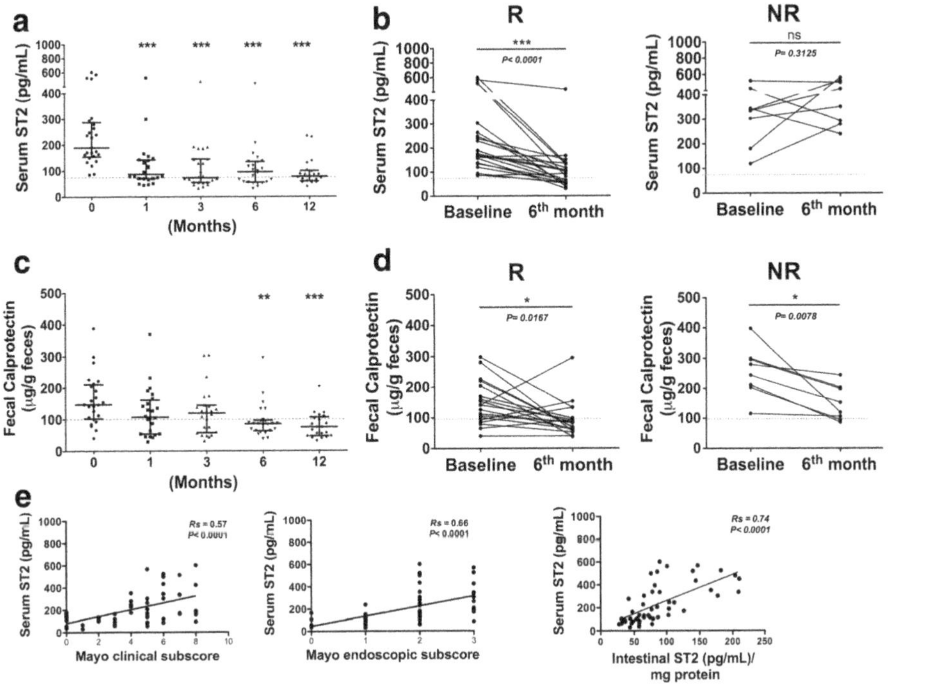

Fig. 2 Distribution of serum ST2 according to response to therapy. **a** Serum ST2 levels during the follow-up period were determined in each patient and are shown as one symbol in the scatter plot. Horizontal lines indicate medians and whiskers (interquartile ranges). Differences were assessed using Kruskal-Wallis test (*** $p < 0.0001$). **b** Serum ST2 levels at baseline and 6 months in responders (R) and non-responders (NR) in relation to therapy decreased only in responders. Differences were assessed using Wilcoxon signed rank test (*** $p < 0.0001$). **c** FC levels in the 1-year follow-up and (**d**) at baseline and 6 months in R and NR in relation to therapy decreased in both subgroups. Panel E shows the correlation between serum ST2 levels and Mayo clinical subscore, Mayo endoscopic subscore, and total ST2 intestinal mucosa content, with a trend line for each correlation. Discontinuous line indicates cut-off value. Rs: Spearman's rank correlation coefficient

was detected in samples incubated with isotype antibody. Epithelial ST2 expression was absent in all responder and non-responder patients analyzed.

Discussion

In this prospective study of UC patients with active disease, we consecutively measured sST2 levels during a 1-year follow-up and compared those with FC, the canonically defined biomarker of activity in IBD patients [23–25]. Our results demonstrate for first time that sST2 is an easily detectable marker of UC evolution and effectiveness of therapy.

Several studies reporting the association of the IL-33/ST2 signalling pathway with IBD pathogenesis in patients and animal models have attempted to address the actual contribution of each component of the pathway [26, 27]. In this context, the sST2 variant, acting as a decoy receptor for IL-33, is increased in UC [10, 15].

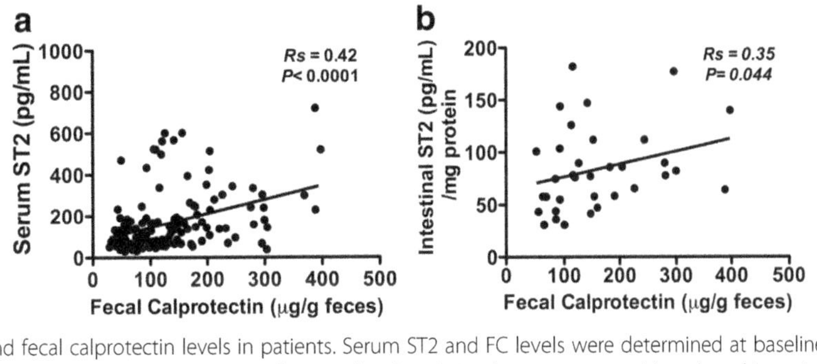

Fig. 3 Correlation of ST2 and fecal calprotectin levels in patients. Serum ST2 and FC levels were determined at baseline, 1, 3, 6 and 12 months of follow-up. Total ST2 intestinal was measure at baseline and 6 months. Correlation between serum (**a**) and total intestinal ST2 (**b**) according to FC levels were assessed. Each symbol in the scatter plot represents the measurement in individual patients, with a trend line for this association. Rs: Spearman's rank correlation coefficient ($p < 0.05$)

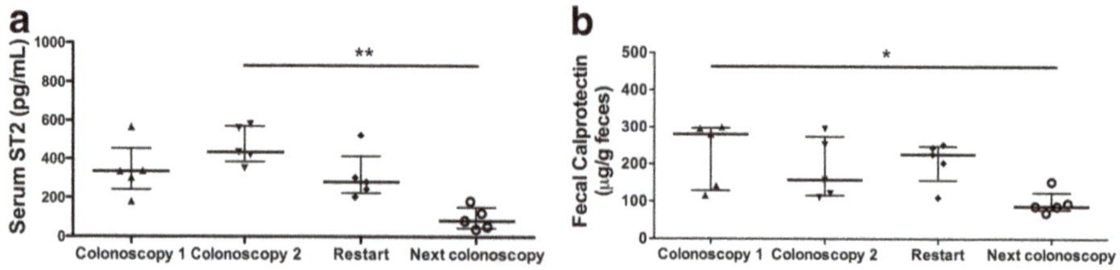

Fig. 4 Distribution of serum ST2 and fecal calprotectin in patients rescued with biological therapy. Serum sST2 (**a**) and fecal calprotectin (**b**) levels are shown for patients non-responsive to conventional therapy or with reactivation but rescued with biological therapy. Each symbol in the scatter plot represents the measurement in individual patients; horizontal lines indicate medians and whiskers (the interquartile ranges). Differences were assessed using Kruskal-Wallis test with Dunn's multiple comparison post-test (*$p < 0.05$ and **$p < 0.01$)

We proposed ST2 as a potential activity biomarker, with a cut-off value of 74.87 pg/mL, that might allow distinction between active and inactive disease with 83 % sensitivity and specificity [15]. At this cut-off value, we found a lower specificity (44 vs 83 %), suggestive of a poorer discrimination of the group of inactive patients or those with sST2 levels <74.87 pg/mL. The higher sST2 levels at baseline and from unresponsive patients/reactivations (endoscopic score ≥ 2) in the vast majority of all detections might explain the lower specificity.

sST2 has also been considered a biomarker of diseases that affect different tissues undergoing deep inflammatory reactions and necrosis; a cut-off of 150 pg/mL and 5.8 ng/mL was determined to predict sudden cardiac death in patients with chronic heart failure and left

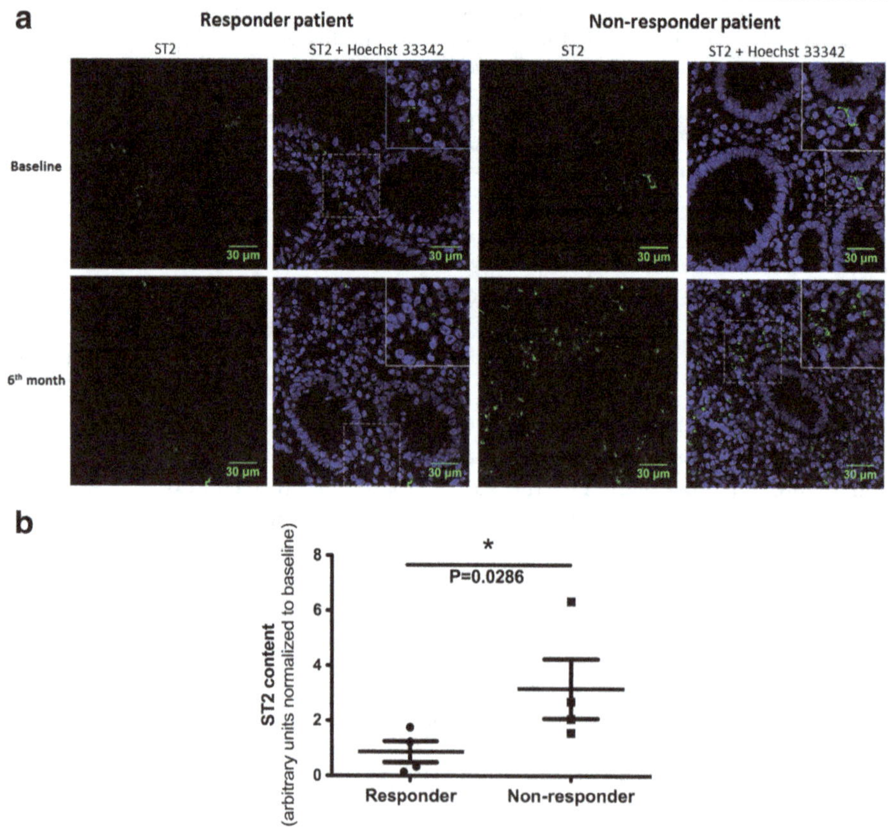

Fig. 5 Immunolocalization of ST2 in colonic tissue from responder and non-responder patients during baseline and 6-month follow-up. **a** Total ST2 immunoreactivity was restricted to the cellular infiltrate in the lamina propria at 6 months in responder patients (right), while in patients showing reactivation, total ST2 was increased in inflamed mucosa, also confined to the cellular infiltrate (left); baseline examination revealed extensive immune cell infiltration of the intestinal mucosa and damaged tissue with loss of architecture. **b** Total ST2 immunoreactivity at 6 months expressed as arbitrary units (A.U.) and normalized to baseline levels in responders and non-responders ($n = 4$ in each group) was higher in the non-responders. Hoechst 33342/ ST2 (blue/green) (60X)

ventricular systolic dysfunction, as well as in patients with rheumatoid arthritis, respectively [28, 29].

In our follow-up study, patients in biological remission showed normalization of sST2, with values close to the cut-off previously determined [15], suggesting that low sST2 levels predict improvement in the inflammatory state. Moreover, we find that increased sST2 levels in UC patients with active disease directly correlate with higher expression of total ST2 in intestinal mucosa, including sST2 and ST2L, consistent with previous observations [15] and suggesting that the increased total ST2 immunoreactivity in non-responder patients is mostly at the expense of newly produced sST2 by cells infiltrating the mucosa. In responder patients, we found no conclusive evidence of a decrease in total ST2 immunoreactivity, possibly reflecting the inability of the technique used to distinguish between the two protein isoforms and its limitation in assessing protein quantity. Moreover, in responder patients, ST2+ cells infiltrating the mucosa might be less effective than those present in non-responders, although additional cell markers are needed to support this hypothesis. The components of this inflammatory microenvironment, including TNF-α, IL-33 and IL-1β produced by infiltrating and resident cells (neutrophils, mast cells and fibroblasts) have been shown to upregulate sST2 expression in vitro [30], although the current lack of a differential tool to detect ST2 variants limits the interpretation of tissue immunodetection of total ST2. On the other hand, studies of intestinal inflammation in murine models have reported that IL-33 itself can play a beneficial or harmful role in IBD depending on the induction of mucosal damage (acute or chronic) or the colitogenic used, arguing against a precise role of the IL-33/ST2 axis. Indeed, IL 33 serum levels did not correlate with the activity score in UC patients [15] and in the present cohort, we found no association between IL33 serum levels with therapy response.

The difficulty in evaluating disease activity in UC patients using clinical, endoscopic and histological approaches has led to greater interest in identifying new biochemical markers that directly reflect intestinal inflammation. Recently, the usefulness of FC as a biomarker has been explained by the fact that inflammation causes neutrophil activation, resulting in a proportional release-to-damage ratio. Yamamoto et al. [31] showed that consecutive measurements of FC in UC patients with proctitis were able to monitor relapse during maintenance therapy with mesalazine suppositories. A cut-off value of 55 μg/g was used to assign those patients who maintained clinical remission, although the optimal cut-off for defining activity in IBD remains controversial [32, 33]. Indeed, FC cut-off values ranging from 50 to 250 μg/g have been used [23, 34] that differ depending on the test used [35, 36]. In our study, we used quantitative ELISA and defined a cut-off of 99.26 μg/g with an AUC of 0.87 to distinguish individuals with an inactive endoscopic score (0–1) from those with activity indices (2–3) [37]. The cut-off value obtained for our cohort is similar to that previously described [38].

In 7 of 8 reactivations in non-responders from our cohort, FC levels showed a decrease despite detectable endoscopic inflammation, although FC values were above the cut-off defined in the current analysis. Unexpectedly, FC did not correlate with the endoscopic score, possibly related to the treatment received or presence of liquid stool [39]. Moreover, an inverse association between FC and neutrophil infiltration has been reported in patients under remission, with high protein levels in stool [40]. Finally, daily fluctuations of up to 40 % have been described for FC determined in four independent stool samples from active patients [41], suggesting that a single FC detection in active patients is not sufficient for a therapeutic decision.

In contrast, the increased inflammatory state of the mucosa in 5 of 8 reactivations of non-responders simultaneous with augmented sST2 levels indicates that this protein can predict lack of response to the therapy used. The direct association between endoscopic score and sST2 might reflect an inflammatory process related to mucosal damage, while the production and secretion of FC requires massive infiltration of neutrophils into the lamina propria [42, 43]. While no test can replace colonoscopy with biopsy to determine the inflammatory condition of the intestinal mucosa, the ability of sST2 levels to predict inflammatory status identifies the need to incorporate analysis of sST2 in selecting patients who require control for reactivation through colonoscopy.

sST2 levels have been also identified as a biomarker in heart failure, efficiently assessing cardiac remodelling and fibrosis; sST2 has been shown to efficiently monitor the effectiveness of an optimized treatment in chronic heart failure patients [44], with increased levels that may be a good predictor of cardiac decompensation as well as worsening renal function.

To date, there are few reports on the behavior of sST2 according to the medication used in IBD patients. We found some association of sST2 with the use of systemic steroids [15], and others have reported the effect of infliximab on this molecule [10]. However, no study has demonstrated how ST2 levels fluctuate in serial and continuous follow-up in relation to endoscopic index.

Based on our previous finding [15], we recruited patients who at baseline had a moderate or severe endoscopic index (≥2) in any analyzed section of the colon. During the follow-up, serial ST2 measurements decreased in those patients with a reduced endoscopic index at

6 months, indicating a positive response to therapy. In those patients, FC levels were also significantly decreased in direct correlation to sST2 levels. Further association studies between sST2 and FC in a larger cohort of UC patients are needed, as well as such analyses in CD and in IBD pediatric patients. Correlation studies between sST2, histologic scores and disease risk might also provide additional information about the strength of this biomarker as has been demonstrated with FC [45].

Our analyses of a one-bounded cohort of UC patients during a 1-year follow-up revealed a direct correlation between sST2 levels and inflammatory activity, strongly suggesting that sST2 is a reliable biomarker of active UC. It will be interesting to examine the predictive role of sST2 for reactivation risk in a cohort of inactive patients or undergoing clinical and endoscopic remission (Mayo subscore 0) and identifying serum levels of this biomarker in a follow-up every 4 months, a protocol in which FC was shown to predict disease recurrence [31]. Finally, it will be interesting to monitor both the behavior of sST2 in a cohort of severe UC patients and the relevance of elevated sST2 content in predicting colectomy risk in a 1-year follow-up, as shown for FC [46].

Conclusions

The accuracy of sST2 in endoscopic detection of UC strongly suggests its usefulness in monitoring relapse and outcome, as well as in identifying patients likely to benefit from a particular treatment.

Acknowledgments

We thank Fabiola Werlinger (Profesor Asistente, Departamento de Tecnología Médica, Facultad de Medicina, Universidad de Chile) and Claudio Molina (Profesor Asociado, Facultad de Odontología, Universidad Mayor, Chile) for their help in statistical analysis.

Funding

This study was supported by research grants from FONDECYT 1110381 (RQ), 1120577 (MAH), 3150328 (MD) and DA-CLC grants PI200803 (RQ), PI2013-B002 (RQ) and CONICYT scholarship 2015 (DDJ).

Authors' contributions

DDJ, participated in design of the study, data collection, acquisition, analysis, interpretation and statistical analysis of data, and drafted the manuscript. MDF and GL participated in acquisition, analysis and interpretation of immunofluorescence and confocal images. KD and MJG participated in acquisition, analysis and interpretation of data. DS and JF participated in patient enrollment, obtaining written consent from patients willing to participate in the protocol, collected the data and their interpretation. TP performed colonoscopic procedures and participated in design of the study. MAH participated in design of the study, data collection, interpretation of data, and drafted the manuscript. RQ participated in design of the study, data collection, interpretation of data, drafted the manuscript and performed colonoscopic procedures. All authors read and approved the final manuscript.

Competing interests

The authors declare that they have no competing interests.

Author details

[1]Programa Disciplinario de Inmunología, Instituto de Ciencias Biomédicas, Facultad de Medicina, Universidad de Chile, Santiago, CL 8380453, Chile. [2]Subdirección de Investigación, Dirección Académica, Clínica Las Condes, Santiago, CL 7591018, Chile. [3]Unidad de Hígado y Gastroenterología, Instituto Chileno-Japonés de Enfermedades Digestivas, Hospital San Borja-Arriarán, Santiago, CL, Chile. [4]Programa disciplinario de Biología Celular, Instituto de Ciencias Biomédicas, Facultad de Medicina, Universidad de Chile, Santiago, CL 8380453, Chile. [5]Servicio de Gastroenterología, Clínica Las Condes, Santiago, CL 7591018, Chile.

References

1. Kaser A, Zeissig S, Blumberg RS. Inflammatory bowel disease. Annu Rev Immunol. 2010;28:573–621.
2. Neurath MF. New targets for mucosal healing and therapy in inflammatory bowel diseases. Mucosal Immunol. 2014;7:6–19.
3. Vermeire S, Van Assche G, Rutgeerts P. Laboratory markers in IBD: useful, magic, or unnecessary toys? Gut. 2006;55:426–31.
4. Annese V, Daperno M, Rutter MD, Amiot A, Bossuyt P, East J, Ferrante M, Götz M, Katsanos KH, Kießlich R, Ordás I, Repici A, Rosa B, Sebastian S, Kucharzik T, Eliakim R. European evidence based consensus for endoscopy in inflammatory bowel disease. J Crohns Colitis. 2013;7:982–1018.
5. Hamilton MJ. The valuable role of endoscopy in inflammatory bowel disease. Diagn Ther Endosc. 2012;2012:467979.
6. Pineton de Chambrun G, Peyrin-Biroulet L, Lémann M, Colombel J-F. Clinical implications of mucosal healing for the management of IBD. Nat Rev Gastroenterol Hepatol. 2010;7:15–29.
7. Colombel JF, Rutgeerts P, Reinisch W, Esser D, Wang Y, Lang Y, Marano CW, Strauss R, Oddens BJ, Feagan BG, Hanauer SB, Lichtenstein GR, Present D, Sands BE, Sandborn WJ. Early mucosal healing with infliximab is associated with improved long-term clinical outcomes in ulcerative colitis. Gastroenterology. 2011;141:1194–201.
8. Colombel J-F, Rutgeerts PJ, Sandborn WJ, Yang M, Camez A, Pollack PF, Thakkar RB, Robinson AM, Chen N, Mulani PM, Chao J. Adalimumab induces deep remission in patients with Crohn's disease. Clin Gastroenterol Hepatol. 2014;12:414–22.e5.
9. Beltrán CJ, Núñez LE, Díaz-Jiménez D, Farfan N, Candia E, Heine C, López F, González MJ, Quera R, Hermoso MA. Characterization of the novel ST2/IL-33 system in patients with inflammatory bowel disease. Inflamm Bowel Dis. 2010;16:1097–107.
10. Pastorelli L, Garg RR, Hoang SB, Spina L, Mattioli B, Scarpa M, Fiocchi C, Vecchi M, Pizarro TT. Epithelial-derived IL-33 and its receptor ST2 are dysregulated in ulcerative colitis and in experimental Th1/Th2 driven enteritis. Proc Natl Acad Sci U S A. 2010;107:8017–22.
11. Hayakawa H, Hayakawa M, Kume A, Tominaga S -i. Soluble ST2 Blocks Interleukin-33 Signaling in Allergic Airway Inflammation. J Biol Chem. 2007; 282:26369–80.
12. Verri W a, Souto FO, Vieira SM, Almeida SCL, Fukada SY, Xu D, Alves-Filho JC, Cunha TM, Guerrero ATG, Mattos-Guimaraes RB, Oliveira FR, Teixeira MM, Silva JS, McInnes IB, Ferreira SH, Louzada-Junior P, Liew FY, Cunha FQ. IL-33 induces neutrophil migration in rheumatoid arthritis and is a target of anti-TNF therapy. Ann Rheum Dis. 2010;69:1697–703.
13. Cui G, Qi H, Gundersen MD, Yang H, Christiansen I, Sørbye SW, Goll R, Florholmen J. Dynamics of the IL-33/ST2 network in the progression of human colorectal adenoma to sporadic colorectal cancer. Cancer Immunol Immunother. 2015;64:181–90.
14. Chapuis J, Hot D, Hansmannel F, Kerdraon O, Ferreira S, Hubans C, Maurage CA, Huot L, Bensemain F, Laumet G, Ayral AM, Fievet N, Hauw JJ, DeKosky ST, Lemoine Y, Iwatsubo T, Wavrant-Devrièze F, Dartigues JF, Tzourio C, Buée L, Pasquier F, Berr C, Mann D, Lendon C, Alpérovitch A, Kamboh MI, Amouyel P, Lambert JC. Transcriptomic and genetic studies identify IL-33 as a candidate gene for Alzheimer's disease. Mol Psychiatry. 2009;14:1004–16.
15. Díaz-Jiménez D, Núñez LE, Beltrán CJ, Candia E, Suazo C, Alvarez-Lobos M, González M-J, Hermoso MA, Quera R. Soluble ST2: a new and promising activity marker in ulcerative colitis. World J Gastroenterol. 2011;17:2181–90.

16. Dignass A, Van Assche G, Lindsay JO, Lémann M, Söderholm J, Colombel JF, Danese S, D'Hoore A, Gassull M, Gomollón F, Hommes DW, Michetti P, O'Morain C, Oresland T, Windsor A, Stange EF, Travis SPL, European Crohn's and Colitis Organisation (ECCO). The second European evidence-based Consensus on the diagnosis and management of Crohn's disease: Current management. J Crohns Colitis. 2010;4:28–62.
17. Van Assche G, Dignass A, Panes J, Beaugerie L, Karagiannis J, Allez M, Ochsenkühn T, Orchard T, Rogler G, Louis E, Kupcinskas L, Mantzaris G, Travis S, Stange E. The second European evidence-based Consensus on the diagnosis and management of Crohn's disease: Definitions and diagnosis. J Crohns Colitis. 2010;4:7–27.
18. Limburg PJ, Ahlquist DA, Sandborn WJ, Mahoney DW, Devens ME, Harrington JJ, Zinsmeister AR. Fecal calprotectin levels predict colorectal inflammation among patients with chronic diarrhea referred for colonoscopy. Am J Gastroenterol. 2000;95:2831–7.
19. Tibble J, Sigthorsson G, Foster R, Sherwood R, Fagerhol M, Bjarnason I. Faecal calprotectin and faecal occult blood tests in the diagnosis of colorectal carcinoma and adenoma. Gut. 2001;49:402–8.
20. Gomollón F, García-López S, Sicilia B, Gisbert JP, Hinojosa J, Grupo Espa˜nol de Trabajo en Enfermedad de Crohn y Colitis Ulcerosa. Therapeutic guidelines on ulcerative colitis: a GRADE methodology based effort of GETECCU. Gastroenterol y Hepatol. 2013;36:104–14.
21. D'Haens G, Sandborn WJ, Feagan BG, Geboes K, Hanauer SB, Irvine EJ, Lémann M, Marteau P, Rutgeerts P, Schölmerich J, Sutherland LR. A review of activity indices and efficacy end points for clinical trials of medical therapy in adults with ulcerative colitis. Gastroenterology. 2007;132:763–86.
22. Rutgeerts P, Sandborn WJ, Feagan BG, Reinisch W, Olson A, Johanns J, Travers S, Rachmilewitz D, Hanauer SB, Lichtenstein GR, de Villiers WJS, Present D, Sands BE, Colombel JF. Infliximab for induction and maintenance therapy for ulcerative colitis. N Engl J Med. 2005;353:2462–76.
23. D'Haens G, Ferrante M, Vermeire S, Baert F, Noman M, Moortgat L, Geens P, Iwens D, Aerden I, Van Assche G, Van Olmen G, Rutgeerts P. Fecal calprotectin is a surrogate marker for endoscopic lesions in inflammatory bowel disease. Inflamm Bowel Dis. 2012;18:2218–24.
24. Sipponen T, Savilahti E, Kärkkäinen P, Kolho K-L, Nuutinen H, Turunen U, Färkkilä M. Fecal calprotectin, lactoferrin, and endoscopic disease activity in monitoring anti-TNF-alpha therapy for Crohn's disease. Inflamm Bowel Dis. 2008;14:1392–8.
25. Mooiweer E, Fidder HH, Siersema PD, Laheij RJF, Oldenburg B. Fecal hemoglobin and calprotectin are equally effective in identifying patients with inflammatory bowel disease with active endoscopic inflammation. Inflamm Bowel Dis. 2014;20:307–14.
26. Groβ P, Doser K, Falk W, Obermeier F, Hofmann C. IL-33 attenuates development and perpetuation of chronic intestinal inflammation. Inflamm Bowel Dis. 2012;18:1900–9.
27. Sedhom MAK, Pichery M, Murdoch JR, Foligné B, Ortega N, Normand S, Mertz K, Sanmugalingam D, Brault L, Grandjean T, Lefrancais E, Fallon PG, Quesniaux V, Peyrin-Biroulet L, Cathomas G, Junt T, Chamaillard M, Girard J, Ryffel B. Neutralisation of the interleukin-33/ST2 pathway ameliorates experimental colitis through enhancement of mucosal healing in mice. Gut. 2013;62:1714–23.
28. Pascual-Figal D a, Ordoñez-Llanos J, Tornel PL, Vázquez R, Puig T, Valdés M, Cinca J, de Luna AB, Bayes-Genis A. Soluble ST2 for predicting sudden cardiac death in patients with chronic heart failure and left ventricular systolic dysfunction. J Am Coll Cardiol. 2009;54:2174–9.
29. Shen J, Shang Q, Wong C-K, Li EK, Wang S, Li R-J, Lee K-L, Leung Y-Y, Ying K-Y, Yim C-W, Kun EW, Leung M-H, Li M, Li TK, Zhu TY, Yu S-L, Kuan W-P, Yu C-M, Tam L-S. IL-33 and soluble ST2 levels as novel predictors for remission and progression of carotid plaque in early rheumatoid arthritis: A prospective study. Semin Arthritis Rheum. 2015;45:18–27.
30. Bandara G, Beaven M a, Olivera A, Gilfillan AM, Metcalfe DD. Activated mast cells synthesize and release soluble ST2-a decoy receptor for IL-33. Eur J Immunol. 2015;45:3034–44.
31. Yamamoto T, Shimoyama T, Matsumoto K. Consecutive monitoring of faecal calprotectin during mesalazine suppository therapy for active rectal inflammation in ulcerative colitis. Aliment Pharmacol Ther. 2015;42:549–58.
32. Lin J-F, Chen J-M, Zuo J-H, Yu A, Xiao Z-J, Deng F-H, Nie B, Jiang B. Meta-analysis: fecal calprotectin for assessment of inflammatory bowel disease activity. Inflamm Bowel Dis. 2014;20:1407–15.
33. Boon GJ, Day AS, Mulder CJ, Gearry RB. Are faecal markers good indicators of mucosal healing in inflammatory bowel disease? World J Gastroenterol. 2015;21:11469–80.
34. Kristensen V, Klepp P, Cvancarova M, Røseth A, Skar V, Moum B. Prediction of endoscopic disease activity in ulcerative colitis by two different assays for fecal calprotectin. J Crohns Colitis. 2015;9:164–9.
35. Schoepfer AM, Beglinger C, Straumann A, Trummler M, Vavricka SR, Bruegger LE, Seibold F. Fecal calprotectin correlates more closely with the Simple Endoscopic Score for Crohn's disease (SES-CD) than CRP, blood leukocytes, and the CDAI. Am J Gastroenterol. 2010;105:162–9.
36. Labaere D, Smismans A, Van Olmen A, Christiaens P, D'Haens G, Moons V, Cuyle P-J, Frans J, Bossuyt P. Comparison of six different calprotectin assays for the assessment of inflammatory bowel disease. United Eur Gastroenterol J. 2014;2:30–7.
37. Sandborn WJ, Feagan BG, Marano C, Zhang H, Strauss R, Johanns J, Adedokun OJ, Guzzo C, Colombel J-F, Reinisch W, Gibson PR, Collins J, Järnerot G, Hibi T, Rutgeerts P. Subcutaneous Golimumab Induces Clinical Response and Remission in Patients With Moderate-to-Severe Ulcerative Colitis. Gastroenterology. 2014;146:85–95.
38. García-Sánchez V, Iglesias-Flores E, González R, Gisbert JP, Gallardo-Valverde JM, González-Galilea A, Naranjo-Rodríguez A, de Dios-Vega JF, Muntané J, Gómez-Camacho F. Does fecal calprotectin predict relapse in patients with Crohn's disease and ulcerative colitis? J Crohns Colitis. 2010;4:144–52.
39. Vestergaard T a, Nielsen SL, Dahlerup JF, Hornung N. Fecal calprotectin: assessment of a rapid test. Scand J Clin Lab Invest. 2008;68:343–7.
40. Yamaguchi S, Takeuchi Y, Arai K, Fukuda K, Kuroki Y, Asonuma K, Takahashi H, Saruta M, Yoshida H. Fecal calprotectin is a clinically relevant biomarker of mucosal healing in patients with quiescent ulcerative colitis. J Gastroenterol Hepatol. 2016;31:93–8.
41. Calafat M, Cabré E, Mañosa M, Lobatón T, Marín L, Domènech E. High within-day variability of fecal calprotectin levels in patients with active ulcerative colitis: what is the best timing for stool sampling? Inflamm Bowel Dis. 2015;21:1072–6.
42. Sacco R, Tanaka T, Yamamoto T, Bresci G, Saniabadi AR. Adacolumn leucocytapheresis for ulcerative colitis: clinical and endoscopic features of responders and unresponders. Expert Rev Gastroenterol Hepatol. 2015;9:327–33.
43. Saniabadi AR, Tanaka T, Ohmori T, Sawada K, Yamamoto T, Hanai H. Treating inflammatory bowel disease by adsorptive leucocytapheresis: a desire to treat without drugs. World J Gastroenterol. 2014;20:9699–715.
44. Piper SE, Sherwood R a, Amin-Youssef GF, Shah, McDonagh T a. Serial soluble ST2 for the monitoring of pharmacologically optimised chronic stable heart failure. Int J Cardiol. 2015;178:284–91.
45. Diamanti a, Colistro F, Basso MS, Papadatou B, Francalanci P, Bracci F, Muraca M, Knafelz D, De Angelis P, Castro M. Clinical role of calprotectin assay in determining histological relapses in children affected by inflammatory bowel diseases. Inflamm Bowel Dis. 2008;14:1229–35.
46. Ho GT, Lee HM, Brydon G, Ting T, Hare N, Drummond H, Shand a G, Bartolo DC, Wilson RG, Dunlop MG, Arnott ID, Satsangi J. Fecal calprotectin predicts the clinical course of acute severe ulcerative colitis. Am J Gastroenterol. 2009;104:673–8.

11

Endovascular management of hemosuccus pancreaticus, a rare case report of gastrointestinal bleeding

Hye Ryoung Sul[1], Hyun Woong Lee[1*], Jeong Wook Kim[1], Sung Jae Cha[2], Yoo Shin Choi[2], Gi Hyeon Kim[3] and Byung Kook Kwak[3]

Abstract

Background: Hemorrhage from the pancreatic duct, or hemosuccus pancreaticus (HP), is an unusual cause of intermittent gastrointestinal bleeding. HP is most often diagnosed in patients with chronic pancreatitis, and is usually due to the rupture of an aneurysm in the splenic artery. The traditional treatment for HP is surgery, although most cases can be managed by angioembolization.

Case Presentation: We present a case of HP in a patient with no history or evidence of chronic pancreatitis. Repeated endoscopy revealed fresh bleeding from the papilla of Vater. Angiography revealed an aneurysm of the splenic artery, which was the suspected cause of the intermittent bleeding from the pancreatic duct. Angiography demonstrated extravasation of contrast from the aneurysm. A peripheral Jostent stent-graft was hand-mounted on an angioplasty balloon and then inserted into the aneurysm. Arteriography revealed successful occlusion of the aneurysm with the stent-graft. No recurrent gastrointestinal bleeding was observed during the five years follow-up periods.

Conclusion: HP should be included in the differential diagnosis of intermittent gastrointestinal bleeding in patients with histories of chronic alcoholism, even when they do not have a history of chronic pancreatitis. We recommend an interventional procedure with a metal stent for the initial treatment of HP.

Keywords: Hemosuccus pancreaticus, Aneurysm, Splenic artery, Stent

Background

Several terms have been used to describe hemorrhage from the pancreatic duct, including wirsumgorrhagia, proposed by Van Kemmel in 1969, the common terminology used in France, or the equivalent hemowirsungia. Hemosuccus pancreaticus (HP) was proposed by Sandblom in 1970, and hemoductal pancreatitis by Longmire and Rose in 1973. All of these terms describe the emission of red blood along the pancreatic duct through the papilla. Mentions of HP in the medical literature remain mostly limited to case reports [1, 2]. Hemorrhage from abdominal vessels other than the splenic artery, such as the hepatic artery, leading to HP is rare [3]. Aneurysm and chronic pancreatitis are often associated, but no causal relationship has been established. Local inflammation with or without a concomitant pseudocyst, possibly combined with local release of elastase or even pressure necrosis from ductal calculi, induce pseudocyst formation. Other pancreatic causes of HP are rare and include pancreatolithiasis, ectopic pancreas, and pancreas divisum [4, 5].

HP caused by arterial aneurysm is conventionally treated surgically, although interventional radiological procedures are now being utilized. However, implantation of a metal stent may be an effective procedure for the treatment of HP. We report on a case of a peripheral Jostent stent-graft insertion for the management of a HP.

* Correspondence: lhwdoc@hanmail.net
[1]Department of Internal Medicine, Chung-Ang University College of Medicine, 224-1 Heuk Seok-Dong, Dongjak-Ku, Seoul 156-755, Republic of Korea
Full list of author information is available at the end of the article

Case Presentation

A 48-year-old male was referred to our institution with a primary complaint of six months of intermittent relapsing melena of unknown origin. He had no additional symptoms and did not have a history of abdominal surgery. Although the patient was a chronic alcoholic, he did not have a history of pancreatitis. Several times of upper and lower endoscopies revealed melena with multiple diverticulae in the ascending colon, but failed to identify a source of the relapsing melena.

On examination, the patient exhibited pallor, his blood pressure was 120/70 mmHg, and pulse was 78/min. His abdominal examination revealed no pathological findings, except for black, tarry stool on digital rectal examination. Laboratory studies revealed a normocytic normochromic anemia (hemoglobin 9.8 mg/dl, hematocrit 30.1 %, mean corpuscular volume 89.9 fl, mean corpuscular hemoglobin 29.3 pg). Folate and vitamin B12 levels were normal, and the peripheral blood smear was compatible with chronic blood loss. Other laboratory tests were normal. Upper abdominal ultrasonography did not show any pathological findings. On abdominal computerized tomography (CT), a 6.0 mm × 10.4 mm saccular aneurysm was evident in the pancreatic segment of the splenic artery at the body-tail junction of pancreas. The aneurysm was out-pouching from the splenic artery perpendicularly down to the pancreas parenchyma, and the aneurysm contacted the pancreatic duct. The pancreatic duct proximal to the aneurysm was not dilated; however, the distal pancreatic duct was slightly dilated up to 4.0 mm (Fig. 1a). There was no extravasation of contrast media into the pancreatic duct, pancreatic parenchyma, or the bowel lumen. The surrounding pancreas, especially distal to the aneurysm, was slightly lower in density after the administration of contrast, probably due to swelling. Additionally, there was no parenchymal calcification, pancreaticolith, or peripancreatic fluid collection on CT.

On the ninth day after admission, the patient experienced sudden hematemesis and melena. An emergency esophagogastroduodenoscopy (EGD) was performed and revealed fresh blood in the stomach and duodenum with active hemorrhage from the major papilla, a finding suggestive of hemosuccus pancreaticus (Fig. 1b). Follow-up abdominal CT showed that the aneurysm was slightly increased in size (6.3 mm × 11.0 mm). Otherwise, there were no interval changes in the pancreatic duct dilatation and lower pancreatic enhancement. No extravasation of contrast media was observed.

Because the EGD findings were suggestive of hemosuccus pancreaticus (HP), angiography of the celiac artery as well as the upper and lower mesenteric arteries was performed. Under local anesthesia and conscious sedation, by catheterization through the right groin, a catheter was positioned in the proximal part of the abdominal aorta. Angiography confirmed the splenic artery aneurysm (SAA) in the pancreatic segment (Fig. 2a). An 8-F Mach 1 guide catheter (Boston Scientific, Natick, MA, USA) was inserted over a stiff-type, 0.035-in., 260-cm Radifocus Terumo guidewire (Terumo, Tokyo, Japan) up to the proximal splenic artery without an arterial sheath. A 4- to 9-mm-diameter and 28-mm-long peripheral Jostent stent-graft (Jostent Graftmaster, Abbott, Rangendingen, Germany) was hand-mounted on a 6-mm-wide and 4-cm-long angioplasty balloon (Ultra-Thin Diamond, Boston Scientific, Watertown, MA, USA). Through the 8-F Mach 1 guide catheter over the stiff-type, 0.035-in., 260-cm Radifocus Terumo guidewire (Terumo), the stent-graft was inserted to the SAA and deployed by inflating the balloon. Arteriography performed immediately after the procedure revealed successful occlusion of the aneurysm with the stent-graft (Fig. 2b).

On a contrast-enhanced abdominal angiography CT scan obtained 10 days after the procedure, the SAA was

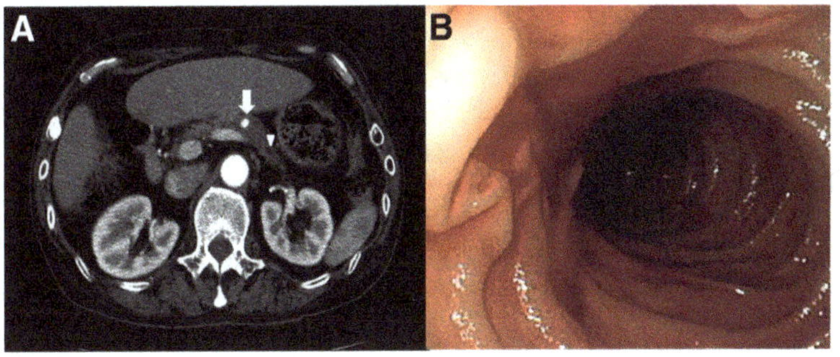

Fig. 1 Abdominal CT scan and Endoscopic findings. **a** 6.0 mm × 10.4 mm saccular aneurysm was evident in the splenic artery (pancreatic segment of the splenic artery) at the body-tail junction of the pancreas (arrow). The aneurysm was out-pouching from the splenic artery perpendicularly down to the pancreas parenchyma. The aneurysm contacted the pancreatic duct, and the pancreatic duct proximal to the aneurysm was not dilated. However, the distal pancreatic duct was slightly dilated (up to 4.0 mm) (arrow head). The surrounding pancreas, especially distal to the aneurysm, was slightly lower in density after contrast enhancement. This finding suggests swelling. **b** On admission day 9, esophagogastroduodenoscopy showed active hemorrhage from the major papilla

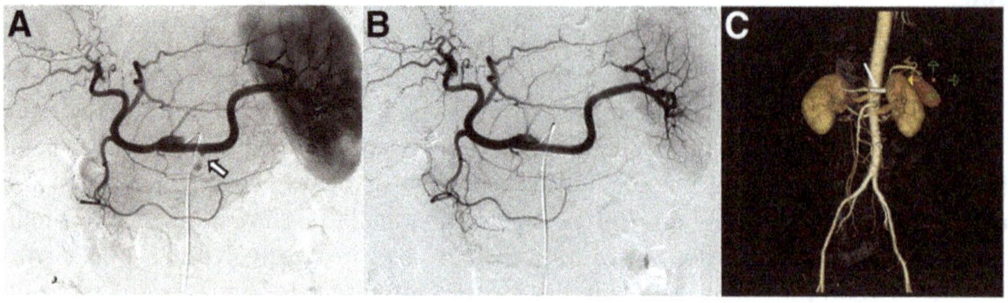

Fig. 2 Angiographic finding and endovascular treatment. **a** Angiography of the splenic artery revealed a 5-mm saccular aneurysm of the splenic artery (arrow). **b** The splenic artery aneurysm after implantation of a 28-mm Jostent. **c** On a contrast-enhanced abdominal angiography CT scan obtained 10 days after the procedure, the splenic artery aneurysm was completely excluded (Stent, arrow)

completely excluded, but the affected artery and spleen were preserved (Fig. 2c). Additionally, the patient's gastrointestinal bleeding was improved. At the time of clinical follow-up four year after the procedure, the patient reported no further episodes of bleeding, and his hemoglobin levels remained stable.

Discussion

The key symptom of HP is melena. Hematemesis is less frequent, and rupture into the abdominal cavity or the retroperitoneum is rare [6]. It is difficult to diagnose HP because the bleeding is usually intermittent. An endoscopic examination of the upper gastrointestinal tract may reveal bleeding from the pancreatic duct. EGD can also show normal findings, and other causes of upper digestive bleeding (erosive gastritis, peptic ulcer, esophageal, and gastric fundus varices) should be ruled out. While the coexistence of chronic, calcifying pancreatitis with HP is the norm, this case report shows that HP is possible in a patient without a history of pancreatitis. Although our patient did not have chronic pancreatitis, he was a chronic alcoholic, and his pancreas may have shown histological signs suggestive of chronic pancreatitis if biopsied. Thus, pancreatic enzyme may erode pancreatic parenchyma and cross tissue boundaries, resulting in connection with adjacent aneurysm. Other uncommon causes of the splenic arterial aneurysm are fibromuscular dysplasia, segmental arterial mediolysis and systemic vasculitis. However, there were no clinical or laboratory findings suggestive of vascular disease.

Once the patient is hemodynamically stable, interventional procedures are effective as an initial treatment in 67 % to 100 % of cases [7]. However, embolization procedures, in which the splenic artery is embolized by platinum spirals or gel foam, may lead to splenic infarction. Coil embolization techniques provoke a thrombus in the aneurysm but also obliterate the artery [6]. Ischemia can develop in the tissue supplied by the artery if the collateral circulation is not sufficient. Embolization of the celiac trunk, the common hepatic artery, or the superior mesenteric artery is thus contraindicated. Yet another possible complication of these procedures is aneurysm infection. Although the embolization of splenic artery is also effective technology, spleen abscess or septic complication would be developed.

Benz et al. recently used an interventional procedure to treat HP, in which an uncoated metal Palmaz stent was placed across the aneurysmic segment of the splenic artery [8]. This report suggests that implantation of a metal stent may be an effective treatment for HP with low rates of recurrence and complications. Nevertheless, stent graft of aneurysms should be avoided in these cases. (1) vessel tortuosity, (2) small caliber size, (3) proximal and distal neck size mismatch. In other words, accessibility to stent grafts in an emergency situation may not be possible. The alternate modes of treatment other than surgery (e.g. EUS guided thrombin injection or coiling of the segment of splenic artery or use of glue to fill the sac of pseudoaneurysm) would be also helpful.

Surgical treatment is indicated in uncontrolled hemorrhage, persistent shock, and when embolization is not feasible. Surgical procedures consist of resection, laparoscopic in part, or ligature of bleeding vessels [9]. Most surgical series have documented a success rate of 70 % to 85 %, with mortality rates of 20 % to 25 %, and rebleeding rates of 0 % to 5 % [10, 11].

This case report suggests that even if a patient does not have any evidence of chronic pancreatitis, HP must be included in the differential diagnosis for chronic alcoholics with intermittent upper gastrointestinal bleeding. In this patient, the treatment was successful without complication or rebleeding for five years after therapy.

Conclusion

Repeated examinations and careful observation should be performed to find obscure sources of repeated upper gastrointestinal bleeding. HP should be included in the differential diagnosis of intermittent gastrointestinal bleeding in patients with histories of chronic alcoholism, even when they do not have a history of chronic pancreatitis. Moreover, as HP may be caused by small aneurysms, it is important to utilize imaging that affords appropriate diagnostic accuracy when trying to rule out HP. We recommend an interventional procedure for the initial treatment of HP, and feel that surgical treatment should only be considered when the patient is unstable, when angiography shows no abnormal findings, or when the interventional therapy is not successful. Furthermore, implantation of a metal stent appears to be an effective treatment for HP.

Consent

Written informed consent was obtained from the patient for publication of this Case report and any accompanying images. A copy of the written consent is available for review by the Editor of this journal.

Abbreviations

HP: Hemosuccus pancreaticus; CT: Computerized tomography; EGD: Esophagogastroduodenoscopy; SAA: Splenic artery aneurysm.

Competing interests

The authors have no conflicts of interest to disclose.

Authors' contributions

HR and HW drafted the manuscript. BK underwent the radiologic procedure and BK and GH provided the radiologic images. SJ and YS reviewed the manuscript. SJ provided the clinical details and reviewed the manuscript. All authors read and approved the final manuscript.

Author details

[1]Department of Internal Medicine, Chung-Ang University College of Medicine, 224-1 Heuk Seok-Dong, Dongjak-Ku, Seoul 156-755, Republic of Korea. [2]Department of Surgery, Chung-Ang University College of Medicine, Seoul, Republic of Korea. [3]Department of Radiology, Chung-Ang University College of Medicine, Seoul, Republic of Korea.

References

1. Etienne S, Pessaux P, Tuech JJ, Lada P, Lermite E, Brehant O, et al. Hemosuccus pancreaticus: a rare cause of gastrointestinal bleeding. Gastroenterol Clin Biol. 2005;29(3):237–42.
2. Panackel C, Kumar A, Subhalal N, Krishnadas D, Kumar KR. Education and imaging. Hepatobiliary and pancreatic: hemosuccus pancreaticus complicating calcific chronic pancreatitis. J Gastroenterol Hepatol. 2007;22(10):1691.
3. De Mas R, Kohler B, Ante D, Schonleben K, Riemann JF. Hemosuccus pancreaticus following rupture of a hepatic artery aneurysm. Z Gastroenterol. 1989;27(12):736–8.
4. Jakobs R, Riemann JF. Hemosuccus pancreaticus due to a pressure ulcer in pancreatolithiasis. Dtsch Med Wochenschr. 1992;117(51–52):1956–61.
5. Meneu JA, Fernandez-Cebrian JM, Alvarez-Baleriola I, Barrasa A, Morales V, Carda P. Hemosuccus pancreaticus in a heterotopic jejunal pancreas. Hepatogastroenterology. 1999;46(25):177–9.
6. Kuhn R, Janocha F, Lazar A, Rambach W, Paquet KJ. Ruptured pseudoaneurysm of the splenic artery. A complication of chronic pancreatitis. Dtsch Med Wochenschr. 1996;121(50):1567–70.
7. Gambiez LP, Ernst OJ, Merlier OA, Porte HL, Chambon JP, Quandalle PA. Arterial embolization for bleeding pseudocysts complicating chronic pancreatitis. Arch Surg. 1997;132(9):1016–21.
8. Benz CA, Jakob P, Jakobs R, Riemann JF. Hemosuccus pancreaticus–a rare cause of gastrointestinal bleeding: diagnosis and interventional radiological therapy. Endoscopy. 2000;32(5):428–31.
9. Saw EC, Ku W, Ramachandra S. Laparoscopic resection of a splenic artery aneurysm. J Laparoendosc Surg. 1993;3(2):167–71.
10. Bender JS, Bouwman DL, Levison MA, Weaver DW. Pseudocysts and pseudoaneurysms: surgical strategy. Pancreas. 1995;10(2):143–7.
11. Heath DI, Reid AW, Murray WR. Bleeding pseudocysts and pseudoaneurysms in chronic pancreatitis. Br J Surg. 1992;79(3):281.

Comparison of sedation between the endoscopy room and operation room during endoscopic submucosal dissection for neoplasms in the upper gastrointestinal tract

Daisuke Yamaguchi[1,3*], Naoko Yamaguchi[2], Yuki Takeuchi[1,3], Takahiro Yukimoto[1,3], Kei Ikeda[1], Kosuke Matsumoto[1], Rikako Kinoshita[1], Saori Kamachi[1], Kyosuke Sugiyama[2], Tomohito Morisaki[1], Keisuke Ario[1], Hisako Yoshida[4], Ryo Katsuki[2], Seiji Tsunada[1] and Kazuma Fujimoto[3]

Abstract

Background: The present study was performed to compare the safety of sedation during endoscopic submucosal dissection (ESD) in the endoscopy room versus operation room.

Methods: In total, 297 patients with gastrointestinal tumors who underwent ESD from January 2011 to December 2016 were retrospectively reviewed. The patients were divided into two groups: those who underwent ESD in the endoscopy room without propofol (Group E) versus operation room with propofol (Group O). The patient, tumor, and procedure characteristics; adverse events; and treatment outcomes were compared between the two groups.

Results: The patient and tumor characteristics, including age (73.6 ± 8.2 vs. 72.5 ± 9.1 years), comorbidities, and tumor size and histology, were not different between Groups E and O. The ESD procedure time was comparable between Groups E and O (105.4 ± 70.4 vs. 106.5 ± 64.4 min), and the anesthesia time was equivalent (138.3 ± 78.1 vs. 148.4 ± 68.8 min). There were no significant differences in adverse events between the two groups. During the ESD procedure, desaturation occurred significantly more often in Group E than O (12.9% vs. 4.0%, $P = 0.021$, odds ratio: 3.53, 95% CI: 1.17–14.4). The recovery time after ESD was significantly longer in Group E than O (180 (100–360) vs. 90 (0–180) min, $P < 0.001$).

Conclusions: A decreased desaturation rate and shorter recovery time after ESD were the advantages of sedation in the operation room with propofol compared with sedation in the endoscopy room. These findings warrant further exploration of the advantages of safe and effective ESD for upper gastrointestinal neoplasms in the operation room.

Keywords: Propofol, Anesthesia, Desaturation, Perforation, Adverse events

* Correspondence: daisukehawks@gmail.com
[1]Department of Gastroenterology, National Hospital Organization Ureshino Medical Center, Ureshino 843-0301, Japan
[3]Department of Internal Medicine and Gastrointestinal Endoscopy, Saga Medical School, Saga 849-8501, Japan
Full list of author information is available at the end of the article

Background

Endoscopic submucosal dissection (ESD) is performed to obtain en bloc specimens of early gastric cancer [1–3]. Because ESD involves a longer operation time than conventional endoscopic mucosal resection, multiple doses of anesthetics are required to provide an adequate level of sedation [4]. Sedation methods vary among countries. In Japan, ESD for gastric cancer is usually performed under sedation provided by the endoscopist in the gastrointestinal endoscopy room as described in the Japan Gastroenterological Endoscopy Society guidelines for sedation during gastroenterological endoscopy [5]. ESD usually requires moderate sedation for maintenance of stable sedation levels while avoiding associated complications [6].

The American Society of Anesthesiologists guidelines for sedation by non-anesthesiologists recommend accurate titration of sedation at the level of consciousness for patients undergoing upper endoscopy [7]. In Japan, the endoscopist and/or nursing staff without assistance of the anesthesiologist usually introduces sedation for pain relief in the endoscopy room without expert technical knowledge. In most institutes in Japan, sedation during ESD is performed by intravenous administration of benzodiazepines in combination with opioids [5]. However, this combination often results in over-sedation and/or difficulty maintaining a stable sedation level. The unstable sedation level disturbs the endoscopist, who must concentrate on the ESD procedure [8, 9].

Propofol, a short-acting sedative characterized by rapid recovery, has several advantages including induction of an appropriate sedation level and relative ease of safely maintaining this level. These advantages have led to a worldwide increase in the application of propofol for standard endoscopic procedures [10–14]. Although administration of propofol for ESD, endoscopic retrograde cholangiography, and endoscopic ultrasonography has been described in several reports [6, 8–14], propofol should be administered for sedation only with the permission of the anesthesiologist in Japan.

The aim of the present study was to compare the outcome and complications of gastric ESD under two sedation conditions: i) sedation by benzodiazepines in combination with analgesic agents (opioids) in the endoscopy room; and ii) sedation by propofol in the operation room with the anesthesiologist.

Methods

Patients

From January 2011 to December 2016, 297 consecutive patients with early upper gastrointestinal tumors who underwent ESD procedures at the National Hospital Organization Ureshino Medical Center were included in the present retrospective chart review. Patients aged >20 years who fulfilled the following criteria were candidates for the study: i) clinical indications for ESD of early esophageal cancer diagnosed as intramucosal squamous cell carcinoma and ii) diagnosis of early gastric cancer according to the absolute indications and expanded indications in the Gastric Cancer Treatment Guidelines [15]. The exclusion criteria were circumferential lesions of early esophageal cancer and suspected early gastric cancer falling outside of the indications for ESD.

Informed consent for the procedures was obtained from all patients. This retrospective study was conducted according to the Ethical Guidelines for Medical and Health Research Involving Human Subjects. The present study was approved by the Ethics Review Committee of National Hospital Organization Ureshino Medical Center (approval number 16–25).

Sedation in the endoscopy room

During the observation period, seven endoscopists performed the ESD procedures in either the endoscopy room or operation room based on their judgment. The distribution of the endoscopists was not different between the endoscopy room and the operation room. In the endoscopy room, sedation for the ESD procedures was introduced by the combination of benzodiazepines and opioids. Specifically, diazepam or midazolam was used as a sedative agent, and buprenorphine, pentazocine, or pethidine hydrochloride was used as an analgesic agent. The sedative and analgesic drugs were selected by the individual endoscopist in charge of the patient's condition.

A dose of 5 to 10 mg of diazepam was infused intravenously [5]. An initial bolus of 3 mg of midazolam for patients with a body weight of <50 kg and 4 mg for patients weighing >50 kg was administered through an intravenous catheter as the main sedative drug, followed by incremental doses (2 mg) when the patient showed signs of discomfort, restlessness, agitation, and/or a response to verbal commands [5]. A midazolam reversal agent was administered after the ESD procedure as necessary. For analgesia, a dose of 0.2 mg of buprenorphine, 15 mg of pentazocine, or 35 mg of pethidine hydrochloride was intravenously injected at the start of ESD. All medications were administered by the physician in the endoscopy division, who did not participate in the actual endoscopic procedure. At least one physician with advanced training in basic and cardiac life support supported the ESD procedure. The anesthesiologist was on standby in case of an emergency but did not support the ESD procedure. Resuscitation devices were equipped in the endoscopy room.

Sedation in the operation room

In the operation room, the medical agents for sedation during the ESD procedure (propofol for sedation and fentanyl for analgesia) were administered under the anesthesiologist's supervision. The patient received an initial intravenous bolus of 0.8 mg/kg of 1% propofol emulsion (10 mg/ml). Additional intravenous boluses of 0.5 mg/kg of 1% propofol emulsion were administered until the patient was fully sedated. An automatic infusion pump was applied to maintain a continuous infusion of 3 mg/kg/h and thus maintain the patient's sedation. The objective was to maintain a sedation level between moderate (proper response to verbal commands either alone or accompanied by light tactile stimulation) and deep (proper response only to repeated or painful stimulation) [6]. As an adjuvant to the sedation, fentanyl was given intravenously at a dose of 1 to 3 μg/kg.

Monitoring and management of adverse events

In the endoscopy room and operation room, the patient received supplemental oxygen (2 L/min) by a nasal cannula while his or her vital signs and oxygen saturation were continuously monitored and recorded every 5 min using standard three-lead electrocardiography, pulse oximetry, and automatic blood pressure equipment. Chest excursions and the respiratory rate were monitored visually, and the consciousness level was assessed initially after induction of sedation and throughout the ESD procedure. With respect to adverse events, desaturation was defined as a decrease in the oxygen saturation to <90%, hypotension was defined as a decrease in the systolic blood pressure to <80 mmHg, and bradycardia was defined as a decrease in the heart rate to <60 bpm. When oxygen desaturation occurred for >10 s, the supplemental oxygen flow was immediately increased to the >95% saturation level. When the supplemental oxygen did not improve the patient's oxygenation condition within 3 min, the ESD procedure was interrupted to secure the airway with administration of the reversal agent as necessary. If hypotension developed, the intravenous drip rate was increased by bolus intravenous injection of 8 mg of ephedrine. For treatment of bradycardia, 0.5 mg of atropine sulfate was injected intravenously. In the operation room, these adverse events were managed by the anesthesiologist.

Patients were discharged from the endoscopy room or operation room after the ESD procedure when they showed stable vital signs (blood pressure, oxygen saturation, and heart rate). Vital signs were recorded at the beginning of the ESD procedure until the patient showed sufficient alertness and activity.

Evaluation of data

The patients were divided into two groups: those who underwent ESD in the endoscopy room (Group E) and those who underwent ESD in the operation room (Group O). The χ^2 test was used to compare the two groups' clinical characteristics, including sex, current drinking and smoking habits, American Society of Anesthesiologists classification, and comorbidities (e.g., cardiovascular diseases, cerebrovascular diseases, chronic liver damage, chronic kidney diseases, diabetes mellitus, and hypertension). Continuous variables were summarized as the mean ± standard deviation for a normal distribution, or median [IQR] for a skewed distribution. The patients' mean age and body mass index were evaluated by Student's *t*-test. The tumor characteristics, including the location, number, historical classification, macroscopic classification, and depth of invasion, were compared between the two groups by the χ^2 test. In patients with multiple tumors, the largest tumor was evaluated based on the underlying assumption of statistically independent observations. Anesthetic outcomes (intubation, desaturation, hypotension, bradycardia, and aspiration pneumonia) and treatment outcomes (en bloc resection, delayed hemorrhage, perforation, and mortality) were evaluated by the χ^2 test. The mean ESD procedure time and anesthesia time were analyzed using Student's *t*-test. The recovery time was analyzed using the Mann–Whitney U test. The economic outcome including the hospitalization period and cost of hospitalization was analyzed using Student's *t*-test. Differences were considered statistically significant at $P < 0.05$. Statistical analyses were performed with the statistical analysis software EZR version 1.26 [16].

Results

Among the 297 patients who underwent ESD procedures, 196 were allocated to Group E and 101 were allocated to Group O. The patients' baseline characteristics were not significantly different between the two groups (Table 1). The median age of the patients in Groups E and O was 73.6 ± 8.2 and 72.5 ± 9.1 years, respectively. In total, 138 (70.4%) and 78 (77.2%) patients in Groups E and O were male, and 187 (95.4%) and 97 (96.0%) patients in Groups E and O had an American Society of Anesthesiologists physical status of I or II, respectively. Comorbidities included hypertension (58.6%), diabetes mellitus (23.4%), and cardiovascular disease (23.4%).

Table 2 lists the characteristics of the gastrointestinal tumors in the two groups. The average tumor size was 17.3 ± 10.5 mm in Group E and 19.7 ± 17.0 mm in Group O, and the ratios of 0-IIc tumors (46.9% vs. 47.5%) and tub1 tumors (58.1% vs. 57.4%) were the highest among all histological subtypes in both groups. There were no significant differences in the baseline tumor characteristics between the two groups.

With respect to sedation during the ESD procedures, diazepam (58.2%) or midazolam (44.4%) with buprenorphine (50.5%) was mainly selected for anesthesia in Group E, and propofol with fentanyl was selected for all patients in Group O (Table 3). The anesthesia time was comparable between the two groups (138.3 ± 78.1 vs.

Table 1 Characteristics of patients in the two groups

	Group E	Group O	*P* value
Number of patients (*N*)	196	101	
Age (years)	73.6 ± 8.2	72.5 ± 9.1	0.26
Sex, male	138 (70.4%)	78 (77.2%)	0.22
Drinking	64 (32.6%)	34 (33.7%)	0.90
Smoking	59 (30.1%)	39 (38.6%)	0.15
BMI (kg/m2)	22.2 ± 3.1	22.9 ± 3.1	0.06
ASA classification I-II	187 (95.4%)	97 (96.0%)	1.00
Comorbidity			
Cardiovascular diseases	33 (16.8%)	18 (17.8%)	0.87
Cerebrovascular diseases	23 (11.7%)	12 (11.9%)	1.00
Chronic kidney diseases	6 (3.1%)	8 (7.9%)	0.08
Chronic liver damage	9 (4.6%)	4 (4.0%)	1.00
Diabetes mellitus	40 (20.4%)	29 (28.7%)	0.11
Hypertension	113 (57.6%)	62 (61.4%)	0.62

Group E: patients who underwent endoscopic submucosal dissection in the endoscopy room, Group O: patients who underwent endoscopic submucosal dissection in the operation room, *BMI* body mass index, *ASA* American Society of Anesthesiologists. Values presented as mean ± standard deviation or n (%)

Table 2 Characteristics of tumors in the two groups

	Group E	Group O	*P* value
Size of tumors (mm)	17.3 ± 10.5	19.7 ± 17.0	0.14
Location of tumors			0.10
Esophagus	0 (0%)	2 (2.0%)	
Stomach	196 (100%)	99 (98.0%)	
Upper third	28 (14.3%)	12 (11.9%)	
Middle third	83 (42.3%)	52 (51.5%)	
Lower third	85 (43.4%)	35 (34.7%)	
Number of tumors			0.07
Single	185 (94.4%)	89 (88.1%)	
Multiple	11 (5.6%)	12 (11.9%)	
Histological classification			0.65
0-I	5 (2.6%)	4 (4.0%)	
0-IIa	82 (41.8%)	38 (37.6%)	
0-IIb	5 (2.6%)	6 (5.9%)	
0-IIc	92 (46.9%)	48 (47.5%)	
0-IIa + IIc	11 (5.6%)	5 (5.0%)	
SMT	1 (0.5%)	0 (0%)	
Macroscopic classification			0.25
Adenoma	55 (28.1%)	28 (27.7%)	
Tub1	114 (58.1%)	58 (57.4%)	
Tub2	18 (9.2%)	6 (5.9%)	
por	1 (0.5%)	4 (4.0%)	
Others	8 (4.1%)	5 (5.0%)	
Depth of invasion			0.97
m	174 (88.8%)	91 (90.1%)	
sm	22 (11.2%)	10 (9.9%)	

Group E: patients who underwent endoscopic submucosal dissection in the endoscopy room, Group O: patients who underwent endoscopic submucosal dissection in the operation room. Values are presented as mean ± standard deviation or n (%)

148.4 ± 68.8 min), as indicated in Table 4. The treatment, anesthetic, and economic outcomes of the ESD procedures are shown in Table 4. During ESD, 99.3% of the patients underwent en bloc resection (99.5% in Group E and 99.0% in Group O), and the procedure time was equivalent between Groups E and O (105.4 ± 70.4 vs. 106.5 ± 64.4 min, respectively). There were no significant differences in the outcomes or complications of the ESD procedures between Groups E and O. Specifically, delayed hemorrhage occurred in 5.1 and 1.0% of patients and perforation occurred in 1.5 and 3.0%, respectively. No mortality within 1 month occurred in either group.

In terms of anesthetic outcomes, the anesthesia time was almost identical in the two groups, and most of the patients (99.7%) underwent the ESD procedure without intubation; 0 and 1 patient in Groups E and O required intubation. Desaturation occurred significantly more often in Group E than O (12.8% vs. 4.0%, respectively; $P = 0.021$), whereas there was no significant difference in the occurrence of hypotension or bradycardia between the two groups. The recovery time after the ESD procedure was significantly longer in Group E than O [180 (100–360) vs. 90 (0–180) min, respectively; $P < 0.001$]. There was no significant difference in the occurrence of aspiration pneumonia after the ESD procedures.

In terms of economic outcomes, there were no differences in the hospitalization period for the ESD procedures between Groups E and O (11.3 ± 5.0 vs. 10.3 ± 4.6 days, respectively). The mean cost of hospitalization was significantly lower in Group E than O (583,806.4 ± 273,117.0 vs. 649,415.7 ± 160,137.3 yen, respectively; $P = 0.027$).

Discussion

In this study, the safety of sedation during ESD in the esophagus and stomach was compared between two sedation conditions: sedation in the endoscopy room and sedation in the operation room. Although ESD has been introduced to obtain en bloc specimens of early-stage gastric cancer in Japan [1, 2, 17–19], ESD requires fine, complicated operative maneuvers with a long period of intraoperative sedation, which might exacerbate the risks of serious complications including perforation and/or bleeding. The present study indicated that sedation with continuous infusion of propofol during ESD in the operation room allows for stable performance of the procedure with a short recovery time. A previous study

Table 3 Medications and doses administered during endoscopic submucosal dissection

Anesthesia drug	Group E	Group O
Diazepam	114 (58.2%)	
Mean diazepam dose (mg)	16.1 ± 9.4	
Midazolam	87 (44.4%)	
Mean midazolam dose (mg)	14.1 ± 6.1	
Buprenorphine	99 (50.5%)	
Mean buprenorphine dose (mg)	0.2 ± 0.1	
Pentazocine	52 (26.5%)	
Mean pentazocine dose (mg)	12.7 ± 4.3	
Pethidine hydrochiloride	55 (28.1%)	
Mean pethidine dose (mg)	73.2 ± 24.3	
Propofol		101 (100%)
Mean propofol dose (mg)		633.6 ± 320.0
Fentanyl		101 (100%)
Mean fentanyl dose (μg)		125.0 ± 52.6

Group E: patients who underwent endoscopic submucosal dissection in the endoscopy room, Group O: patients who underwent endoscopic submucosal dissection in the operation room. Values are presented as mean ± standard deviation or n (%)

Table 4 Anesthetic and treatment outcomes of endoscopic submucosal dissection

	Group E	Group O	*P* value
Treatment outcome			
Procedure time (min)	105.4 ± 70.4	106.5 ± 64.4	0.89
En bloc resection	195 (99.5%)	100 (99.0%)	1.00
Delayed hemorrhage	10 (5.1%)	1 (1.0%)	0.11
Perforation	3 (1.5%)	3 (3.0%)	0.41
Mortality	0 (0%)	0 (0%)	1.00
Anesthetic outcome			
Anesthesia time (min)	138.3 ± 78.1	148.4 ± 68.8	0.27
Intubation case	0 (0%)	1 (1.0%)	0.34
Desaturation	25 (12.8%)	4 (4.0%)	0.02
Hypotension	26 (13.3%)	8 (7.9%)	0.25
Bradycardia	8 (4.1%)	3 (3.0%)	0.76
Recovery time (min)[a]	180 (100–360)	90 (0–180)	<0.001
Aspiration pneumonia	2 (1.0%)	2 (2.0%)	0.61
Economic outcome			
Hospitalization period (day)	11.3 ± 5.0	10.3 ± 4.6	0.09
Cost of hospitalization (1,000yen)	583.8 ± 273.1	649.4 ± 160.1	0.03

Group E: patients who underwent endoscopic submucosal dissection in the endoscopy room, Group O: patients who underwent endoscopic submucosal dissection in the operation room
[a]Median [interquartile range]; other values are mean ± standard deviation or *n* (%)

reported that sedation with propofol for endoscopic procedures leads to a decrease in complications [6, 13, 20]; this was due to the rapid onset and offset of sedation associated with the continuous infusion of propofol.

Sedation for ESD in the operation room might be ideal. ESD procedures in Japan are mainly performed under sedation provided by the endoscopist in the endoscopy room because of space limitations in the operation room and the cost of maintaining a high number of available anesthesiologists. A previous study revealed that administration of propofol by the gastroenterologist did not increase the complication rate [20]. The American Society for Gastrointestinal Endoscopy recommends additional training by the anesthesiologist to ensure safe administration of propofol by non-anesthesiologists during endoscopic procedures [21]. As demonstrated in the present study, sedation with propofol might ideally be administered either by the anesthesiologist or under supervision of the anesthesiologist.

Perforation during ESD is a serious and relatively common complication with an incidence of 3.0 to 4.8% in the stomach [22, 23]. Unstable sedation might result in perforation due to an unexpected gag reflex, hiccups, and/or body movement. In the present study, the en bloc resection rate was 99.3%, the incidence of perforation was 2.0%, and no mortality occurred, and these results were not different between the two sedation groups.

In the present study, desaturation during the ESD procedure occurred significantly more often in the endoscopy room than in the operation room. The increased incidence of desaturation in the endoscopy room might have been due to saliva flowing into the airway, requiring suction of the saliva from the oral cavity during the ESD procedure. The recovery time after ESD was significantly longer in the endoscopic than operation room, although the occurrence of aspiration pneumonia was not different between the two groups. These two factors (desaturation and the recovery time) might be advantages of sedation with propofol in the operation room.

A disadvantage of sedation in the operation room is the high hospitalization fee for ESD in patients with early esophageal or gastric cancers. This high cost is mainly due to the use of general anesthesia, not the duration of hospitalization. Economic evaluation has revealed that ESD performed in the endoscopy room is cost-effective, which might be a problem in terms of health insurance coverage in Japan.

Limitations of this study were the small number of participants, and the fact that it was a single-institution study. In addition, this study was a retrospective nature of the chart review. Consequently, there would have been selection bias of participants by the endoscopists performed the ESD procedures. Further studies involving multiple institutes might be required to accumulate more data on ESD procedures.

Conclusions

Although decreases in the desaturation rate and recovery time after ESD were the only advantages of sedation with propofol in the operation room, sedation in the operation room might be required to ensure safer application of ESD for tumors of the gastrointestinal tract.

Abbreviations

ESD: Endoscopic submucosal dissection; Group E: Patients who underwent ESD in the endoscopy room; Group O: Patients who underwent ESD in the operation room

Acknowledgements

Not applicable.

Funding

No specific grants from any funding agencies in the public, commercial, or not-for-profit sectors were received for this research.

Authors' contributions

DY, NY and KF designed the research; DY, YT, TY, KI, KM, RK, SK, TM, KA and ST performed the endoscopic submucosal dissection procedure and interpreted the patient data; NY, KS and RK performed the sedation during endoscopic submucosal dissection and acquired of data; DY and HY analyzed the data; DY and KF wrote the paper; KF was a major contributor in writing the manuscript. All authors read and approved the final manuscript.

Competing interests

The authors declare that they have no competing interests.

Author details

[1]Department of Gastroenterology, National Hospital Organization Ureshino Medical Center, Ureshino 843-0301, Japan. [2]Department of Anesthesiology, National Hospital Organization Ureshino Medical Center, Ureshino 843-0301, Japan. [3]Department of Internal Medicine and Gastrointestinal Endoscopy, Saga Medical School, Saga 849-8501, Japan. [4]Clinical Research Center, Saga Medical School, Saga 849-8501, Japan.

References

1. Ono H, Kondo H, Gotoda T, et al. Endoscopic mucosal resection for treatment of early gastric cancer. Gut. 2001;48:225–9.
2. Watanabe K, Ogata S, Kawazoe S, et al. Clinical outcomes of EMR for gastric tumors: historical pilot evaluation between endoscopic submucosal dissection and conventional mucosal resection. Gastrointest Endosc. 2006;63:776–82.
3. Kakushima N, Fujishiro M. Endoscopic submucosal dissection for gastrointestinal neoplasms. World J Gastroenterol. 2008;14:2362–7.
4. Oda I, Gotoda T, Hamanaka H, et al. Endoscopic submucosal dissection for early gastric cancer: technical feasibility, operation time and complications from a large consecutive series. Dig Endosc. 2005;17:54–8.
5. Obara K, Haruma K, Irisawa A, et al. Guidelines for sedation in gastroenterological endoscopy. Dig Endosc. 2015;27:435–49.
6. Kiriyama S, Gotoda T, Sano H, et al. Safe and effective sedation in endoscopic submucosal dissection for early gastric cancer: a randomized comparison between propofol continuous infusion and intermittent midazolam injection. J Gastroenterol. 2010;45:831–7.
7. American Society of Anesthesiologists Task Force on Sedation and Analgesia by Non-Anesthesiologists. Practice guidelines for sedation and analgesia by non-anesthesiologists. Anesthesiology. 2002;96:1004–17.
8. Nonaka S, Kawaguchi Y, Oda I, et al. Safety and effectiveness of propofol-based monitored anesthesia care without intubation during endoscopic submucosal dissection for early gastric and esophageal cancers. Dig Endosc. 2015;27:665–73.
9. Seo SI, Ryu JY, Kang SS, et al. Safety of target-controlled propofol infusion by gastroenterologists in patients undergoing endoscopic resection. Dig Dis Sci. 2016;61:3199–206.
10. Gotoda T, Kusano C, Nonaka M, et al. Non-anesthesiologist administrated propofol (NAAP) during endoscopic submucosal dissection for elderly patients with early gastric cancer. Gastric Cancer. 2014;17:686–91.
11. Heuss LT, Schnieper P, Drewe J, Pflimlin E, Beglinger C. Safety of propofol for conscious sedation during endoscopic procedures in high-risk patients: a prospective, controlled study. Am J Gastroenterol. 2003;98:1751–7.
12. Buxbaum J, Roth N, Motamedi N, et al. Anesthetist-directed sedation favors success of advanced endoscopic procedures. Am J Gastroenterol. 2017;112:290–6.
13. Ominami M, Nagami Y, Shiba M, et al. Comparison of propofol with midazolam in endoscopic submucosal dissection for esophageal squamous cell carcinoma: a randomized controlled trial. J Gastroenterol 2017 [Epub ahead of print].
14. Tohda G, Higashi S, Wakahara S, Morikawa M, Sakumoto H, Kane T. Propofol sedation during endoscopic procedures: safe and effective administration by registered nurses supervised by endoscopists. Endoscopy. 2006;38:360–7.
15. Japanese Gastric Cancer Association. Japanese classification of gastric carcinoma: 3rd English edition. Gastric Cancer. 2011;14:101–12.
16. Kanda Y. Investigation of the freely available easy-to-use software 'EZR' for medical statistics. Bone Marrow Transplant. 2013;48:452–8.
17. Mannen K, Tsunada S, Hara M, et al. Risk factors for complications of endoscopic submucosal dissection in gastric tumors: analysis of 478 lesions. J Gastroenterol. 2010;45:30–6.
18. Miyahara K, Iwakiri R, Shimoda R, et al. Perforation and postoperative bleeding of endoscopic submucosal dissection in gastric tumors: analysis of 1190 lesions in low- and high-volume centers in Saga, Japan. Digestion. 2012;86:273–80.
19. Yamanouchi K, Ogata S, Sakata Y, et al. Effect of additional surgery after noncurative endoscopic submucosal dissection for early gastric cancer. Endosc Int Open. 2016;4:E24–9.
20. Wadhwa V, Issa D, Garg S, Lopez R, Sanaka MR, Vargo JJ. Similar risk of cardiopulmonary adverse events between Propofol and traditional anesthesia for gastrointestinal endoscopy: a systematic review and meta-analysis. Clin Gastroenterol Hepatol. 2017;15:194–206.
21. Standards ASGE. Of practice committee. Guidelines for the use of deep sedation and anesthesia for GI endoscopy. Gastrointest Endosc. 2002;56:613–7.
22. Oda I, Suzuki H, Nonaka S, Yoshinaga S. Complications of gastric endoscopic submucosal dissection. Dig Endosc. 2013;25:71–8.
23. Yamamoto K, Shimoda R, Ogata S, et al. Perforation and postoperative bleeding associated with endoscopic submucosal dissection in colorectal tumors: analysis of 398 lesions treated in Saga, Japan. Intern Med 2017, in press.

13

High prevalence of advanced colorectal neoplasia in the Thai population: a prospective screening colonoscopy of 1,404 cases

Bunchorn Siripongpreeda[1*], Chulabhorn Mahidol[1,2,3], Navara Dusitanond[1], Tassanee Sriprayoon[1], Bunlung Muyphuag[1], Thaniya Sricharunrat[1], Narongchai Teerayatanakul[1], Watanya Chaiwong[1], Wipra Worasawate[1], Prassanee Sattayarungsee[1], Juthamas Sangthongdee[1], Jirapa Prarom[1], Gaidganok Sornsamdang[1], Kamonwan Soonklang[1], Kasiruck Wittayasak[1] and Chirayu U. Auewarakul[1,3]

Abstract

Background: Increasing morbidity and mortality from colorectal cancer is evident in recent years in the developing Asian nations. Particularly in Thailand and most neighbouring low-income countries, screening colonoscopy is not yet recommended nor implemented at the national policy level.

Methods: Screening colonoscopy was offered to 1,500 healthy volunteers aged 50–65 years old who were registered into the program between July 2009 and June 2010. Biopsy and surgery was performed depending on the identified lesions. Fecal immunochemical tests (FIT) were additionally performed for comparison with colonoscopy.

Results: There were 1,404 participants who underwent colonoscopy. The mean age of the cohort was 56.9 ± 4.2 years and 69.4 % were females. About 30 % (411 cases) of all colonoscopies had abnormal colonoscopic findings, and of these, 256 cases had adenomatous polyps. High risk adenomas (villous or tubulovillous or high grade dysplasia or size > 1 cm or > 3 adenomatous polyps) were found in 98 cases (7 %), low risk adenoma in 158 cases (11.3 %), and hyperplastic polyps in 119 cases (8.5 %). Eighteen cases (1.3 %) had colorectal cancer and 90 % of them (16 cases) were non-metastatic including five stage 0 cases, seven stage I cases, and four stage IIA cases. Only two cases had metastasis: one to regional lymph nodes (stage IIIB) and another to other organs (stage IVA). The most common cancer site was the distal intestine including rectum (7 cases, 38.9 %) and sigmoid colon (7 cases, 38.9 %). Ten colorectal cancer cases had positive FIT whereas 8 colorectal cancer cases were FIT-negative. The sensitivity and specificity of FIT was 55.6 % and 96.2 %, respectively, while the positive predictive value was 16.4 % and negative predictive value was 99.4 %. The overall survival of colorectal cancer cases at 5-year was 83.3 %.

Conclusion: High prevalence of colorectal cancer and high-risk adenoma was found in the Thai population aged 50–65 years old by screening colonoscopy. FIT was not sensitive enough to detect colorectal cancer in this asymptomatic cohort. Integration of screening colonoscopy into the national cancer screening program should be implemented to detect early cases of advanced colorectal neoplasia and improve survival of colorectal cancer patients in Thailand.

Keywords: Colorectal cancer, Adenoma, Advanced colorectal neoplasia, Screening colonoscopy, Fecal immunochemical test, National policy

(Continued on next page)

* Correspondence: bunchorn_sir@yahoo.com
[1]Chulabhorn Hospital, Bangkok, Thailand
Full list of author information is available at the end of the article

(Continued from previous page)

Abbreviations: BMI, Body mass index; CT colonography, Comperized tomographic colonography; FIT, Fecal immunochemical tests; FOB, Fecal occult blood; NCCN, National Comprehensive Cancer Network; NPV, Negative predictive value; PPV, Positive predictive value; UICC, The Union for International Cancer Control

Background

Colorectal cancer is one of the most common causes of cancer death globally each year, along with lung, liver, prostate, and breast cancer [1]. Disease incidence of economically developed countries in Asia such as Japan, Korea and Singapore abruptly approached the level of the Western countries. Data from the National Cancer Institute of Thailand Cancer Registry also showed a gradual increase in the number of new colorectal cancer patients in recent years with increased advance stage cases identified [2]. Colorectal cancer screening can diagnose cases in early stages, decrease cancer mortality and potentially prevent this disease [3, 4]. Detection and proper management of advanced colorectal neoplasia which included malignant and some high risk colorectal lesions that need therapeutic interventions should prevent progression and worse outcomes in the affected cases.

Colonoscopy is one of the cancer screening tests that achieves goals of premalignant and early stage cancer detection and when it is coupled with polypectomy, it can prevent and reduce the incidence of disease, and finally of all results, decrease mortality from colorectal cancer [3–5]. Therefore, colonoscopy is recommended in colorectal cancer screening guideline since 1997 [6]. However, screening colonoscopy is presently not included in the national colorectal cancer screening policy in Thailand nor widely recommended for the Thai population. Most previous studies utilized fecal immuno chemical test (FIT) as a first screening tool although the majority of the Thai population do not undergo such testing on a regular basis [7–9]. This study aimed to provide essential information on consideration of implementation of a nation-wide colorectal cancer screening program in Thailand and developing countries. Screening colonoscopy was performed as a first screening tool in all cases while FIT was done as a comparison.

Methods

Study participants

After the study protocol had been approved by the Human Research Ethical Committee of Chulabhorn Research Institute, we enrolled participants between 50 and 65 years of age with no past medical history of colorectal cancer or poorly controlled underlying diseases in July 2009. In total, 1,612 applicants expressed their willingness to participate in this project. All participants were educated about colorectal cancer and screening methods that were to be used in this study as well as study objectives, details of each procedure including possible complications, and usage of data from the study. Some patients were excluded based on age, poor medical problem control, or the inability to be followed over a long-term period. Finally, 1,404 participants underwent colonoscopy between July 2009 and June 2010 after they provided informed consent. Their demographic data, medical history, physical examination, and pre-operative management were collected.

Screening colonoscopy and pathological diagnosis

Bowel preparation before colonoscopy was established by using 90 mL of sodium phosphate after a low fiber diet for 2 days. All participants underwent colonoscopy under intravenous anaesthesia. The colonoscopic findings in each colonic section were recorded. If abnormal mucosal findings or polyps were found, the removed tissue was sent for pathological diagnosis. We categorized abnormal tissue from colonoscopic findings and pathological reports into malignant, high-risk adenoma, low risk adenoma, and non-adenomatous polyps, for which each group underwent different appropriate management according to National Comprehensive Cancer Network (NCCN) guidelines for colorectal cancer screening. High-risk adenoma cases recommended to have repeat colonoscopy earlier than low risk adenoma cases included one of the following colonoscopic and pathological criteria: size ≥1 cm, ≥3 adenomas, or tubulovillous or villous adenoma or high grade dysplasia. All malignant cases were diagnosed by pathological staging using the Seventh edition of the Union for International Cancer Control (UICC) TNM Classification of Malignant Tumours [10]. Patients with colorectal cancer were treated according to the NCCN Guidelines [11]. Participants without malignancy were seen annually in the clinic for general evaluation, and FIT and follow-up colonoscopy was to be performed based on clinical findings and colorectal cancer risks. The second screening colonoscopy was respectively performed at 3, 4, and 5 years follow-up for high risk adenoma cases, low risk adenoma/hyperplastic polyp cases, and normal colonoscopy cases.

Screening fecal immunochemical test (FIT)

FIT was performed in parallel to screening colonoscopy by fecal occult blood (FOB) one-step test device, a rapid chromatographic immunoassay (Abon Biopharm Hangzhou, China) with relative sensitivity of 93.6 % and relative specificity of 99.1 % [12, 13]. The FOB one-step test can detect fecal blood as low as 50 ng/mL or 6 μg/g feces and is specific for human hemoglobin at a concentration of 1.0 mg/mL. Fecal specimens were self-collected from the first bowel movement in the morning of the appointed date for FIT test which occurred before the start of bowel preparation for screening colonoscopy. The specimens were stored in a clean and dry container and brought in to the hospital by the participants at environmental temperature. The participants were instructed to hand in the samples to the laboratory within 6 h of collection.

Statistical analysis

Statistical analyses were performed with STATA version 12.1. Data of the participants were reported as means and standard deviation for continuous variables and as proportions and absolute counts for categorical variables. We also estimated FIT sensitivity, specificity and predictive values in detecting colorectal cancer.

Results

Demographic characteristics of the study cohort

Of the 1,404 participants, there were 429 males and 975 females, with a mean age of 56.9 ± 4.2 years. Most (81.8 %) of the participants lived in Bangkok Metropolitan and connective territorial provinces during the time of the colonoscopy. Overall, 96.1 % of participants had no lower gastrointestinal symptoms, i.e. bowel habit changes or lower gastrointestinal bleeding or decreased stool calibre or anemia, and the majority (91.7 %) did not have a family history of colorectal cancer, respectively (Table 1). Complete colonoscopy was accomplished in 99.6 % (1,399) of cases. In five incomplete colonoscopy cases, patients were further investigated by CT colonography, all of which produced normal findings.

Table 1 Demographic data of the study cohort (N = 1,404)

Variable	N (%)
Sex	
Male	429 (30.6)
Female	975 (69.4)
Age	56.9 ± 4.2
BMI	
> 25	640 (45.6)
≤ 25	764 (54.4)
Area	
Bangkok and territories	1148 (81.8)
Other	256 (18.2)
Lower gastrointestinal tract symptoms	
Yes	55 (3.9)
No	1349 (96.1)
Family history of colorectal cancer	
Yes	117 (8.3)
No	1287 (91.7)

Screening colonoscopy findings

About 30 % (411 cases) of all colonoscopies had abnormal colonoscopic findings. Malignancy was found in 1.3 % (18 cases) of all cases. Of all colonoscopies, 18.2 % (256 cases) had adenomatous polyps, of which 7 % (98 cases) were high risk adenoma. The other 9.8 % (137 cases) had abnormal tissue, of which 8.5 % (119 cases) were hyperplastic polyps (Fig. 1). The pathological diagnosis of malignant tissue in this study showed two cases of carcinoid tumor out of 18 cases. Others were adenocarcinoma with stages varying from stage 0 to stage 4 (Table 2). Nearly 90 % (16 cases) were non-metastatic colorectal cancer; five stage 0 cases, seven stage I cases, and four stage IIA cases. Only two cases from our study had metastasis: one to regional lymph nodes (stage IIIB) and another to other organs (stage IVA). Most abnormalities that required tissue diagnosis were found in the left side of the colon (Fig. 2). The most common cancer site was rectum (7 cases, 38.9 %) and sigmoid colon (7 cases, 38.9 %). Also, the most common site for high risk adenoma and low risk adenoma was sigmoid colon (30 % and 35 %, respectively) and the second most common sites were ascending and transverse colon. Most adenoma had only low grade dysplasia. Only one case of high grade dysplasia was detected in a tubulovillous adenoma case. The gender proportion in 256 cases of adenoma group was 117 males (45.7 %) and 139 females (54.3 %). For colorectal cancer cases, they were 8 males (44.4 %) and 10 females (55.6 %).

Table 3 summarizes histopathology findings of 55 cases with complaining symptoms that may have suggested cancer at the outset of screening and 117 cases with a family history of colorectal cancer. Among 55 cases, 3 developed colorectal cancer (5.5 %) as compared with 15 cases in asymptomatic cases (1.1 %) (p = 0.031). Various types of adenomas and polyps were also found in symptomatic cases. If symptomatic cases were excluded, high risk adenoma and colorectal cancer accounted for 8.15 % (110/1,349 cases). Four colorectal cancer cases developed in participants with a family history of colorectal cancer (3.4 %) whereas 14 colorectal cancer cases (1.1 %) were found in a no family history group (p = 0.056). Hyperplastic polyps tended to be more common in participants with a family history of colorectal cancer.

Sensitivity and specificity of FIT in diagnosis of colorectal cancer

As shown in Table 4, 10/18 colorectal cancer cases had positive FIT whereas 8 colorectal cancer cases were FIT-negative. The sensitivity and specificity of FIT in detection of colorectal cancer was 55.6 % and 96.2 %, respectively, while the positive predictive value (PPV) was 16.4 % and

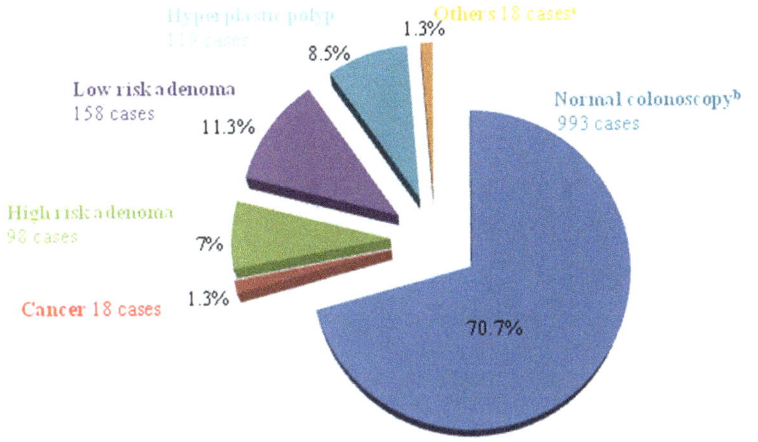

Fig. 1 Pathological diagnosis from screening colonoscopy; [a]including inflammatory polyp, colitis, lipoma and loss specimens; [b]including diverticulosis without biopsied tissues and hemorrhoids

the negative predictive value (NPV) was 99.4 %. Table 5 shows the distribution of FIT-positivity among participants with various histopathology findings. Most of adenoma cases were FIT-negative. FIT-positive non-cancer cases included6 high risk adenoma, 3 low risk adenoma, 8 hyperplastic polyps, and 33 cases with normal colonoscopy results.

Follow-up of study participants and survival of colorectal cancer cases

In the follow-up period after colonoscopic screening, there were three additional new cases of colorectal cancer. Two cases of intramucosal carcinoma of sigmoid colon and another case with stage 1 anal canal adenocarcinoma were found in the second year from the group previously identified as high risk adenoma, low risk adenoma and hyperplastic polyp, respectively. The mortality due to colorectal cancer cases in this study was 3/18 cases: 1 case with stage IV disease died in the first year, 1 case with stage IIA in the fourth year, and another case in stage I died from unrelated primary hepatobiliary cancer. The overall survival of colorectal cancer cases at 5 year was 83.3 % (88.9 % if excluded 1 death from unrelated cancer).

Table 2 Staging and 5-year survival rates of 18 colorectal cancer cases diagnosed by screening colonoscopy

Variable	N (%)
Screening colonoscopy	
Cancer	18 (100)
Stage	
0	5 (27.8)
I	7 (38.9)
IIA	4 (22.2)
IIIB	1 (5.6)
IVA	1 (5.6)
5-year survival rate	15 (83.3)[a]

[a]One case died from unrelated hepatobiliarycancer

Discussion

The discovery rate of high risk adenoma and invasive colorectal cancer in this study (8.15 %) was nearly twice that of advanced colorectal neoplasia in the asymptomatic population (4.5 %) as reported from multiple studies in Asia but comparable to that of the symptomatic population (7.8 %) [14]. These patients should receive therapeutic intervention before progression to more advanced disease. When we excluded the amount criteria from the high risk adenoma group, the prevalence of advanced colorectal neoplasia in our study (3 %) and also adenocarcinoma (1.3 %) were still comparable to the country with a high incidence of colorectal cancer [14, 15]. Prior hospital-based reports and retrospective

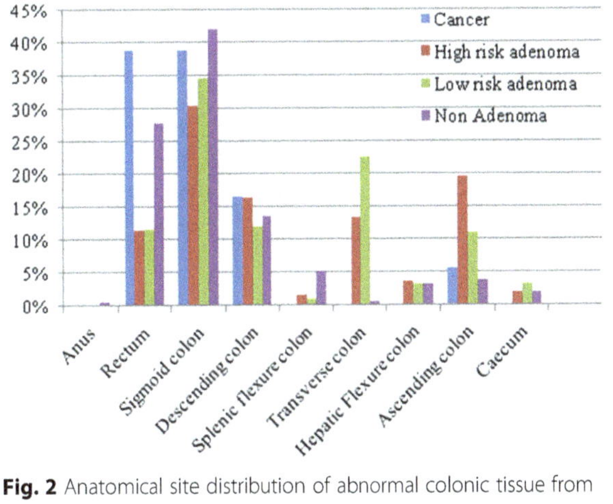

Fig. 2 Anatomical site distribution of abnormal colonic tissue from screening colonoscopy

Table 3 Histological comparison between cases with or without symptoms at screening day 0 visit and between cases with or without family history of colorectal cancer

	Symptoms that may suggest colorectal cancer at the outset			Family history of colorectal cancer		
	Yes 55 cases	No 1,349 cases	*P*-value	Yes 117 cases	No 1,287 cases	*P*-value
Screening colonoscopy						
Colorectal cancer	3 (5.5)	15 (1.1)	0.031[b]	4 (3.4)	14 (1.1)	0.056[b]
Stage						
0	1	4		2	3	
I	0	6		0	6	
IIA	1	4		1	4	
IIIB	0	1		1	0	
IVA	1	0		0	1	
High risk adenoma	3 (5.5)	95 (7.0)		0 (0.0)	98 (7.6)	
Low risk adenoma	10 (18.2)	148 (11.0)		13 (11.1)	145 (11.3)	
Hyperplastic polyp	3 (5.5)	116 (8.6)		14 (12.0)	105 (8.2)	
Other pathological diagnosis[a]	0 (0.0)	18 (1.3)		2 (1.7)	16 (1.2)	
No colorectal tumor	36 (65.5)	957 (70.9)		84 (71.8)	909 (70.6)	

[a]Inflammatory polyp, colitis, and lipoma
[b]Fisher Exact Test

studies from Thailand also showedcancer detection rate by colonoscopy of 0.6–7.1 % in different studied population [7–9, 16, 17]. These previous studies utilized FIT as a first screening tool and were unlike our study whereby colonoscopy was performed as a first screening tool.

The abnormal colonic tissue (29.3 %) findings from our screening colonoscopy study are in the range of polyp detection rates (25–37 %) reported in other studies from within and outside Thailand [16–20]. Both adenomatous polyp and hyperplastic polyposis can accumulate worse genetic changes and become malignant [21, 22]. Therefore, colorectal cancer screening would benefit this population. Although most abnormalities that required tissue diagnosis were found in the left side of the colon, complete colonoscopy should be done to include low and high risk adenomas in the second most common locations, the transverse and ascending colon.

There are some key differences in the selection of subjects for our study compared with others: our study included screening criteria for an age group at high risk of colorectal cancer [23], while others included data from a symptom-related group. Moreover, this result might not represent the incidence of colorectal cancer from all regions in Thailand because most (81.8 %) of the participants were from the Bangkok metropolitan region and territories. If this finding represented the real incidence of colorectal cancer in our population, or perhaps even in urban and suburban areas, launching a national colorectal cancer screening policy should be considered for specific groups. Other factors that might affect a high yield of colorectal cancer findings include public information that may stimulate awareness and access to reluctant cancer patients.

Problems related to colonoscopy screening include its invasiveness, complications, high financial cost, and need of specialized endoscopists; these reasons were reported as causes of low colorectal screening adherence in well

Table 4 Diagnostic value of FIT in the diagnosis of colorectal cancer

FIT	Colonoscopy	
	Malignancy	No malignancy[a]
Positive	10	51
Negative	8	1,295
Total	18	1,346

[a]FIT not done in 40 cases
Sensitivity (55.6 %), Specificity (96.2 %), PPV (16.4 %), NPV (99.4 %)

Table 5 Histopathology characteristics of cases with FIT-positive and FIT-negative results

Histopathology	FIT[a]	
	Positive *N* (%)	Negative *N* (%)
Colorectal cancer	10 (16.4)	8 (0.6)
High risk adenoma	6 (9.8)	87 (6.7)
Low risk adenoma	3 (4.9)	152 (11.7)
Hyperplastic polyp	8 (13.1)	106 (8.1)
Other pathological diagnosis[b]	1 (1.6)	17 (1.3)
No colorectal tumor	33 (54.1)	933 (71.6)

[a]FIT not done in 40 cases
[b]Inflammatory polyp, colitis, lipoma

developed countries [24, 25]. Therefore, other more practical screening methods were utilized instead of colonoscopy. The sensitivity of FIT for cancer detection in our study (55 %) was comparable to Guaiac fecal occult blood test (37–79 %) but somewhat lower than results of FIT in other studies (79 %) [26, 27]. In some resource-limited countries, fecal-based screening may play a major role in decreasing colorectal cancer mortality with high subject acceptance rates [28, 29]. However, in our study, the sensitivity of FIT of 55.6 % was deemed inadequate to detect colorectal cancer cases and 8/18 cancer cases had negative FITs.

There are no recommendations for any other surveillance procedure after screening colonoscopy, but endoscopic management after colonoscopic and pathologic findings have been suggested [30–34]. However, in this study, cases of colorectal cancer were found before the recommended period of surveillance colonoscopy, which were similar to the findings of other studies [5, 24, 35–39]. Moreover, some cases also suffered from unrelated types of cancer. Thus, some individual risk criteria such as smoking, a family history of biliary tract cancer which are common in Thailand should be concerned for improvement of screening benefits in specific groups of patients [40, 41]. Quality indices [42, 43], technology of colonoscopy [44] and other predictors [45–48] should be included for detection of these interval cancers. Particularly, with the aging population in Thailand, proper screening and surveillance programsneed to be further evaluated [3].

The mortality caused by colorectal cancer in our study after monitoring for 5 years was only two cases from colorectal cancer. Another case died from unrelated hepatobiliary cancer. So the 5-yearsurvival rate after screening colonoscopy and standard treatment of detected colorectal cancer cases in this study, even including five cases (27.8 %) with stage IIA and IIIB, was excellent at 88.9 %. This survival rate was comparable to survival of stage I colorectal cancer (87–92 %) after standard staging and treatment [49].

Conclusions

In our study population aged 50–65 years old, 30 % of colonoscopically screened cases had abnormal colonic lesions that needed further pathological diagnosis. The colorectal cancer detection rate was 1.3 % and the overall prevalence of advanced colorectal neoplasia was 3 % by screening colonoscopy. Tissue abnormalities were found more in the distal part than the proximal part of the large intestine. The overall survival of colorectal cancer patients diagnosed by colonoscopic screening was 83 %. FIT was inadequate to detect advanced colorectal neoplasia and missed almost half of the colorectal cases. We suggest that screening colonoscopy should be implemented as part of the National Colorectal Cancer Screening Program in Thailand.

Acknowledgements
We appreciated all volunteer participants and Chulabhorn Hospital staff, particularly the Colorectal Cancer Care Team, the Nursing Division and the Data Management Unit, who generously spared their time for the accomplishment and fulfillment of this project.

Funding
This study was funded by Chulabhorn Hospital Research Grant.

Authors' contributions
BS performed colonoscopy, data collection and manuscript drafting. CM was responsible for the initiation and execution of the entire project. ND, BM and TS performed colonoscopy. TSr and NT reviewed and reported pathological results. WC and WW were responsible for anesthesia of the participants. PS, JJ and JP helped coordinating the appointment and follow-ups of the participants and patients. GS was responsible for FIT analysis. KW and KS performed data collection, data management and statistical analysis. CA reviewed the study design, monitored the project, and critically revised the final manuscript. All authors approved to the final manuscript.

Competing interests
The authors declare that they have no competing interests.

Author details
[1]Chulabhorn Hospital, Bangkok, Thailand. [2]Chulabhorn Research Institute, Bangkok, Thailand. [3]Faculty of Medicine Siriraj Hospital, Mahidol University, Bangkok, Thailand.

References

1. Ferlay J, Shin HR, Bray F, Forman D, Mathers C, Parkin DM. Estimates of worldwide burden of cancer in 2008: GLOBOCAN 2008. Int J Cancer. 2010;127(12):2893–917.
2. Hospital based cancer registry National Cancer Institute of Thailand. 2002–2011. http://www.nci.go.th/en/cancer_record/cancer_rec1.html. Accessed 20 July 2012
3. Zauber AG, Winawer SJ, O'Brien MJ, Lansdorp-Vogelaar I, van Ballegooijen M, Hankey BF, et al. Colonoscopic polypectomy and long-term prevention of colorectal-cancer deaths. N Engl J Med. 2012;366(8):687–96.
4. Winawer SJ. The history of colorectal cancer screening: a personal perspective. Dig Dis Sci. 2015;60(3):596–608.
5. Friedrich K, Gruter L, Gotthardt D, Eisenbach C, Stremmel W, Scholl SG, et al. Survival in patients with colorectal cancer diagnosed by screening colonoscopy. Gastrointest Endosc. 2015;82(1):133–7.
6. Winawer SJ, Fletcher RH, Miller L, Godlee F, Stolar MH, Mulrow CD, et al. Colorectal cancer screening: clinical guidelines and rationale. Gastroenterology. 1997;112(2):594–642.
7. Khuhaprema T, Sangrajrang S, Lalitwongsa S, Chokvanitphong V, Raunroadroong T, Ratanachu-ek T, et al. Organised colorectal cancer screening in Lampang Province, Thailand: preliminary results from a pilot implementation programme. BMJ Open. 2014;4(1):1–11.
8. Aniwan S, Rerknimitr R, Kongkam P, Wisedopas N, Ponuthai Y, Chaithongrat S, et al. A combination of clinical risk stratification and fecal immunochemical test results to prioritize colonoscopy screening in asymptomatic participants. Gastrointest Endosc. 2015;81(3):719–27.
9. Lohsiriwat V. Accuracy of self-checked fecal occult blood testing for colorectal cancer in Thai patients. Asian Pac J Cancer Prev. 2014;15(18):7981–4.
10. Sobin LH, Wittekind C, M. G. TNM classification of malignant tumours (UICC S.). 7th ed. New York: Wiley-Blackwell; 2009. p. 73–7.
11. Network NCC. NCCN Guidelines, Colorectal Cancer, Version I 2010. 2010.
12. Simon JB. Occult blood screening for colorectal carcinoma: a critical review. Gastroenterology. 1985;88(3):820–37.
13. Blebea J, McPherson RA. False-positive guaiac testing with iodine. Arch Pathol Lab Med. 1985;109(5):437–40.

14. Sung JJ, Lau JY, Young GP, Sano Y, Chiu HM, Byeon JS, et al. Asia Pacific consensus recommendations for colorectal cancer screening. Gut. 2008;57(8):1166–76.
15. Bae T, Ha Y, Kim C, Lee J, Ha K, Shin S, et al. Distribution of the colonoscopic adenoma detection rate according to age: is recommending colonoscopy screening for koreans over the age of 50 safe? Ann Coloproctol. 2015;31(2):46–51.
16. Rerknimitr R, Ratanapanich W, Kongkam P, Kullavanijaya P. Differences in characteristics of colorectal neoplasm between young and elderly Thais. World J Gastroenterol. 2006;12(47):7684–9.
17. Aswakul P, Prachayakul V, Lohsiriwat V, Bunyaarunnate T, Kachintorn U. Screening colonoscopy from a large single center of Thailand - something needs to be changed? Asian Pac J Cancer Prev. 2012;13(4):1361–4.
18. Wisedopas N, Thirabanjasak D, Taweevisit M. A retrospective study of colonic polyps in King Chulalongkorn Memorial Hospital. J Med Assoc Thai. 2005;88 Suppl 4:S36–41.
19. Arayasakulwong N, Rojborwonwitaya J, Onnom K. Prevalence of colorectal adenomatous polyps in patients undergoing colonosopic examination at rajavithi hospital. Thai J Gastroenterol. 2009;10(1):9–15.
20. Srichan P, Wasutit Y, Suwanthanma W, Euanorasetr C, Sornmayura P, Puanfoong O, et al. Characteristic of mixed hyperplastic-adenomatous polyps at ramathibodi hospital. Thai J Surg. 2009;30:17–21.
21. Leggett BA, Devereaux B, Biden K, Searle J, Young J, Jass J. Hyperplastic polyposis: association with colorectal cancer. Am J Surg Pathol. 2001;25(2):177–84.
22. Hyman NH, Anderson P, Blasyk H. Hyperplastic polyposis and the risk of colorectal cancer. Dis Colon Rectum. 2004;47(12):2101–4.
23. SEER Cancer Statistics Review, National Cancer Institute. 1975–2010. http://seer.cancer.gov/archive/csr/1975_2010/. Accessed 20 July 2012.
24. Young PE, Womeldorph CM. Colonoscopy for colorectal cancer screening. J Cancer. 2013;4(3):217–26.
25. Paskett ED, Khuri FR. Can we achieve an 80 % screening rate for colorectal cancer by 2018 in the United States? Cancer. 2015.
26. Allison JE, Tekawa IS, Ransom LJ, Adrain AL. A comparison of fecal occult-blood tests for colorectal-cancer screening. N Engl J Med. 1996;334(3):155–9.
27. Lee JK, Liles EG, Bent S, Levin TR, Corley DA. Accuracy of fecal immunochemical tests for colorectal cancer: systematic review and meta-analysis. Ann Intern Med. 2014;160(3):171.
28. Giorgi Rossi P, Vicentini M, Sacchettini C, Di Felice E, Caroli S, Ferrari F, et al. Impact of screening program on incidence of colorectal cancer: a cohort study in Italy. Am J Gastroenterol. 2015;110(9):1359–66.
29. Saengow U, Chongsuwiwatvong V, Geater A, Birch S. Preferences and acceptance of colorectal cancer screening in Thailand. Asian Pac J Cancer Prev. 2015;16(6):2269–76.
30. Levin B, Lieberman DA, McFarland B, Andrews KS, Brooks D, Bond J, et al. Screening and surveillance for the early detection of colorectal cancer and adenomatous polyps, 2008: a joint guideline from the American Cancer Society, the US Multi-Society Task Force on Colorectal Cancer, and the American College of Radiology. Gastroenterology. 2008;134(5):1570–95.
31. Cairns SR, Scholefield JH, Steele RJ, Dunlop MG, Thomas HJ, Evans GD, et al. Guidelines for colorectal cancer screening and surveillance in moderate and high risk groups (update from 2002). Gut. 2010;59(5):666–89.
32. Lieberman DA, Rex DK, Winawer SJ, Giardiello FM, Johnson DA, Levin TR. Guidelines for colonoscopy surveillance after screening and polypectomy: a consensus update by the US Multi-Society Task Force on colorectal cancer. Gastroenterology. 2012;143(3):844–57.
33. Fairley KJ, Li J, Komar M, Steigerwalt N, Erlich P. Predicting the risk of recurrent adenoma and incident colorectal cancer based on findings of the baseline colonoscopy. Clin Transl Gastroenterol. 2014;5:e64.
34. Provenzale D, Jasperson K, Ahnen DJ, Aslanian H, Bray T, Cannon JA, et al. Colorectal cancer screening, version 1.2015. J Natl Compr Canc Netw. 2015;13(8):959–68.
35. Imperiale TF, Glowinski EA, Lin-Cooper C, Larkin GN, Rogge JD, Ransohoff DF. Five-year risk of colorectal neoplasia after negative screening colonoscopy. N Engl J Med. 2008;359(12):1218–24.
36. Leung WK, Lau JY, Suen BY, Wong GL, Chow DK, Lai LH, et al. Repeat-screening colonoscopy 5 years after normal baseline-screening colonoscopy in average-risk Chinese: a prospective study. Am J Gastroenterol. 2009;104(8):2028–34.
37. Brenner H, Chang-Claude J, Seiler CM, Hoffmeister M. Long-term risk of colorectal cancer after negative colonoscopy. J Clin Oncol. 2011;29(28):3761–7.
38. Chung SJ, Kim YS, Yang SY, Song JH, Kim D, Park MJ, et al. Five-year risk for advanced colorectal neoplasia after initial colonoscopy according to the baseline risk stratification: a prospective study in 2452 asymptomatic Koreans. Gut. 2011;60(11):1537–43.
39. Shergill AK, Conners EE, McQuaid KR, Epstein S, Ryan JC, Shah JN, et al. Protective association of colonoscopy against proximal and distal colon cancer and patterns in interval cancer. Gastrointest Endosc. 2015;82(3):529–37. e1.
40. Brenner H, Chang-Claude J, Seiler CM, Hoffmeister M. Interval cancers after negative colonoscopy: population-based case–control study. Gut. 2012;61(11):1576–82.
41. Itatsu K, Yokoyama Y, Ebata T, Igami T, Sugawara G, Uehara K, et al. The value of preoperative screening colonoscopies in patients with biliary tract cancer. J Gastroenterol. 2016;51(2):138–43.
42. Robertson DJ, Kaminski MF, Bretthauer M. Effectiveness, training and quality assurance of colonoscopy screening for colorectal cancer. Gut. 2015;64(6):982–90.
43. Ross WA, Thirumurthi S, Lynch PM, Rashid A, Pande M, Shafi MA, et al. Detection rates of premalignant polyps during screening colonoscopy: time to revise quality standards? Gastrointest Endosc. 2015;81(3):567–74.
44. Hassan C, Gralnek IM. Cost-effectiveness of "full spectrum endoscopy" colonoscopy for colorectal cancer screening. Dig Liver Dis. 2015;47(5):390–4.
45. Singh H, Turner D, Xue L, Targownik LE, Bernstein CN. Risk of developing colorectal cancer following a negative colonoscopy examination: evidence for a 10-year interval between colonoscopies. J Am Med Assoc. 2006; 295(20):2366–73.
46. Bressler B, Paszat LF, Chen Z, Rothwell DM, Vinden C, Rabeneck L. Rates of new or missed colorectal cancers after colonoscopy and their risk factors: a population-based analysis. Gastroenterology. 2007;132(1):96–102.
47. Lakoff J, Paszat LF, Saskin R, Rabeneck L. Risk of developing proximal versus distal colorectal cancer after a negative colonoscopy: a population-based study. Clin Gastroenterol Hepatol. 2008;6(10):1117–21. quiz 064.
48. Singh H, Nugent Z, Demers AA, Bernstein CN. Rate and predictors of early/missed colorectal cancers after colonoscopy in Manitoba: a population-based study. Am J Gastroenterol. 2010;105(12):2588–96.
49. Colorectal Cancer Facts & Figures 2014–2016. American Cancer Society, Atlanta. 2014. http://www.cancer.org/acs/groups/content/documents/document/acspc-042280.pdf. Accessed 8 Oct 2015.

Food IgG_4 antibodies are elevated not only in children with wheat allergy but also in children with gastrointestinal diseases

Grażyna Czaja-Bulsa[1,2*], Michał Bulsa[1] and Aneta Gębala[2,3]

Abstract

Background: Food sIgG and $sIgG_4$ are highly individually versatile. We put a hypothesis that one of the responsible factors is the presence of gastrointestinal inflammatory diseases. The objectives were: 1. An analysis of wheat and rice sIgG and $sIgG_4$ in healthy children, children with IgE-mediated wheat allergy (WA), coeliac disease (CD) and Helicobacter pylori infection (HP). 2. Usability of wheat sIgG and $sIgG_4$ in the WA diagnostics.

Methods: We compared 388 each wheat and rice sIgG and $sIgG_4$ in a group of 200 children: 50 WA (diagnosis, diet treatment, tolerance), 50 CD (diagnosis and remission), 50 HP and 50 healthy. SIgE, sIgG, $sIgG_4$ were determined with the FEIA method (Pharmacia CAP System).

Results: In healthy children food sIgG were the lowest; no $sIgG_4$ were found. In the CD diagnosis group wheat and rice sIgG and rice $sIgG_4$ were the most common and their concentrations were the highest ($p < .001$, $p < .05$). Wheat $sIgG_4$ were the highest in WA children (diagnosis and tolerance) to fall during the elimination diet ($p < .05$). Wheat and rice sIgG remained the same in all allergy phases. Rice sIgG also did not differ in the class G_4.

Conclusions: 1. Serum concentrations of wheat and rice sIgG and $sIgG_4$ are elevated in children with CD, HP and WA. 2. Sub-clinical incidence of some gastrointestinal inflammatory diseases may be responsible for high individual versatility of food sIgG and $sIgG_4$ concentrations in serum. 3. Wheat sIgG and $sIgG_4$ in children do not correlate with WA clinical picture.

Keywords: Children, Coeliac disease, Helicobacter pylori infection, Specific IgG, Specific IgG_4, Wheat allergy

Background

Along with the recent development of diagnostic techniques it has become increasingly popular to use serum concentration levels of specific IgG (sIgG) and IgG_4 ($sIgG_4$) as markers of food hypersensitivity. Vast popularity of these diagnostically incorrect tests provoked EAACI to issue an official statement which was later supported by AAAAI and CSACI [1–3]. Scientific associations do not recommend using sIgG and $sIgG_4$ assays in the food hypersensitivity diagnostics. They point out that many individuals have their elevated levels which do not correspond to clinical symptoms of the disease.

The research has shown that in humans the presence of food sIgG and $sIgG_4$ is highly individual. The sIgG appear in half of the population, usually as a response to the most common foods [4]. The $sIgG_4$ is only in the case of some food allergens of cow's milk and egg protein. It has not been resolved so far why in healthy people the frequency and the titers of food sIgG and $sIgG_4$ show such substantial individual variations. Does it depend merely on the frequency of food consumption and the nature of the antigen? Or are there any additional factors?

In this paper we make a hypothesis that these factors can be gastrointestinal inflammatory diseases. One of them is coeliac disease (CD) which can be asymptomatic [5]. The adults with untreated CD showed higher sIgG activity for gliadin, casein and ovalbumin [6, 7]. There have been no research in this respect into other

* Correspondence: grazyna.bulsa@wp.pl
[1]Pediatrics and Pediatric Nursery Unit of The Pomeranian Medical University in Szczecin, ul. Żołnierska 48, 71-210 Szczecin, Poland
[2]Division of Paediatrics, Gastroenterology and Rheumatology of The „Zdroje" Hospital in Szczecin, Szczecin, Poland
Full list of author information is available at the end of the article

gastrointestinal diseases, hence the question arises if in their case the titers of food sIgG and $sIgG_4$ are different from normal. Some of these diseases, e.g. the infection with Helicobacter pylori (HP), are very common and can take a non-symptomatic or mildly symptomatic form or its symptoms may be non-specific.

The purpose of this paper is a comparative analysis of the frequency and titers of wheat and rice sIgG and $sIgG_4$ in healthy children and the children with IgE-mediated wheat allergy (WA), with CD and HP. Moreover, we evaluate the usefulness of assays of wheat sIgG and $sIgG_4$ in the WA diagnostics. Although wheat is one of the most common food allergens in children, the presence of food sIgG and $sIgG_4$ in WA has'nt been discussed in the literature.

Methods

We compared 338 assays each of wheat and rice sIgG and $sIgG_4$ antibodies determined in 200 children in four groups: 50 children with WA (50 assays each at the time of diagnosis and during the elimination diet; 38 assays during the tolerance); 50 children with CD (diagnosis – aCD, remission - rCD), 50 children with HP and 50 children from the control group (Table 1). Information was collected about the subjects' consumption of wheat and rice (a questionnaire). The course of WA in a group of 50 children described in this paper (clinical picture over the years, tolerance development age and its factors, specific IgE and IgE on diagnosis, during diet treatment and tolerance) were specified earlier in References #8.

WA was diagnosed in children with positive food challenge results (double-blind placebo-controlled food challenge, DBPCFC) with symptoms occurring within 2 h after wheat consumption and positive SPT as well as with the levels of wheat sIgE higher than 0.7 kU/L. The first challenge test was performed as the open food challenge (OFC), the second - always as the DBPCFC followed by the OFCs. DBPCFC has been described in detail before [8]. 38 children developed tolerance. The subjects were diagnosed with other food allergies, most frequently to cow's milk, egg protein and peanuts. During the observation the majority of children were diagnosed with atopic dermatitis (78 %), asthma (48 %) and allergic rhinitis (34 %). The progress of WA has been described in detail in References #8. The sIgG and $sIgG_4$ assays were made at the time of diagnosis (the median age was 13 months: 2–22 months.), after 2 years of treatment with a wheat-free diet (the median age was 36 months: 21–42 months.) and during the period of tolerance - negative OFC with wheat (the median age was 69.5 months: 37–192 months).

Table 1 Characteristics of the study patients

Study groups	No.	Sex	Age (mo.)	
		Male	Median	Range
Control group	50	26	66,4	12 - 197
Wheat allergy				
-Diagnosis -Diet treatment -Tolerance	505038	323220	13,036,069,5	2 - 2221 - 4237 - 192
Coeliac disease				
-Active -Remission	5050	1919	76,398,6	33 - 23057 - 254
Helicobacter pylori infection	50	23	97,4	58 - 212

CD children were examined at the time of diagnosis – aCD (76.3 months: 33 – 230 month.) and remission – rCD (98.6 months: 57 – 254 months). The aCD was made for children with the malabsorption syndrome (Marsh IIIC) and with antibodies to tissue transglutaminase as well as with endomysial antibodies [5]. The rCD was diagnosed when this antibodies were normal. The sIgG and $sIgG_4$ assays were not made until after 12 monthsnths of remission, usually 2 years after the diagnosis.

HP was diagnosed in children (97.4 months: 58 – 212 mo.) with typical endoscopic (gastritis, positive CLO test) and histological picture (chronic gastritis) [9].

The control group (66.4 months: 12 – 197 months.) was composed of patients in whom lesions in the upper part of the digestive tract were ruled out (endoscopic and histological examination). Children had been admitted due to abdominal pains or dwarfism (suspected malabsorption syndrome). They were diagnosed with functional gastrointestinal disorders or constitutional dwarfism.

The inclusion criteria were: diagnosed WA, CD or HP infection and the consent of participants and their guardians.

The criteria for a child to be excluded from observation were other chronic diseases and decreased concentration of total IgG. For children from the CD group, the HP group and the control group an additional elimination factor was atopy which was diagnosed on the basis of an elevated level of tIgE and/or positive sIgE test results for 8 allergens (milk, egg, peanut, cat, Cladosporium herbarum, Dermathophagoides pteronyssinus, grass, sagebrush) and/or a positive SPT (10 air-borne and 10 food allergens). 56 children were lost to follow-up: 52 children with atopy and from WA group: 1 child with ulcerative colitis and 3 children who visited the clinic only once.

All the patients remained under the care of an attending physician (an allergologist or gastroenterologist) throughout the whole observation period. Children were patients of the outpatient clinic and the gastroenterology department. The study was conducted from January 1990 to May 2012.

The titers of tIgE (accuracy 2–9,1 %, sensitivity <2 kU/L, specificity 100 %), sIgE (accuracy 5–11 %, sensitivity <0,35 kU/L, specificity 100 %), sIgG (accuracy 5–10 %, sensitivity <20ug/L, specificity 100 %) and $sIgG_4$ (accuracy 4–7 %, sensitivity <1,5ug/L, specificity >95 %) to wheat and rice were determined by means the FEIA method using the ImmunoCAP System (UniCAP, CAP 100; Pharmacia & Upjohn Diagnostics AB, Uppsala, Sweden). SPTs were performed by means of commercial solutions manufactured by Allergopharma (Germany). The wheal reactions were read after 15 min. (histamine) - 20 min (allergens). Tests were considered positive when the wheal size was ≥ 3 mm in diameter in comparison with the negative control (control solution).

The data were characterized by the median, the minimum and maximum values. The Mann–Whitney test was used to compare sIgG and $sIgG_4$ levels among the patients in the examined groups. The correlation between the selected variables was evaluated with the Spearman rank correlation. A tool used for the statistical analysis was STATA 11, License No 30110532736.

The study was conducted in compliance with the Declaration of Helsinki and following the consent by the Ethical Committee of the Pomeranian Medical University in Szczecin (BN-001/107/90). Sources of funding for the research: State Committee for Scientific Research grant No4 PO5E 086 14 and the clinic in-house research budget.

Results

The children from the control group as well as the ones with WA (diagnosis and tolerance), aCD and HP consumed wheat daily and rice – 1–2 times a week. The children in rCD and the WA children did not consume wheat, but they were given rice at least 4 times a week.

Wheat and rice $sIgG_4$ are not present in children from the control group

In the children from the control group wheat sIgG was found in 66 % of subjects and rice sIgG – in 30 % (Table 2). No wheat or rice $sIgG_4$ was found in any of those children. The median titer of wheat sIgG was 2850 μg/L (0–7250 μg/L), while that of rice sIgG was 0 (0–4780 μg/L) (Fig. 1).

Wheat and rice sIgG and IgG_4 are elevated in children over the three wheat allergy phases

At the time of WA diagnosis, diet treatment and WA tolerance, wheat sIgG and $sIgG_4$ and rice sIgG were

Table 2 Incidence of wheat and rice sIgG and $sIgG_4$ antibodies in children from the study groups

Study groups	Wheat IgG (%)	Wheat IgG_4 (%)	Rice IgG (%)	Rice IgG_4 (%)
Control group	66	0	30	0
Wheat allergy				
-Diagnosis -Diet treatment -Tolerance	969898	928894	949294	504648
Coeliac disease				
-Active -Remission	10084	8654	10084	5016
Helicobacter pylori infection	78	76	56	12

found in the majority of subjects (88–96 %), while rice $sIgG_4$ – in 46–50 % (Table 2). In each of the WA phases the titers of sIgG and $sIgG_4$ were significantly higher for wheat than for rice ($p < .005$ and $p < .001$) (Figs. 1, 2). In the class G they did not differ significantly over the three allergy phases both in the case of wheat and rice (Fig. 1). Rice $sIgG_4$ the titers were also the same over the three allergy phases (Fig. 2). Wheat $sIgG_4$ titers were the same at the time of diagnosis and in the period of tolerance, and decreased during the wheat-free diet ($p < .05$).

Wheat and rice sIgG and IgG_4 are elevated in children with coeliac disease and Helicobacter pylori infection

In the period of aCD wheat and rice sIgG were present in all the subjects, $sIgG_4$ were less common (86 % and 50 %) (Table 2). In the rCD the antibodies were rarer: wheat and rice IgG was found in 84 % of subjects and $sIgG_4$ in 54 % and 16 %. The titers of wheat and rice sIgG and $sIgG_4$ were always more elevated in aCD than in rCD ($p < .001$) (Figs. 3, 4). In aCD the serum concentrations of wheat sIgG and $sIgG_4$ were higher than the rice-specific ones ($p < .05$), to remain the same in rCD.

In the HP children wheat sIgG and $sIgG_4$ were found in 78 % and 76 % respectively, while rice sIgG and $sIgG_4$ were less common (56 % and 12 %). The median wheat sIgG and $sIgG_4$ were higher than that for rice ($p < .05$) (Figs. 3, 4).

In children in aCD wheat and rice sIgG and rice $sIgG_4$ were the most elevated ($p < .001$, $p < .001$ and $p < .05$) (Figs. 3, 4). In the $sIgG_4$ subclass the highest titers for wheat were observed in WA children in the phase of diagnosis and tolerance, while in the period of wheat-free diet they were identical as in aCD (Fig. 2).

Discussion

In our study we examined the frequency and titers of wheat and rice IgG and IgG_4. We compared a group

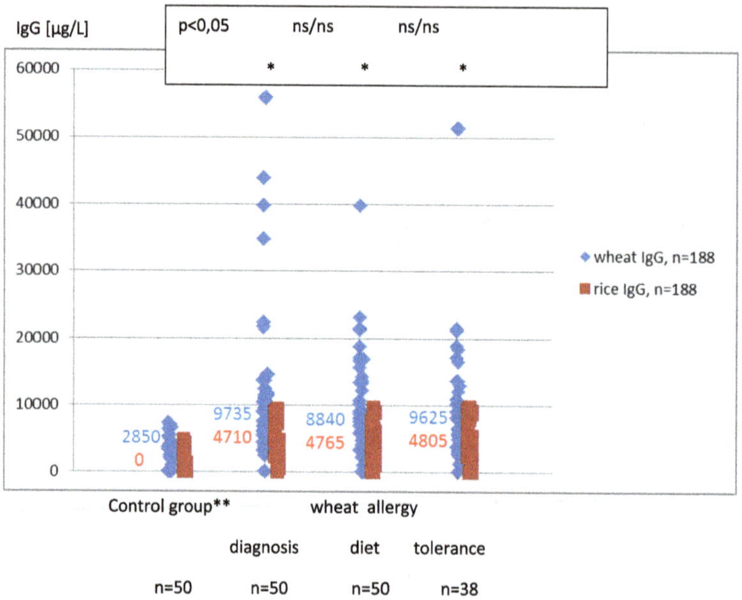

Fig. 1 Serum concentrations and medians of wheat and rice sIgG in children from the control group and in children with IgE mediated wheat allergy. *wheat/rice: $p < 0,05$; Mann–Whitney test, **control group: children not suffering from atopy and gastrointestinal diseases in the upper part of the digestive tract (endoscopic and histological examination). In the control group the median titer of wheat sIgG was 2850 µg/L (0–7250 µg/L), while that of rice sIgG was 0 (0–4780 µg/L). In each of the wheat allergy phases the titers of sIgG were significantly higher for wheat than for rice ($p < .005$). They did not differ significantly over the three allergy phases both in the case of wheat and rice

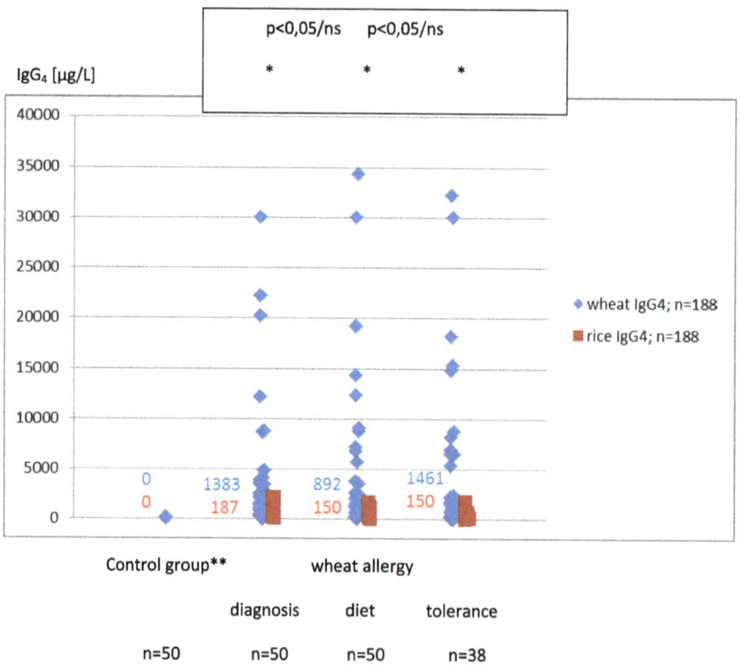

Fig. 2 Serum concentrations and medians of wheat and rice sIgG4 in children from the control group and in children with IgE mediated wheat allergy. *wheat/rice: $p < 0,05$; Mann–Whitney test, **control group: children not suffering from atopy and gastrointestinal diseases in the upper part of the digestive tract (endoscopic and histological examination). In children from the control group wheat or rice sIgG$_4$ were not found. In each of the wheat allergy phases the titers of sIgG$_4$ were significantly higher for wheat than for rice ($p < .001$). Wheat sIgG$_4$ titers were the same at the time of diagnosis and in the period of tolerance, and decreased during the wheat-free diet ($p < .05$). Rice sIgG$_4$ the titers were also the same over the three allergy phases

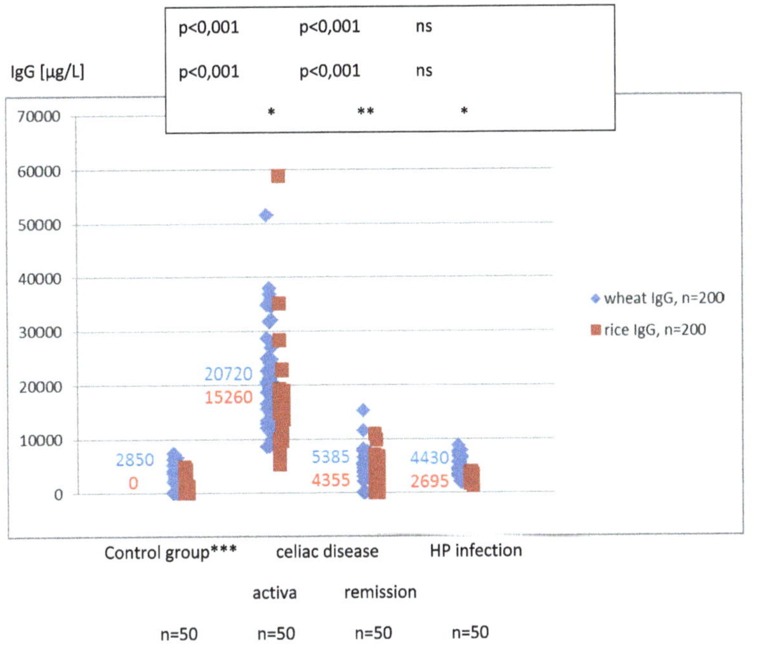

Fig. 3 Serum concentrations and medians of wheat and rice sIgG in children from the control group and in children with coeliac diseases and Helicobacter pylori infection. wheat/rice: *$p < 0{,}05$, **ns; Mann–Whitney test, ***control group: children not suffering from atopy and gastrointestinal diseases in the upper part of the digestive tract (endoscopic and histological examination). The titers of wheat and rice sIgG were always more elevated in children with active celiac disease than in remission of celiac disease ($p < .001$). In active celiac disease the serum concentrations of wheat sIgG were higher than the rice-specific ones ($p < .05$), to remain the same in remission of celiac disease. In the children with Helicobacter infection the median wheat sIgG were higher than that for rice ($p < .05$). Their serum concentrations of wheat sIgG were the same as in children with the remission of celiac disease

children not suffering from atopy and gastrointestinal diseases in the upper part of the digestive tract (control group) to a group of children with WA and with CD and HP, two common and usually mildly symptomatic gastrointestinal diseases. Atopy had been excluded from the study since it is known to predispose to developing food sIgG and sIgG$_4$ [7, 10, 11].

Wheat and rice sIgG are not present in all healthy children (control group) but are more common in children with wheat allergy, coeliac disease and Helicobacter pylori infection

The results confirm other authors' observation that food sIgG do not develop in all healthy children. In addition to that, their incidence and titers vary depending on the food [4]. In this study we detected double as much wheat sIgG as rice IgG (66 % and 30 %) (Table 2). Our research has also shown that wheat sIgG reach higher titers than the ones that are rice specific. In children with WA, CD and HP not only did we observe more common wheat and rice sIgG, but they also reached higher concentration levels in serum (Figs. 1, 3). We did not find the wheat and rice sIgG$_4$ fraction in children from the control group who suffered neither from atopy nor from any gastrointestinal disease (Table 2). The fraction was present in children from the remaining groups: WA, CD and HP (Figs. 2, 4).

The highest concentrations and frequency of wheat and rice sIgG were observed in aCD, while in rCD their frequency was lower and their titer values were smaller (Fig. 2).

Wheat and rice IgG$_4$ don't present in healthy children (control group) but are more common in children with wheat allergy, coeliac disease and Helicobacter pylori infection (Table 2)

The results confirm other authors' observation that food IgG$_4$ do not develop in healthy children as a reaction to all kinds of food. As a prevailing subclass they are synthesized for some food allergens only, mainly to chicken egg protein and cow's milk. They are most common and reach the highest titers for the chicken egg protein ovomucoid, while in the case of cow's milk casein, gliadin and gluten the system first of all synthesizes subclasses 1 and 3 of immunoglobulin G [6].

Wheat sIgG and sIgG$_4$ do not correlate with the wheat allergy clinical picture

In the majority of children with WA and CD the humoral response to wheat in the class sIgG and sIgG$_4$

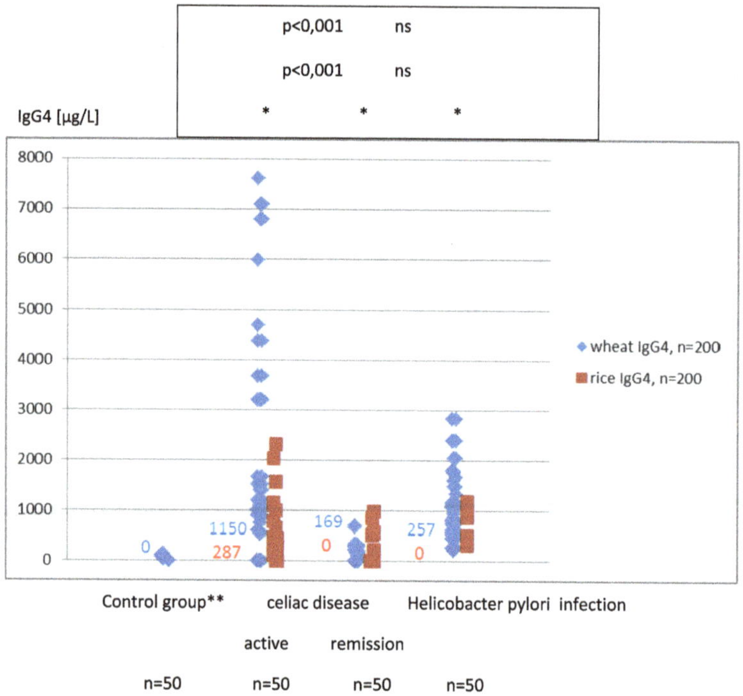

Fig. 4 Serum concentrations and medians of wheat and rice sIgG$_4$ in children from the control group and in children with coeliac diseases and Helicobacter pylori infection. *wheat/rice: $p < 0{,}05$; Mann–Whitney test, **control group: children not suffering from atopy and gastrointestinal diseases in the upper part of the digestive tract (endoscopic and histological examination). The titers of wheat and rice sIgG$_4$ were always more elevated in children with active celiac disease than in children with remission of celiac disease ($p < .001$). In children with active celiac disease the serum concentrations of wheat sIgG$_4$ were higher than the rice-specific ones ($p < .05$), to remain the same in children with remission of celiac disease. In the children with the Helicobacter pylori infection the median wheat of sIgG$_4$ were higher than that for rice ($p < .05$). Their serum concentrations of wheat sIgG$_4$ were the same as in children with the remission of celiac disease

was persistent – specific antibodies were present in serum even after wheat had been eliminated from the diet. In WA they were still found in most of the subjects, sIgG titer did not change and sIgG$_4$ decreased ($p < .05$). In rCD their concentration fell considerably. Persisting long-term highly stable sIgE and sIgG$_4$ epitope-binding patterns were also observed among patients with peanut allergy who were avoiding the allergen [12, 13].

In contrast to children with WA, the elimination of a food from healthy children's diet results in decreased sIgG titers [14]. Also in milk allergic small children being on a milk-free diet a considerable fall in sIgG serum concentration was observed, which had taken place before their tolerance to milk was developed [15, 16]. Infants with longstanding presence of milk or hen's egg sIgG suffered from a persistent allergy to those foods [17].

We also found out that the frequency and titers of wheat sIgG and sIgG$_4$ did not correlate to the WA clinical picture. They were developed by the majority of children, but not in all of them, and their frequency was the same in all the disease phases (Table 2). Rice sIgG was observed in the majority of children in all the WA phases, while rice sIgG$_4$ - in a half of the subjects. This indicates that in WA the immune response is changed. It refers not only to food allergens, but also to tolerated foods.

However, several opposite findings have been published that the sIgG and sIgG$_4$ titers do not differ between healthy individuals and patients with atopy or with food allergy to cow's milk, chicken's egg and kiwi [16, 18, 19]. Tay et al. found that serum concentration of ovalbumin sIgG and sIgG$_4$ is identical in healthy, allergic and tolerant individuals, but in the case of peanut sIgG and sIgG$_4$ the titers are higher in allergic and atopic patients than in healthy subjects [10].

It is generally assumed that in children with food allergy the elevated titers of food sIgG are the effect of their increased intestinal permeability. When an allergen is eliminated from a diet, intestinal permeability normalizes [20]. In our study group, most of the WA children (78 %) suffered from atopic dermatitis as well. As Majamaa and Isolauri have found out, in such patients the transport of food macromolecules is seven times larger than in healthy individuals and it includes 20 % of the absorbed proteins [21, 22].

The development of food tolerance, both natural and in oral immunotherapy, is associated with the increase in food sIgG$_4$ [23–26]. The maintenance of tolerance to cow's milk in atopic individuals is characterized by the fall in sIgE titers and high levels of $sIgG_4$ [27]. Children with egg allergy who have developed tolerance to baked egg also experience lowered sIgE and elevated $sIgG_4$ concentrations [28]. Low titers of $sIgG_4$ in young children with food allergy indicate its longstanding character. High serum concentrations of $sIgG_4$ is characteristic to these food allergic children who develop their tolerance early [29, 30]. Sletten et al. claimed opposite findings that in children with milk allergy high titers of $sIgG_4$ for milk allergens decrease during the tolerance period [31].

In conclusion, the incidence and titers of sIgG and $sIgG_4$ are determined not only by the type of food, but also by the type and the activity of a gastrointestinal disease. Higher incidence and titers of food sIgG and $sIgG_4$ were observed in all the diseases under study, i.e. in WA, CD and HP. This indicates that gastrointestinal diseases, due to its commonness and mildly-symptomatic nature, can be one of the factors responsible for high individual versatility of food sIgG and $sIgG_4$.

The highest concentration of wheat and rice sIgG are in children with coeliac disease

High concentrations of food sIgG in serum are characteristic of CD (Fig. 3). They are elevated also at the time of remission when they reach slightly higher titers than in HP infection. Elevated $sIgG_4$ is not a distinctive feature of CD as it is secondary to the rise in sIgG. Still, in CD these antibodies reach top values that are just slightly lower than in WA where the wheat $sIgG_4$ synthesis is preferential (Figs. 2, 4). What is more, it is worth noting that in WA and CD the enhanced synthesis of sIgG and $sIgG_4$ includes not only the symptom-inducing food (wheat), but also the food which is tolerated (rice). This confirms that in WA, CD and HP the immune response to various foods is changed.

Wheat sIgG and $sIgG_4$ are useless in the wheat allergy diagnostics

The findings of our study also point to the fact that the assays of wheat sIgG and $sIgG_4$ are useless in the WA diagnostics. In WA the concentration of these antibodies increases as a response to not only wheat, but to other foods as well, hence it is impossible to determine the actual allergen. The elevated titers persist throughout all the disease phases, so patients recently diagnosed for allergy cannot be distinguished from those who are being treated with elimination diet or have entered the period of tolerance.

The above findings are burdened by a small size of the sample (50 children in each of the groups). Therefore, it is necessary to confirm the findings in a larger group of patients.

Conclusions

1. Serum concentrations of wheat and rice sIgG and $sIgG_4$ are elevated in children with coeliac disease, Helicobacter pylori infection and IgE-mediated wheat allergy.
2. Sub-clinical incidence of some gastrointestinal inflammatory diseases may be responsible for high individual versatility of food sIgG and $sIgG_4$ concentrations in serum.
3. Wheat sIgG and $sIgG_4$ in children do not correlate with IgE-mediated wheat allergy clinical picture.

Abbreviations

AAAAI: American Academy of Allergy, Asthma & Immunology; aCD: coeliac disease diagnosis; CD: coeliac disease; CLO test: test for Helicobacter pylori diagnosis in tissue; CSACI: Canadian Society of Allergy and Clinical Immunology; DBPCFC: double-blind placebo-controlled food challenge; EAACI: The European Academy of Allergy and Clinical Immunology Organisation; FEIA method: fluoro-immuno-enzymatic method; HP: helicobacter pylori infection; M: male; mo.: months; OFC: open food challenge; rCD: remission of coeliac disease; sIgE: specific immunoglobulin E; sIgG: specific immunoglobulin G; sIgG4: specific immunoglobulin G4; SPT: skin prick test; tIgE: total immunoglobulin E; WA: IgE-mediated wheat allergy.

Competing interests

The authors declare that they have no competing interests.
All the authors have no financial relationships relevant to this article to disclose.

Authors' contributions

GC-B conceptualized and designed the study, designed the data collection instruments, coordinated and supervised data collection, drafted the initial manuscript, and approved the final manuscript as submitted. MB conceptualized the study, supervised data collection, carried out the analyses, drafted the initial manuscript and approved the final manuscript as submitted. AG conceptualized the study, data collection, carried out the analyses, drafted the initial manuscript and approved the final manuscript as submitted.

Authors' information

Grażyna Czaja-Bulsa – Prof Pomeranian Medical University in Szczecin, Poland
- paediatrician, allergologist, gastroenterologist
- head of Pediatrics and Pediatric Nursery Unit of The Pomeranian Medical University
- head of Division of Paediatrics, Gastroenterology and Rheumatology of The „Zdroje" Hospital
Michał Bulsa – MD
Aneta Gębala – MD, PhD, paediatrician, gastroenterologist

Author details

[1]Pediatrics and Pediatric Nursery Unit of The Pomeranian Medical University in Szczecin, ul. Żołnierska 48, 71-210 Szczecin, Poland. [2]Division of Paediatrics, Gastroenterology and Rheumatology of The „Zdroje" Hospital in Szczecin, Szczecin, Poland. [3]Independent Laboratory of Propaedeutics in Paediatrics of The Pomeranian Medical University in Szczecin, Szczecin, Poland.

References

1. Stapel SO, Asero R, Ballmer-Weber BK, Knol EF, Strobel S, Vieths S, et al. EAACI Task Force. Testig for IgG4 against food is not recommended as a diagnostic tool: EAACI Task Force report. Allergy. 2008;63:793–6.
2. Bock SA. AAAAI support of the EAACI Position Paper on IgG_4. J Allergy Clin Immunol. 2010;125:1410.
3. Carr S, Chan E, Lavine E, Moote W. CSACI Position statement on the testing of foo-specific IgG. Allergy, Asthma Clin Immunol. 2012;8:12. doi:10.1186/1710-1492-8-12.

4. Volpi N, Maccari F. Serum IgG Responsens to Food Antigens in the Italian Population Evaluated by Highly Sensitive and Specific ELISA Test. J Immunoass Immunochem. 2009;30:51–69.
5. Husby S, Koletzko S, Korponay-Szabó IR, Mearin ML, Phillips A, Shamir R, et al. ESPGHAN Working Group on Coeliac Disease Diagnosis; ESPGHAN Gastroenterology Committee; European Society for Pediatric Gastroenterology, Hepatology, and Nutrition. European Society for Pediatric Gastroenterology, Hepatology, and Nutrition guidelines for the diagnosis of coeliac disease. J Pediatr Gastroenterol Nutr. 2012;54:136–60.
6. Hvatum M, Scott H, Brandtzaeg P. Serum IgG subclass antibodies to a variety food antigens in patients with coeliac disease. Gut. 1992;33:632–8.
7. Kemeny DM, Urbanek R, Amlot PL, Ciclitira PJ, Richards D, Lessof MH. Sub-class of IgG in allergic disease. I. IgG sub-class antibodies in immediate and non-immediate food allergy. Clin Allergy. 1986;16:571–81.
8. Czaja-Bulsa G, Bulsa M. The natural history of IgE mediated wheat allergy in children with dominant gastrointestinal symptoms. Allergy, Asthma Clin Immunol. 2014;10:12. doi:10.1186/1710-1492-10-12.
9. Koletzko S, Jones NL, Goodman KJ, Gold B, Rowland M, Cadranel S, et al. H pylori Working Groups of ESPGHAN and NASPGHAN. Evidence-based guidelines from ESPGHAN and NASPGHAN for Helicobacter pylori infection in children. J Pediatr Gastroenterol Nutr. 2011;53:230–43.
10. Tay SS, Clark AT, Deighton J, King Y, Ewan PW. Patterns of immunoglobulin G responses to egg and peanut allergens are distinct: Ovalbumin-specific immunoglobulin responses are ubiquitous, but peanut-specific immunoglobulin responses are upregulated in peanut allergy. Clin Exp Allergy. 2007;37:1512–8.
11. Shek LP, Bardina L, Castro R, Sampson HA, Beyer K. Humoral and cellular responses to cow milk proteins in patients with milk-induced IgE-mediated and non-IgE-mediated disorders. Allergy. 2005;60:912–9.
12. Flinterman AE, Knol EF, Lencer DA, Bardina L, den Hartog Jager CF, Lin J, et al. Peanut epitopes for IgE and IgG_4 in peanut-sensitized children in relation to severity of peanut allergy. J Allergy Clin Immunol. 2008;121:737–43.
13. Vickery BP, Lin J, Kulis M, Fu Z, Steele PH, Jones SM, et al. Peanut oral immunotherapy modifies IgE and IgG_4 responses to major peanut allergens. J Allergy Clin Immunol. 2013;131:128–34.
14. Vance GH, Grimshaw KE, Briggs R, Lewis SA, Mullee MA, Thornton CA, Warner JO. Serum ovalbumin – specific immunoglobulin G responses during pregnancy reflect maternal intake of dietary egg and relate to the development of allergy in early infancy. Clin Exp Allergy. 2004;34:1855–61.
15. Orivuori L, Mustonen K, Roduit C, Braun-Fahrländer C, Dalphin JC, Genuneit C, et al. PASTURE Study Group. Immunoglobulin A and immunoglobulin G antibodies against β-lactoglobulin and gliadin at age 1 associate with immunoglobulin E sensitization at age 6. Pediatr Allergy Immunol. 2014; 25:329–37.
16. Hidvegi E, Cserhati E, Kereki E, Savilahti E, Arato A. Serum immunoglobulin E, IgA, and IgG antibodies to different cow's milk proteins in children with cow's milk allergy: association with prognosis and clinical manifestations. Pediatr Allergy Immunol. 2002;13:255–61.
17. Vance GH, Thornton CA, Bryant TN, Warner JA, Warner JO. Ovalbumin-specific immunoglobulin G and subclass responses through the first 5 years of life in relation to duration of egg sensitization and the development of asthma. Clin Exp Allergy. 2004;34:1542–9.
18. Bublin M, Dennstedt S, Buchegger M, Antonietta Ciardiello M, Bernardi ML, Tuppo L. The performance of a component-based allergen microarray for the diagnosis of kiwifruit allergy. Clin Exp Allergy. 2011;41:129–36.
19. Ahrens B, de Oliveira LC L, Schulz G, Borres MP, Niggemann B, Wahn U, Beyer K. The role of hen's egg-specific IgE, IgG and IgG_4 in the diagnostic procedure of hen's egg allergy. Allergy. 2010;65:1554–7.
20. Yu LC. Intestinal Epithelial Barrier Dysfunction in Food Hypersensitivity. J Allergy (Cairo). 2012;2012:96081. doi:10.1155/2012/596081.
21. Majamaa H, Isolauri E. Evaluation of the gut mucosal barrier. Evidence for increased antigen transfer in children with atopic eczema. J Allergy Clin Immunol. 1996;97:985–90.
22. Caffarelli C, Cavagni G, Menzies IS, Bertolini P, Atherton DJ. Elimination diet and intestinal permeability in atopic eczema: a preliminary study. Clin Exp Allergy. 1993;23:28–31.
23. Akdis M, Akdis CA. Mechanisms of allergen-specific immunotherapy: multiple suppressor factors at work in immune tolerance to allergens. J Allergy Clin Immunol. 2014;133:621–31.
24. Lee JH, Kim WS, Kim H, Hahn YS. Increased cow's milk protein-specific IgG_4 levels after oral desensitization in 7- to 12-month-old infants. Ann Allergy Asthma Immunol. 2013;111:523–8.
25. Savilahti EM, Savilahti E. Development of natural tolerance and induced desensitization in cow's milk allergy. Pediatr Allergy Immunol. 2013;24:114–21.
26. Hofmaier S, Comberiati P, Matricardi PM. Immunoglobulin G in IgE-mediated allergy and allergen-specific immunotherapy. Eur Ann Allergy Clin Immunol. 2014;46:6–11.
27. Merras-Salmio L, Kolho KL, Pelkonen AS, Kuitunen M, Mäkelä MJ, Savilahti E. Markers of gut mucosal inflammation and cow's milk specific immunoglobulins in non-IgE cow's milk allergy. Clin Transl Allergy. 2014;4:8. doi:10.1186/2045-7022-4-8.
28. Leonard SA, Sampson HA, Sicherer SH, Noone S, Moshier EL, Godbold J, Nowak-Węgrzyn A. Dietary baked egg accelerates resolution of egg allergy in children. J Allergy Clin Immunol. 2012;130:473–80.
29. Tomicić S, Norrman G, Fälth-Magnusson K, Jenmalm MC, Devenney I, Böttcher MF. High levels of IgG_4 antibodies to foods during infancy are associated with tolerance to corresponding foods later in life. Pediatric Allergy Clin Immunol. 2009;20:35–41.
30. Jenmalm MC, Björkstén B. Cord blood levels of immunoglobulin G subclass antibodies to food and inhalant allergens in relation to maternal atopy and the development of atopic disease during the first 8 years of life. Clin Exp Allergy. 2000;30:34–40.
31. Sletten GB, Halvorsen R, Egaas E, Halstensen TS. Changes in humoral responses to beta-lactoglobulin in tolerant patients suggest a particular role for IgG_4 in delayed, non –IgE-medated cow's milk allergy. Pediatr Allergy Immunol. 2006; 17:435–43.

15

The cut-off value of tumor size and appropriate timing of follow-up for management of minimal EUS-suspected gastric gastrointestinal stromal tumors

Zhidong Gao[1†], Chao Wang[1†], Qian Xue[2], Jingtong Wang[2], Zhanlong Shen[1], Kewei Jiang[1], Kai Shen[1], Bin Liang[1], Xiaodong Yang[1], Qiwei Xie[1], Shan Wang[1] and Yingjiang Ye[1*]

Abstract

Backgroud: The detectable rate of minimal gastric GISTs has continuously increased. While the surveillance and management of GIST <2 cm have been deemed controversial or lack evidence-based approaches. The aim of the current study is to propose a cut-off value of tumor size for treatment policy and the appropriate timing for endoscopic ultrasonography (EUS) follow-up in the minimal EUS-suspected gastric GIST patients.

Methods: A single-institution retrospective study was performed. 69 patients with EUS-suspected gastric GISTs were studied from November 2008 to March 2015. 69 patients with minimal gastric GISTs ≤2 cm diagnosed by EUS were followed for a mean period of 29 months (range, 12 to 70). An at least 20% increase of the maximal diameter of the tumors was set as a significant change.

Results: During follow-up, Of the 69 minimal EUS-suspected GISTs, 16 (23.2%) showed significant changes in size. 11 out of 69 GISTs (15.9%), 6 out of 43 GISTs (14.0%), 7 out of 30 GISTs (23.3%) showed significant changes in size, at 1 year, 2 years, and more than 3 years respectively. The receiver operating characteristic curve analysis showed that the tumor size cut-off was 9.5 mm. Only 4.7 and 3.7% of gastric EUS-suspected GISTs of <9.5 mm in size showed significant changes at 1 year and 2 years, while 9.5% at more than 3 years. 34.6, 31.3 and 55.6% of gastric EUS-suspected GISTs of ≥ 9.5 mm in size showed significant changes at 1 year, 2 years and more than 3 years.

Conclusions: Minimal EUS-suspected GISTs, larger than 9.5 mm may be associated with significant progression. The patients with a ≥ 9.5 mm GIST should have a EUS 6–12months, while <9.5 mm GIST may have a EUS extended to every 2–3 years.

Keywords: Endoscopic ultrasound (EUS), Stomach, Gastrointestinal stromal tumor (GIST)

Background

Gastrointestinal stromal tumors (GISTs) are the most common primary mesenchymal tumors in the gastrointestinal tract and span a clinical spectrum from benign to malignant. GISTs occur anywhere along the gastrointestinal tract, but they are most common in the stomach (50–60%) [1]. Owing to the popularization of EUS, the detectable rate of gastric GISTs has continuously increased, specifically for minimal gastric GISTs (diameter less than 2 cm). Surgery is the treatment for primary, local gastric GISTs larger than 2 cm, while conservative follow-up is suggested for lesions less than 2 cm. In fact, the National Comprehensive Cancer Network (NCCN) and the European Society of Medical Oncology (ESMO) guidelines for the surveillance and management of GIST <2 cm have been deemed controversial or lack evidence-based approaches. Endoscopic ultrasonography (EUS) has been utilized to diagnose gastric GISTs with high accuracy, sensibility, and specificity (87, 95, 72%, respectively) [2, 3]. The typical

* Correspondence: yeyingjiang@pkuph.edu.cn
Zhidong Gao and Chao Wang own equal first authorship
[†]Equal contributors
[1]Department of Gastrointestinal Surgery, Peking University People's Hospital, Beijing 100044, People's Republic of China
Full list of author information is available at the end of the article

EUS finding of a gastric GIST is a hypoechoic lesion arising from the fourth layer of the gastric wall. The goal of this study was to evaluate the malignant potential of minimal gastric GISTs to determine the best cut-off value for tumor size and appropriate timing for EUS follow-up, in order to provide clinical evidence for malignant potential in the management of minimal gastric GISTs.

Methods

Study design and population

This retrospective study was approved by our institutional ethics committee and meets the guidelines of our responsible governmental agency. It reviewed data from patients with minimal gastric GISTs diagnosed by using EUS at Peking University People's Hospital between November 2008 and March 2015.

Tumor size was determined with the maximum diameter obtained by using EUS. The criterion of minimal gastric GISTs diagnosed by using EUS is a hypoechoic lesion arising from the fourth layer of the gastric wall. Every patient had signed a consent form before EUS inspection. All EUS image files were reviewed by a single experienced EUS endoscopist (JW).

Inclusion criteria for this study were: (1) tumor size ≤ 2 cm; (2) patients were followed by using EUS at least twice over a period of 12 months; (3) EUS follow-up period of more than 1 year. The exclusion criteria were: (1) cancer patients; (2) diagnosis changed during follow-up. A flow diagram of the enrolled patients is shown in Fig. 1.

Definitions and study procedure

All enrolled patients were divided into two subgroups based on the criteria: patients with at least a 20% increase in the initial maximal diameter of the tumors during follow-up were included in the progressive disease group; the other patients were assigned to the stable disease group. We compared patient demographics, initial tumor size, tumor location, ultrasonographic features, and growth rate between the two groups at 1 year, 2 years and more than 3 years respectively. In the receiver operating characteristic (ROC) curve analysis, the progressive disease cases were defined as the true positives, and the stable disease cases were defined as the true negatives when determining the cut-off value of the optimal initial size for medical intervention.

Statistical analysis

All statistical analyses were performed with SPSS statistical software (version 20.0 for Windows; SPSS, Chicago, IL, USA). Numerical variables were expressed as the mean ± SD unless otherwise stated. Discrete variables were analyzed using the Chi-square test or Fisher's exact test. The optimal cut-off values for tumor size as a prognostic variable were chosen from a ROC curve with the criterion variable "tumor size" and "progressive disease" as condition variables. We considered P values <0.05 to be statistically significant for a two-sided test.

Results

Patient characteristics

A total of 74 patients were diagnosed with minimal gastric GISTs by using EUS meeting the included criteria; 5 patients were excluded for diagnoses changed during the follow-up. Finally, 69 patients met the criteria for enrolment (see Table 1). The average age was 59 (range, 27–84) years. There were 17 (21.8%) men and 52

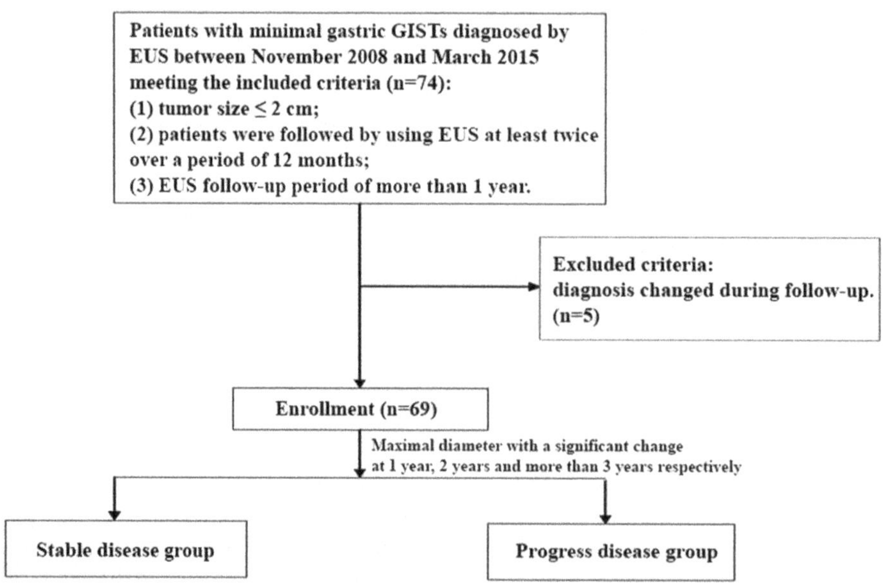

Fig. 1 Flow diagram of enrollment patients

Table 1 Clinical characteristics of patients

Characteristics	Cases ($n = 69$)
Age (years)	58 (59, 27–84)[a]
Gender, n (%)	
Male	17 (21.8%)
Female	52 (66.7%)
Tumor location	
Cardia	7 (9.0%)
Fundus	43 (55.1%)
Body	18 (23.1%)
Antrum	1 (1.3%)
Initial diameter (mm)	8 (8.8, 3–20)[a]
Initial EUS features, n (%)	
Low-risk features	65 (94.2%)
High-risk features	4 (5.8%)
Follow-up duration (mo)	23 (28, 12–70)[a]
≥ 12 months, n (%)	69 (100%)
≥ 24 months, n (%)	43 (62.3%)
≥ 36 months, n (%)	30 (43.5%)

[a]Median (mean, range)

(66.7%) women. Tumors were located at the cardia in 7 patients (9.0%), at the fundus in 43 (55.1%) patients, at the body in 18 (23.1%) patients, and at the pylori in 1 (1.3%) patient. The mean initial tumor size was 8.8 (range, 3–20) mm. Only 4 cases' (5.8%) initial EUS features have the high risk feature, such as heterogeneous echo texture, irregular extraluminal border, echogenic foci, and anechoic space. 5 cases (7.2%) were identified by successfully performing pathological examination of EUS-FNA. The mean EUS follow-up period was 28 months (range 12–70 months). Of the 69 EUS-suspected GISTs, 16 (23.2%) showed significant changes in size (see Table 2). The tumors were mainly located in the gastric body (9 cases, 56.3%) and fundus (7 cases, 43.7%). Among the cases, 11 patients underwent resection, and all their tumors proved to be GISTs. While the other 5 patients refused surgery and were followed up. Out of 11 patients, 4 patients had lesions with higher malignant potential, reflected by mitotic rates of more than 5 per 50 high-power fields (HPFs). Molecular analysis revealed KIT exon 11 mutation in 10 cases, and wild type in 1 cases. Moreover, of the 69 EUS-suspected GISTs, significant change in echo patterns was observed in 8 patients (11.6%). 6 cases (75%) showed significant changes in size.

Analysis of the two groups

Out of all, 69, 43 and 30 patients had been followed up more than 1 year, 2 years and 3 years respectively. When all the patients were followed up to 1 years, according to the criteria, there were 58 (84.1%) patients in the stable disease group and 9 (15.9%) patients in the progressive disease group (see Table 3). Both groups were similar in gender, tumor location, and initial EUS features. The mean age (67.9 vs. 57.6, $p = 0.012$), initial diameter (12.6 mm vs. 8.1 mm, $p = 0.000$), and follow-up EUS high risk features (45.5% vs. 8.6%, $p = 0.001$) significantly predicted progressive disease compared with the stable

Table 2 Characteristics of the GISTs that changed in size

No.	Sex	Age	Site	Initial Size	F/u Size	Initial EUS	F/u EUS	Treatment	Final Diagnosis	Mitotic count	Mutation type
1	M	72	Fundus	6	17	Low risk	Low risk	OP	GIST	7/50HPF	KIT exon 11
2	F	75	Body	16	30	Low risk	High risk	OP	GIST	6/50HPF	KIT exon 11
3	M	71	Body	20	40	Low risk	High risk	OP	GIST	10/50HPF	KIT exon 11
4	F	51	Fundus	8	15	Low risk	High risk	OP	GIST	0/50HPF	KIT exon 11
5	F	83	Fundus	7	15	Low risk	Low risk	Surveillance	Not available	Not available	Not available
6	F	78	Body	11	22	Low risk	High risk	OP	GIST	2/50HPF	KIT exon 11
7	M	67	Body	12	17	Low risk	Low risk	OP	GIST	3/50HPF	KIT exon 11
8	M	57	Fundus	10	12	Low risk	Low risk	Surveillance	Not available	Not available	Not available
9	F	51	Fundus	10	13	Low risk	Low risk	Surveillance	Not available	Not available	Not available
10	F	53	Body	11	15	Low risk	Low risk	Surveillance	Not available	Not available	Not available
11	M	84	Body	18	35	Low risk	High risk	OP	GIST	3/50HPF	KIT exon 11
12	F	57	Body	11	14	Low risk	Low risk	Surveillance	Not available	Not available	Not available
13	M	67	Body	15	30	Low risk	Low risk	OP	GIST	6/50HPF	KIT exon 11
14	M	65	Fundus	10	24	Low risk	High risk	OP	GIST	3/50HPF	KIT exon 11
15	F	59	Body	12	15	Low risk	Low risk	OP	GIST	0/50HPF	KIT exon 11
16	F	51	Fundus	8	13	High risk	High risk	OP	GIST	2/50HPF	Wild-type

Abbreviations: *F/u* indicates follow-up, *HR* high risk, *IR* intermediate risk, *LR* low risk, *OP* operation

Table 3 Characteristics of the minimal EUS-suspected GISTs followed up to 1 year

Characterisitics	Stable disease group (*n* = 58)	Progress disease group (*n* = 11)	*P*
Age	57.6 ± 12.3	67.9 ± 11.2	0.012
Gender, *n* (%)			0.053
Male	9 (17.6%)	8 (44.4%)	
Female	42 (82.4%)	10 (55.6%)	
Tumor location, *n* (%)			
Cardia	7 (12.1%)	0	0.587
Fundus	39 (67.2%)	4 (36.4%)	0.087
Body	11 (19.0%)	7 (63.6%)	0.005
Antrum	1 (1.7%)	0	1.000
Initial diameter (mm)	8.07 ± 3.11	12.55 ± 4.16	0.000
Initial EUS, *n* (%)			0.509
Low risk	55 (94.8%)	10 (90.9%)	
High risk	3 (5.2%)	1 (9.1%)	
F/u EUS, *n* (%)			0.001
Low risk	53 (91.4%)	6 (54.5%)	
High risk	5 (8.6%)	5 (45.5%)	
Growth rate per year (%)	−1.2 ± 9.7	50.7 ± 33.6	0.000

Table 4 Characteristics of the minimal EUS-suspected GISTs followed up to 2 years

Characterisitics	Stable disease group (*n* = 37)	Progress disease group (*n* = 6)	*P*
Age	58.0 ± 11.8	70.7 ± 11.6	0.019
Gender, *n* (%)			0.164
Male	8 (17.6%)	3 (44.4%)	
Female	29 (82.4%)	3 (55.6%)	
Tumor location, *n* (%)			
Cardia	6 (16.2%)	0	0.571
Fundus	25 (67.6%)	2 (33.3%)	0.174
Body	6 (16.2%)	4 (66.7%)	0.020
Antrum	0	0	1.000
Initial diameter (mm)	8.14 ± 3.10	13.83 ± 4.83	0.033
Initial EUS, *n* (%)			1.000
Low risk	35 (94.6%)	6 (100%)	
High risk	2 (5.4%)	0	
F/u EUS, *n* (%)			0.007
Low risk	33 (89.2%)	2 (33.3%)	
High risk	4 (10.8%)	4 (66.7%)	
Growth rate per year (%)	−0.8 ± 5.4	37.3 ± 22.1	0.008

disease group. The mean value for the average tumor growth rate per annum in the progressive disease group was 50.7%, which was significantly higher than the −1.2% rate in the stable disease group ($p = 0.000$). The data for the two groups are presented in Table 1. When the patients were followed up to 2 years and more than 3 years (see Tables 4 and 5), we could find similar results that the age, initial diameter and follow-up EUS high risk features were significantly predicted progressive disease.

ROC curve analysis

We generated ROC curves to find best the sensitivity and specificity to detect the optimal cut-off value for predicting potential tumor growth. For 1 year follow-up, The area under the curve (AUC) was 0.818, indicating that the best cut-off value of tumor size was 9.5 mm. The sensitivity, specificity, positive predictive value, negative predictive value, and consistency rates were 81.8, 70.7, 34.6, 95.3, 72.5%, respectively (see Fig. 2a). For 2 years and more than 3 years follow-up, the best cut-off value of tumor size was also 9.5 mm. The AUC, sensitivity, specificity, positive predictive value, negative predictive value, and consistency rates were 0.858, 83.3, 70.3, 31.3, 96.3, 69.8 and 0.786, 82.6, 73.3, 55.6, 90.5, 80.0%, respectively.(see Fig. 2b, c).

Table 5 Characteristics of the minimal EUS-suspected GISTs followed up to more than 3 years

Characterisitics	Stable disease group (*n* = 23)	Progress disease group (*n* = 7)	*P*
Age	59.4 ± 11.8	62.9 ± 10.7	0.487
Gender, *n* (%)			0.345
Male	5 (21.7%)	3 (42.9%)	
Female	18 (78.3%)	4 (57.1%)	
Tumor location, *n* (%)			
Cardia	4 (17.4%)	0	0.548
Fundus	16 (69.6%)	4 (57.1%)	0.657
Body	3 (13.0%)	3 (42.9%)	0.120
Antrum	0	0	1.000
Initial diameter (mm)	7.70 ± 2.79	11.86 ± 4.78	0.007
Initial EUS, *n* (%)			1.000
Low risk	22 (95.7%)	7 (100%)	
High risk	1 (4.3%)	0	
F/u EUS, *n* (%)			0.031
Low risk	22 (95.7%)	4 (57.1%)	
High risk	1 (4.3%)	3 (42.9%)	
Growth rate per year (%)	−0.5 ± 3.1	19.1 ± 9.1	0.001

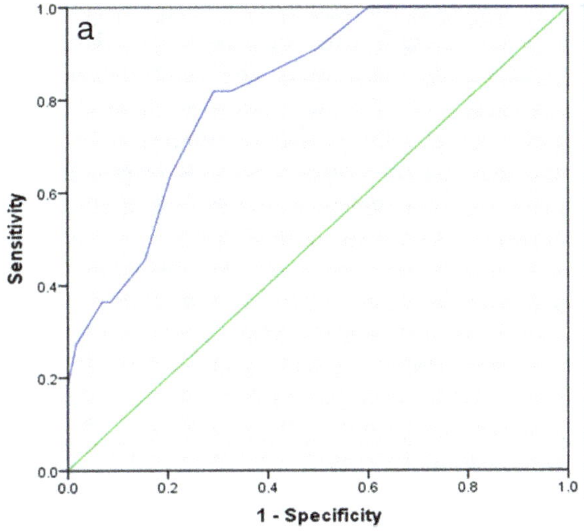

Test Result Variable(s): Initial size

Positive if ≥cm	Sensitivity	1 - Specificity
-.7000	1.000	1.000
.3500	1.000	.983
.4500	1.000	.931
.5500	1.000	.810
.6500	1.000	.603
.7500	.909	.500
.8500	.818	.328
.9500	.818	.293
1.0500	.636	.207
1.1500	.455	.155
1.3000	.364	.086
1.4500	.364	.069
1.5500	.273	.017
1.7000	.182	.000
1.9000	.091	.000
3.0000	.000	.000

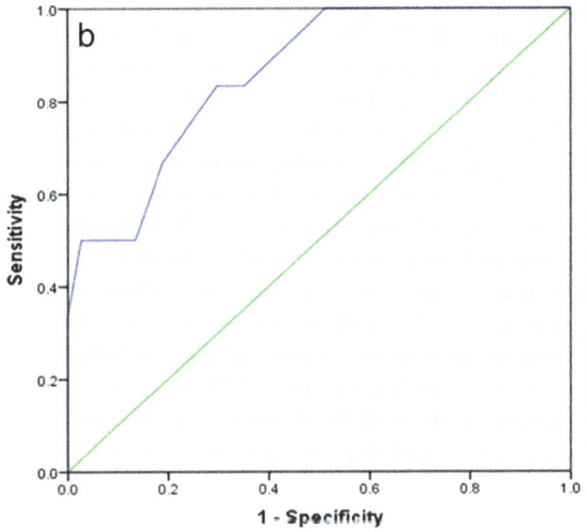

Test Result Variable(s): Initial size

Positive if ≥cm	Sensitivity	1 - Specificity
-.7000	1.000	1.000
.3500	1.000	.973
.4500	1.000	.919
.5500	1.000	.838
.6500	1.000	.649
.7500	1.000	.514
.8500	.833	.351
.9500	.833	.297
1.0500	.667	.189
1.1500	.500	.135
1.3500	.500	.081
1.5500	.500	.027
1.7000	.333	.000
1.9000	.167	.000
3.0000	.000	.000

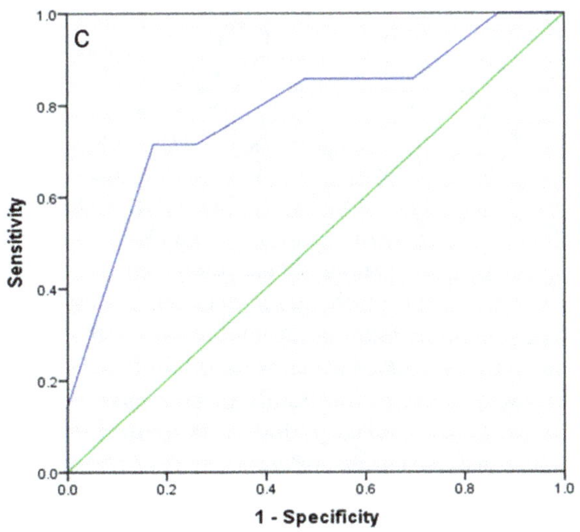

Test Result Variable(s): Initial size

Positive if ≥cm	Sensitivity	1 - Specificity
-.7000	1.000	1.000
.3500	1.000	.957
.5000	1.000	.870
.6500	.857	.696
.7500	.857	.478
.8500	.714	.261
.9500	.714	.174
1.0500	.571	.130
1.1500	.429	.087
1.4000	.286	.043
1.8000	.143	.000
3.0000	.000	.000

Fig. 2 Receiver operating characteristic curve. All the receiver operating characteristic curve analyses showed that the tumor size cut-off was 9.5 mm, at 1 year (**a**), 2 years (**b**), and more than 3 years (**c**)

Surveillance timing

Eleven out of 69 GISTs (15.9%), 6 out of 43 GISTs (14.0%), 7 out of 30 GISTs (23.3%) showed significant changes in size, at 1 year, 2 years, and more than 3 years respectively. With the 9.5 mm cut-off, there was a significant difference between the two subgroups. Only 4.7% (2/43) and 3.7% (1/27) of gastric EUS-suspected GISTs of <9.5 mm in size showed significant changes at 1 year and 2 years, while 9.5% (2/21) at more than 3 years. 34.6% (9/26), 31.3% (5/16) and 55.6% (5/9) of gastric EUS-suspected GISTs of ≥ 9.5 mm in size showed significant changes at 1 year, 2 years and more than 3 years.

Discussion

For a long time, the actual incidence of gastrointestinal stromal tumor (GIST) was underestimated. With the improvements in understanding of this disease and examination methods, the detection rate was increasing. Most recent studies have suggested the incidence of gastric GISTs to be between 10 and 20 cases per million, which is 2–3 times more than the data of 20 years ago [4].This trend was also showed in minimal GIST especially for gastric GIST. Based on the data 20 years ago from Armed Forces Institute of Pathology (AFIP) of US, it has been reported that of the 1687 tumors with size measurements, 127 (7.5%) were 2 cm or smaller [5]. While the data 10 years later from the REGISTER study of Italy showed the rate was up to 18.3%(170/929) [6]. Moreover, A study from Germany showed among the consecutive 98 autopsy cases, miro-GIST (less than 1 cm) were found in 22 patients (22.5%) [7]. A latest population-Based study [8] for milli-GIST (<2 cm) in the National Cancer Institute's SEER database showed that the annual incidence rate of gastric milli-GISTs was 2.6 per 10 million.

Because the natural course of minimal gastric GIST remains largely unknown, the current management policy for gastric GISTs <2 cm is usually conservative, unless tumors grow more than 2 cm or symptoms occur such as bleeding, acute abdomen, etc. [9]. Despite the patients with minimal gastric GIST are recommend for close surveillance, there are some difficulties in clinical works. Firstly, some patients would feel anxiety, depression and stress for survival with tumor. Secondly, some patients could not be followed up regularly for their poor compliance. These cause some patients to choose the two extremes: excision by over-treatment or few surveillance with delayed treatment. Therefore, identification of malignant potential for minimal gastric GIST is very important. Although most milli-GISTs are presumed to have less malignant potential especially which with low mitotic rate. If with high mitotic rate, the metastases rate or tumor-related mortality would be significantly worse. EUS-guided fine needle aspiration (EUS-FNA) has been suggested for the determination of malignant potential in gastric GISTs with high accuracy (91.7–97%) [10, 11]. While in these study, the GISTs evaluated were larger ones >2 cm mostly (80–91%). It would have been difficult to use EUS-FNA for minimal gastric GISTs. Due to the small size, success ratio of puncture maybe low. Moreover there would be insufficient tissues obtained by biopsy to assess mitotic or genetic mutation. Mekky et al. reported adequate samples were obtained in 67.6% of gastric submucosal tumors with size <20 mm [12]. Even the adequate specimens were considered, the reported diagnostic yields for tumors less than 20 mm was 71% [11]. Thus, the diagnosis of miminal GISTs may be mostly diagnosed based on EUS appearance. Ultrasonographic features are another important predictive factor of malignancy. High-risk EUS features include irregular border, cystic spaces, ulceration, echogenic foci, and heterogeneity [13]. However, ultrasonographic features might not have been in smaller lesions as sensitive as for larger ones. In our study, there was no difference between stable disease group and progressive disease group regarding initial malignant ultrasonographic features. While we found 8 cases showed ultrasonographic feature changes. They all occurred after the diameter increased more than 1 cm. Among them 6 (75.0%) showed significant changes in size.

With knowledge of GIST biological behaviours, we gradually realized that the malignancy potential of some minimal gastric GISTs was high, and these need to have medical intervention. Even some experts suggested surgical resection of all minimal gastric GISTs once diagnosed [14]. The growth of the tumor is an important index of malignant potential. There are some studies proposing a cut-off value of initial tumor size, in order to predicting GISTs with significant-sized change. A retrospective analysis by Lachter et al. [15] reported that out of 70 GISTs monitored by EUS, enlargement in size was detected significantly more in GISTs over 17 mm diameter ($P < 0.018$) at averaged follow-up examination 23.2 mm. In another retrospective study by Gill et al. [16], the majority (86.3%) of <3 cm upper gastrointestinal subepithelial tumors (SETs) did not increase in size and/or change in echogenic features during a median of 23 months. In another study by Kim et al. [17], in 989 gastric subepithelial tumors, SETs of 10 to 30 mm in size grew significantly more rapidly than SETs <10 mm over a median period of 24 months when followed up endoscopically or by EUS. Fang et al. [18] followed 50 patients with EUS-suspected gastric GISTs of sizes less than 3 cm over a period of more than 24 months (range 24–101 months), found that the best cutoff size associated with tumor progression was 1.4 cm having an 85.7% sensitivity, 86.1% specificity, and 86.0% accuracy.

While all these studies included the GISTs or SETs >2 cm. These tumors should be resected without controversy. The current surveillance and management policy for gastric minimal GISTs is still controversial. So our study was specific for GISTs ≤2 cm of the stomach. Moreover most studies above followed the patients over much different time (range 3 months to more than 5 years). This may increase select bias, because the possibility of significant increase in tumor size is different over different time. In this study, all the patients were followed up over the same time (1 year, 2 years or more than 3 years). It was also helpful to propose appropriate timing for endoscopic ultrasonography (EUS) follow-up. We found Minimal EUS-suspected GISTs larger than 9.5 mm may be associated with significant progression.

Experts recommend EUS surveillance of gastric milli-GISTs, although there are few data to support surveillance at all. In 2015, NCCN recommended for the patients with gastric minimal GISTs, EUS surveillance at 6–12 moths intervals may be considered [19]. The study cited by NCCN analyzed the data of 37 patients with GISTs, while only 13.5% (5/37) of all GISTs showed <2 cm in size. Due to insufficient evidences, the latest edition of the guide by NCCN [9] modified its recommendation description to "consider periodic endoscopic surveillance". This new study cited by NCCN was designed as an online survey from all 413 members of the American Society for Gastrointestinal Endoscopy (ASGE) EUS Special Interest Group. It showed for lesions not resected, 70% survey annually, 19% less than annually, 10% more than annually, and 1% do not survey [20]. While this studies also included a lot of GISTs >2 cm. Based on experts' preferences, ASGE recommended annual surveillance is commonly practiced [21]. In our study, 15.9, 14.0 and 23.3% GISTs showed significant changes in size, at 1 year, 2 years, and more than 3 years respectively. So we also recommend endoscopic surveillance annually for all gastric milli-GISTs. In addition, with the 9.5 mm cut-off, few of GISTs <9.5 mm (<5%) showed significant size changes in the first 2 years. On the contrary, numerous GISTs ≥ 9.5 mm showed significant changes even in the first year. So ≥ 9.5 mm GIST maybe need a EUS less than annually. For the patients with <9.5 mm GIST, EUS surveillance at 2–3 years interval may be considered. This strategy may increase the quality of life and enhance the compliance for patients with smaller milli-GIST.

Some limitations existed in our study. First, few cases (5/69) enrolled in the study were identified by successfully performing pathological examination of EUS-FNA, due to technical difficulty or insufficient material to make diagnosis. Although the accuracy of GIST diagnosed by using EUS is as high as 87%, [2, 3] this would influence the results of our study because of some them might have had benign submucosal tumors, such as leiomyoma. While in our data, out of 16 tumors with significant increase in tumor size located in the fourth layer on EUS, 11 underwent surgical resection and final pathological diagnosis was all GISTs. Second, this is a single-institution retrospective study. Further confirmation of these findings is needed in a larger, multicentre cohort.

Conclusions

In conclusion, an initial tumor size larger than 9.5 mm was associated with significant tumor progression and was valuable for predicting the malignant potential GIST. According to our results, the patients with a <9.5 mm GIST may have a EUS extended to every 2–3 years, while ≥ 9.5 mm GIST should have a EUS 6–12 months.

Abbreviations

AFIP: Armed Forces Institute of Pathology; ASGE: American Society for Gastrointestinal Endoscopy; AUC: Area under the curve; ESMO: European Society of Medical Oncology; EUS: Endoscopic ultrasonography; FNA: Fine needle aspiration; GIST: Gastrointestinal stromal tumor; HADS: Hospital anxiety depression scale; NCCN: National Comprehensive Cancer Network; ROC: Receiver operating characteristic; SET: Subepithelial tumor

Acknowledgements

The authors extend thanks to the staff on the Endoscopic unit at Peking University People's Hospital, Beijing, China.

Funding

From the Specialized Research Fund for the Doctoral Program of Higher Education (20130001120064) and the Capital Health Development Research Project (TG-2015-002) of China.

Authors' contributions

There are the authors' contributions as follows: study concepts (YY & SW); study design (ZG, YY & JW); data acquisition (CW, QX, KS & BL); quality control of data and algorithms (ZG, KJ & YY); data analysis and interpretation (ZG & YY); statistical analysis (ZG & CW); manuscript preparation (ZG, CW & ZS); manuscript editing (ZG, KS & XY); manuscript review (YY & QX).
All authors have read and approved the final version of this manuscript.

Competing interests

The authors declare that they have no competing interests.

Author details

[1]Department of Gastrointestinal Surgery, Peking University People's Hospital, Beijing 100044, People's Republic of China. [2]Department of Gastroenterology and Endoscopy, Peking University People's Hospital, Beijing 100044, People's Republic of China.

References

1. Joensuu H, Vehtari A, Riihimäki J, et al. Risk of recurrence of gastrointestinal stromal tumor after surgery: an analysis of pooled population-based cohorts. Lancet oncol. 2012;13:265–74.
2. Brand B, Oesterhelweg L, Binmoeller KF, et al. Impact of endoscopic ultrasound for evaluation of submucosal lesions in gastrointestinal tract. Dig liver dis. 2002;34:290–7.

3. Rösch T, Kapfer B, Will U, et al. Accuracy of endoscopic ultrasonography in upper gastrointestinal submucosal lesions: a prospective multicenter study. Scand j gastroenterol. 2002;37:856–62.
4. Søreide K, Sandvik OM, Søreide JA, et al. Global epidemiology of gastrointestinal stromal tumours (GIST): a systematic review of population-based cohort studies. Cancer epidemiol. 2016;40:39–46.
5. Miettinen M, Sobin LH, Lasota J. Gastrointestinal stromal tumors of the stomach: a clinicopathologic, immunohistochemical, and molecular genetic study of 1765 cases with long-term follow-up. Am j surg pathol. 2005;29:52–68.
6. Rossi S, Gasparotto D, Toffolatti L, et al. Molecular and clinicopathologic characterization of gastrointestinal stromal tumors (GISTs) of small size. Am j surg pathol. 2010;34:1480–91.
7. Agaimy A, Wünsch PH, Hofstaedter F, et al. Minute gastric sclerosing stromal tumors (GIST tumorlets) are common in adults and frequently show c-KIT mutations. Am j surg pathol. 2007;31:113–20.
8. Coe TM, Fero KE, Fanta PT, et al. Population-based epidemiology and mortality of small malignant gastrointestinal stromal tumors in the USA. J gastrointest surg. 2016;20:1132–40.
9. von Mehren M, Randall RL, Benjamin RS, et al. Soft tissue sarcoma, version 2. 2016, NCCN clinical practice guidelines in oncology. J natl compr canc netw. 2016;14:758–86.
10. Ando N, Goto H, Niwa Y, et al. The diagnosis of GI stromal tumors with EUS-guided fine needle aspiration with immunohistochemical analysis. Gastrointest endosc. 2002;55:37–43.
11. Akahoshi K, Sumida Y, Matsui N, et al. Preoperative diagnosis of gastrointestinal stromal tumor by endoscopic ultrasound-guided fine needle aspiration. World j gastroenterol. 2007;13:2077–82.
12. Mekky MA, Yamao K, Sawaki A, et al. Diagnostic utility of EUS-guided FNA in patients with gastric submucosal tumors. Gastrointest endosc. 2010;71:913–9.
13. Palazzo L, Landi B, Cellier C, et al. Endosonographic features predictive of benign and malignant gastrointestinal stromal cell tumours. Gut. 2000;46: 88–92.
14. Yang J, Feng F, Li M, et al. Surgical resection should be taken into consideration for the treatment of small gastric gastrointestinal stromal tumors. World j surg oncol. 2013;11:273.
15. Lachter J, Bishara N, Rahimi E, et al. EUS clarifies the natural history and ideal management of GISTs. Hepatogastroenterology. 2008;55:1653–6.
16. Gill KR, Camellini L, Conigliaro R, et al. The natural history of upper gastrointestinal subepithelial tumors: a multicenter endoscopic ultrasound survey. J clin gastroenterol. 2009;43:723–6.
17. Kim MY, Jung HY, Choi KD, et al. Natural history of asymptomatic small gastric subepithelial tumors. J clin gastroenterol. 2011;45:330–6.
18. Fang YJ, Cheng TY, Sun MS, et al. Suggested cutoff tumor size for management of small EUS-suspected gastric gastrointestinal stromal tumors. J formos med assoc. 2012;111:88–93.
19. Sepe PS, Moparty B, Pitman MB, et al. EUS-guided FNA for the diagnosis of GI stromal cell tumors: sensitivity and cytologic yield. Gastrointest endosc. 2009;70:254–61.
20. Ha CY, Shah R, Chen J, et al. Diagnosis and management of GI stromal tumors by EUS-FNA: a survey of opinions and practices of endosonographers. Gastrointest endosc. 2009;69:1039–44.
21. ASGE Standards of Practice Committee, Evans JA, Chandrasekhara V, et al. The role of endoscopy in the management of premalignant and malignant conditions of the stomach. Gastrointest endosc. 2015;82:1–8.

16

Fecal calprotectin level correlated with both endoscopic severity and disease extent in ulcerative colitis

Kousaku Kawashima[1], Shunji Ishihara[1*], Takafumi Yuki[1], Nobuhiko Fukuba[1], Naoki Oshima[1], Hideaki Kazumori[2], Hiroki Sonoyama[1], Noritsugu Yamashita[1], Yasumasa Tada[1], Ryusaku Kusunoki[1], Akihiko Oka[1], Yoshiyuki Mishima[1], Ichiro Moriyama[1,3] and Yoshikazu Kinoshita[1]

Abstract

Background: The relationship between fecal calprotectin (FC) and disease extent in ulcerative colitis (UC) has not been fully elucidated. The aim of this study was to clarify the correlation of FC with disease extent and severity in UC patients.

Methods: UC patients scheduled to undergo an ileocolonoscopy were enrolled and fecal samples for FC measurement were collected prior to the procedure. A Mayo endoscopic subscore (MES) was determined for each of 5 colonic segments. To evaluate the association of FC with extent of affected mucosa as well as disease severity, we assessed the correlation of FC level with the sum of MES (S-MES) for the 5 colonic segments as compared to the maximum score of MES (M-MES).

Results: FC measurements in conjunction with findings from 136 complete colonoscopies in 102 UC patients were evaluated. FC level showed a stronger correlation with S-MES (correlation coefficient $r = 0.86$, $p < 0.001$) as compared to M-MES ($r = 0.79$, $p < 0.001$). In patients with an M-MES of 1, 2, and 3, FC level showed a significant correlation with S-MES ($r = 0.67$, $p < 0.001$; $r = 0.70$, $p < 0.001$; $r = 0.47$, $p = 0.04$, respectively). Our findings indicate that FC level is elevated in patients with greater areas of affected mucosa even in those with the same M-MES value.

Conclusions: FC level was shown to be correlated with the extent of affected mucosa as well as severity in UC patients, thus it is useful for precise assessment of mucosal inflammation.

Keywords: Ulcerative colitis, Fecal calprotectin, Disease extent

Background

Ulcerative colitis (UC) is a chronic idiopathic disorder characterized by mucosal inflammation in the colon and rectum. In recent years, management of UC has substantially changed, with newly introduced treatments such as biologics and tacrolimus shown to result in significant endoscopic improvement as well as clinical remission in some cases [1–8]. Therefore, endoscopic mucosal healing (MH), which is associated with sustained clinical remission and reduced rates of hospitalization and surgical resection, has emerged as a major treatment goal for UC patients [9–11]. Although an endoscopy is recognized as the most reliable method for evaluating MH, that examination is relatively invasive and sometimes painful, while a colonoscopy procedure may exacerbate UC [12]. As a result, it is difficult to perform frequent endoscopic assessments of affected mucosa in clinical practice and alternative noninvasive methods are necessary for assessment of mucosal inflammation associated with UC.

Calprotectin is a 36-kDa calcium- and zinc-binding protein that represents most of the cytosolic proteins of granulocytes [13]. Measurement of fecal calprotectin (FC), which is stable for up to 3 days at room temperature and resistant to degradation [14], is useful, as its level reflects migration of neutrophils through the

* Correspondence: si360405@med.shimane-u.ac.jp
[1]Department of Internal Medicine II, Shimane University Faculty of Medicine, 89-1, Enya-cho, Izumo, Shimane 693-8501, Japan
Full list of author information is available at the end of the article

inflamed bowel wall to the mucosa and has been widely utilized to clarify its correlation with endoscopically proven UC activity [15–21]. Based on previously reported data showing a strong correlation with endoscopic activity, noninvasive measurement of FC level has been proposed to provide a reliable surrogate marker of mucosal inflammation associated with UC [22].

Numerous scoring systems have been developed for assessment of endoscopic activity in UC patients, of which the Mayo endoscopic subscore (MES) is one of the most widely employed endoscopic indices [23]. MES is divided into 4 points (0–3) based on proctosigmoiddoscopic appearance. When an ileocolonoscopy is performed, MES is often regarded as the maximum score for the parts of the colorectum examined. In addition, most other endoscopic indices also use such a maximum score for assessment of colonic mucosal activity [24–27]. In previous reports of the correlation of FC with mucosal activity, the endoscopic scores used were those obtained for the most severe level of inflammation in the colorectum and disease extent was not considered to be related to UC for evaluating the clinical usefulness of FC. In this regard, the correlation of FC with disease extent in UC has not been fully investigated.

In the present study, we assessed the sum of MES (S-MES) for the 5 colonic segments in patients with UC who underwent a complete colonoscopy. To clarify the correlation of FC with extent of affected mucosa as well as disease severity, we investigated the correlation of FC level with S-MES as compared to the maximum score of MES (M-MES).

Methods

This study was prospectively conducted from February 2013 to December 2014 at Shimane University Hospital and Matsue Seikyo General Hospital in Japan. The protocol was approved by the ethical committees of both hospitals and all patients gave written informed consent, and the study was performed in adherence to the Helsinki Declaration.

Patients

Patients with a previously established diagnosis of UC and scheduled to undergo an ileocolonoscopy were enrolled. For those who were outpatients, we asked them to obtain fecal samples within 7 days before the ileocolonoscopy, which were brought to the hospital or sent by postal mail immediately after collection. Fecal samples from inpatients were obtained the day before the ileocolonoscopy and examined in the hospital laboratory. Patients who previously underwent a sigmoidoscopy, or with a history of colorectal surgery, acute infectious enterocolitis, or regular intake of aspirin and/or other nonsteroidal anti-inflammatory drugs (NSAIDs) were excluded from this study. Those unable to provide a fecal sample were also excluded. When exacerbation of symptoms such as diarrhea and melena were noted prior to the ileocolonoscopy examination, we performed a stool culture for diagnosis of pathogenic bacteria infection including *Clostridium difficile*, as well as serum and histological examinations to exclude CMV infection, as necessary. For patient demographics, age, sex, duration of disease, clinical activity, extent type of UC, and concomitant medications being taken at each colonoscopic examination were noted. The extent type of UC was determined according to the Montreal classification based on previous colonoscopic findings, unless the extent of affected mucosa based on the present colonoscopic findings revealed more extensive involvement [28, 29].

Fecal calprotectin measurement

Collected fecal samples used for FC measurements were stored at −20 °C until shipment to the laboratory (SRL Inc., Tokyo, Japan), where the FC level was determined with the examiner blinded to the endoscopic findings using a quantitative enzyme-linked immunosorbent assay (PhiCal®, Immundiagnostik, Germany), with a standard method. The detection limits of this ELISA kit for FC range from 5.3 to 2100 μg/g.

Colonoscopic findings and clinical disease activity

Patients with UC received a magnesium citrate- or polyethylene glycol-based electrolyte solution for bowel preparation prior to the ileocolonoscopy. All of the procedures (EVIS 260 series, Olympus, Tokyo, Japan) were performed by 2 of the authors (K.K. and T.Y.). Patients who underwent an incomplete colonoscopy examination (cecum not reached) were excluded, as some with UC had maximum inflammation in the right colon [30]. Colonoscopic findings were finally determined according to the MES for each of the 5 portions of the colorectum (cecum to ascending colon, transverse, descending, sigmoid colon, rectum). Those determinations were made by the first 5 authors of this study (K.K., S.I., T.Y., N.F., N.O.), each an experienced gastroenterologist, within 1 week after the colonoscopy. When endoscopic grading differed among them, the final grade was decided based on consensus. We precisely defined the maximum score of MES as M-MES, while the sum of MES for the 5 colonic segments, which ranged from 0 to 15 was determined as S-MES. Clinical disease activity was evaluated on the day of the ileocolonoscopy using Rachmilewitz' clinical activity index (CAI) consisting of 7 subscores, as previously reported [27]. Clinical remission was defined as a CAI value of 4 or less.

Statistical analysis

Statistical analysis was performed using the SPSS statistical package (version 19.0, SPSS, Chicago, USA). Parametric numerical results are presented as the mean ± standard deviation (SD), while nonparametric data are presented as the median and interquartile range (IQR). A Mann-Whitney test was used to investigate differences between nonparametric data. Correlation analyses were performed using Spearman's rank correlation test. All P-values are two-sided and $P < 0.05$ was considered to be statistically significant.

Results

Patients

The clinical characteristics of the present UC patients are shown in Table 1. A total of 136 complete colonoscopies that were accompanied by fecal sample examinations were performed in 102 UC patients. Of those, 32 (24 %) were performed in patients with clinical activity (CAI ≥5), while the other 104 (76 %) were performed in those with clinical remission (CAI ≤4). Of the 136 colonoscopies, 68 (50.0 %) were performed for pancolitis, 36 (26.4 %) for left-sided colitis, and 32 (23.6 %) for proctitis.

Correlation of FC level with both M-MES and S-MES

As shown in Fig. 1, the median FC level in patients with an M-MES of 0 ($n = 35$), 1 ($n = 33$), 2 ($n = 47$), and 3 ($n = 21$) was 35.2 (IQR 17.3-76.6), 103.3 (55.2-336.4), 295.0 (162.9-1000.0), and 751.9 (632.8-1685.6) μg/g, respectively. FC was significantly elevated in accordance with endoscopic severity and showed a significant correlation with M-MES (Spearman's rank correlation coefficient $r = 0.79$; $p < 0.001$). Furthermore, FC demonstrated a strong correlation with S-MES ($r = 0.86$, $p < 0.001$), as shown in Fig. 2. In patients with an M-MES of 1, 2, and 3, FC demonstrated a significant correlation with S-MES ($r = 0.67$, $p < 0.001$; $r = 0.70$, $p < 0.001$; $r = 0.47$, $p = 0.04$, respectively), as shown in Fig. 3a–c. These results indicated that FC level is correlated with the extent of affected mucosa even in patients with the same M-MES value as well as endoscopic severity.

FC levels in patients with the same S-MES, but different extent of affected mucosa

We also compared FC levels in patients with the same S-MES, but different extent of affected mucosa. Of 22 with an S-MES of 2, an MES of 1 in 2 segments (S-MES = 1 + 1 = 2 points) was seen in 6 and an MES of 2 in only 1 segment (S-MES = 2 points) was seen in 16, with FC level in the former at 272.2 ± 144.0 μg/g and at 256.7 ± 192.2 μg/g in the latter, not a significant difference ($p = 0.86$).

Discussion

An important element of the present study is that MES was determined in each of the 5 colonic segments to evaluate the extent of affected mucosa as well as endoscopic severity. Our results clearly showed that FC level is significantly correlated with both endoscopic severity and the extent of affected mucosa in patients with UC, revealing the importance of its measurement as an indicator of mucosal inflammation.

Table 1 Characteristics of study patients and colonoscopic findings

Patients	
Total	102
Gender	
Male	65 (64 %)
Female	47 (36 %)
Number of colonoscopy	
Once	71 (70 %)
Twice	28 (27 %)
3 times	3 (3 %)
Complete colonoscopy	
Total number	136
Median age in years (IQR)	44.5 (31.0-63.5)
Median duration of disease in years (IQR)	7.0 (4.0-12.5)
Clinical activity	
Remission	104 (76 %)
Active	32 (24 %)
Purpose of colonoscopy	
Evaluation of disease	46 (34 %)
Surveillance	90 (66 %)
Concomitant medications	
Aminosalicylate	129 (95 %)
Topical aminosalicylate	35 (26 %)
Corticosteroids	23 (17 %)
Topical steroids	8 (6 %)
Azathioprine/Mercaptopurine	37 (27 %)
Tacrolimus	11 (8 %)
Biologics	13 (10 %)
Colonoscopic findings (maximum score in colorectum)	
Mayo endoscopic subscore 0	35 (26 %)
Mayo endoscopic subscore 1	33 (24 %)
Mayo endoscopic subscore 2	47 (35 %)
Mayo endoscopic subscore 3	21 (15 %)
Biochemical Results	
Median C-reactive protein (mg/l) (IQR)	0.05 (0.03-0.12)
Median serum albumin (g/l) (IQR)	4.4 (4.0-4.6)
Median white blood cell count (10^3×/μL) (IQR)	5.88 (4.86-7.52)
Median hemoglobin (g/dL) (IQR)	13.8 (12.2-14.9)
Median platelet count (10^4×/μL) (IQR)	24.7 (20.8-29.3)

IQR interquartile range

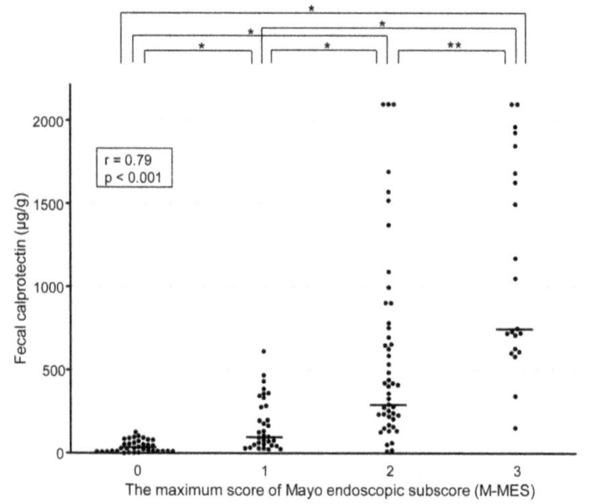

Fig. 1 Scatterplot showing correlation of fecal calprotectin (FC) level with maximum of Mayo endoscopic subscore (M-MES). The median and interquartile range (IQR) for FC levels in patients with an M-MES of 0 ($n = 35$), 1 ($n = 33$), 2 ($n = 47$), and 3 ($n = 21$) were 35.2 (17.3-76.6), 103.3 (55.2-336.4), 295.0 (162.9-1000.0), and 751.9 (632.8-1685.6) μg/g, respectively. *$p < 0.001$, **$p < 0.01$

FC level has been widely examined in regard to its correlation with endoscopic activity in UC patients, with correlation coefficients between FC level and UC endoscopic activity reported to range from 0.51 to 0.83 [15–21]. In those studies, the endoscopic index for UC was determined by examining the part of the colorectum with the most severe inflammation. Similarly, in the present study, we evaluated mucosal severity in UC patients using M-MES, and found that the correlation coefficient between FC level and M-MES was 0.79, which correlated well with those previous reports. Thus, our findings confirmed that FC level is correlated

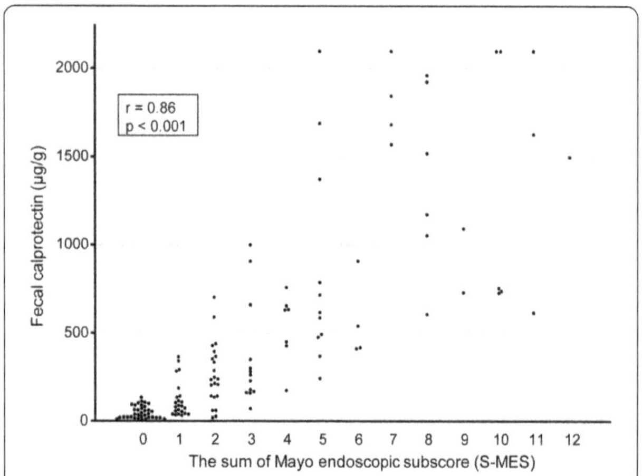

Fig. 2 Scatterplot showing correlation of fecal calprotectin (FC) level with sum of Mayo endoscopic subscore (S-MES) for 5 colonic segments

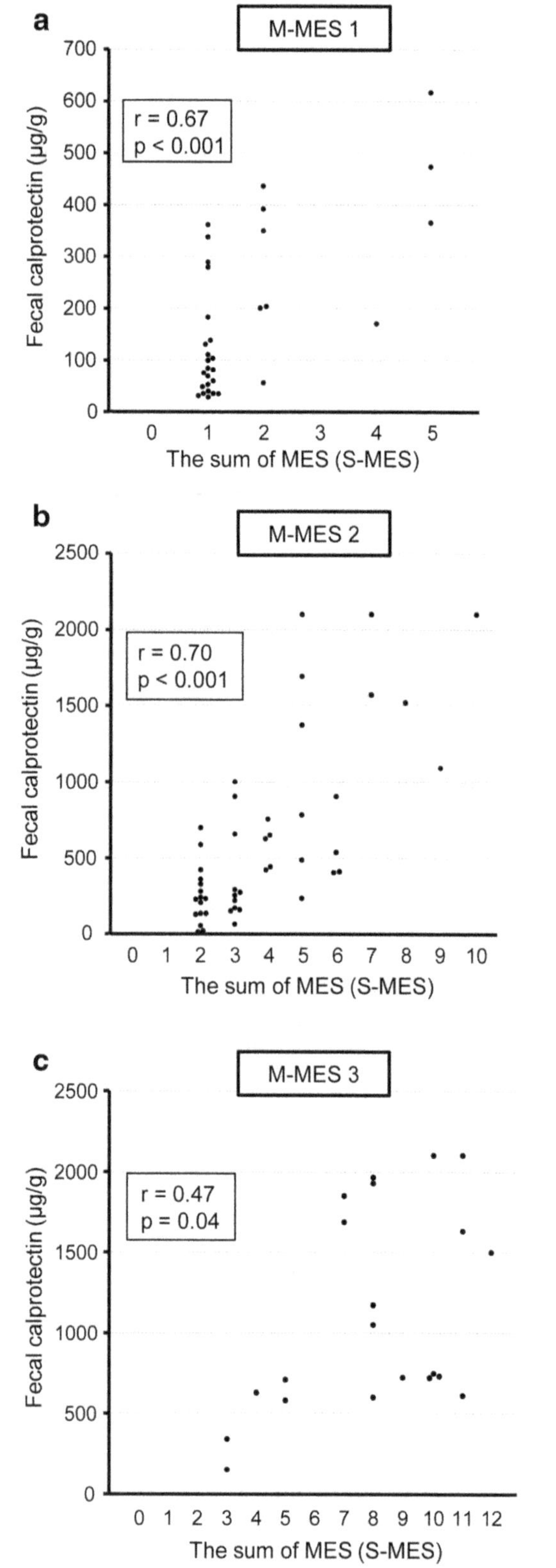

Fig. 3 Scatterplot showing correlation of fecal calprotectin (FC) level with sum of Mayo endoscopic subscore for 5 colonic segments (S-MES) in patients with a maximum MES (M-MES) of 1, 2, and 3. **a** M-MES 1. **b** M-MES 2. **c** M-MES 3

with endoscopic severity in the most severely affected segment of the colorectum.

In most previous reports, the UC endoscopic index was determined using the most severely affected segment in the colorectum [23–27]. However, segmental colonic assessment is becoming increasingly important in cases of UC according to the United States Food and Drug Administration [30, 31]. Furthermore, the recent proposed definition of mucosal healing by the International Organization for the study of Inflammatory Bowel Disease includes absence of friability, blood, erosions, and ulcers in all gastrointestinal mucosa segments [31]. Another report also noted that the recently developed UC colonoscopic index of severity (UCCIS) is relevant as an endoscopic index, because of its scoring system, which evaluates all colonic segments [32]. Thus, endoscopic assessment of all segments of the colorectum is recommended for investigating disease extent as well as severity in UC patients.

To investigate the correlation between FC level and extent of affected mucosa, we used the sum of MES (S-MES) in all 5 colonic segments in the preset study, as MES is the most widely used endoscopic index for UC and considered to be highly reliable. Very recently, Lobaton T, et al. proposed a modified Mayo endoscopic score as a new endoscopic index for UC, which is calculated based on analysis of the MES for each of the 5 colonic segments [33]. In our study, the correlation coefficient value for the correlation of FC with S-MES was 0.86, nearly as high as the value (0.73) reported in their study. Furthermore, we found that FC level had a stronger correlation with S-MES ($r = 0.86$) as compared to M-MES ($r = 0.79$), also similar to that previous study. Based on these results, we concluded that FC level likely has a stronger correlation with the sum of MES for the 5 colonic segments as compared to the maximum score of MES.

A novel finding presented in our study that differentiates it from other previous reports is clarification of the significant correlation of FC level with S-MES, even in UC patients with the same M-MES value (Fig. 3). Our results also indicate that FC is elevated in conjunction with a greater area of affected mucosa even in UC patients with the same classification of endoscopic severity. Therefore, we concluded that FC level in UC patients is important for precise assessment of mucosal inflammation by showing the extent of affected mucosa as well as severity. In addition, the correlation coefficient of FC with S-MES in patients with an M-MES of 3 was comparatively low at 0.47 as compared to those in patients with an M-MES of 1 or 2, though those cannot be directly compared. FC level in patients with an M-MES of 3 is higher due to excessive mucosal severity, while the influence of the extent of affected mucosa on FC level might be relatively low in those patients.

In addition, we compared FC levels in patients with the same S-MES, but different extent of affected mucosa. The result suggests that FC level is similar between patients with mild activity in a greater extent of mucosa and those with moderate activity in a limited extent. However, to clearly show this point, examinations of a larger number of enrolled subjects will be necessary.

Our study has some limitations. First, it was conducted at 2 different hospitals in Japan. To reduce interobserver variations as much as possible, before performing the FC measurement, all colonoscopic findings were finally determined by 5 experienced gastroenterologists, each of whom had at least 10 years of experience with performing colonoscopic examinations. However, additional investigations that include a greater number of institutions will be necessary. Second, our cohort included few UC patients with an M-MES of 3, as some of those had difficulty with providing an adequate fecal sample due to lack of consistency. In addition, an incomplete colonoscopy may easily occur in UC patients with an M-MES of 3 due to their severe condition and pain related to the procedure. Finally, we did not perform histological examinations of colonic biopsy samples. Further investigations based on histological examination findings obtained from all 5 colonic segments including endoscopically non-inflamed mucosa are necessary for understanding the correlations of those results with endoscopic findings and FC level.

Conclusions

The present results revealed that FC level is significantly correlated with the extent of affected mucosa as well as disease severity in patients with UC, and its measurement is important for precise assessment of mucosal inflammation.

Abbreviations

CAI: clinical activity index; FC: fecal calprotectin; IQR: interquartile range; MES: Mayo endoscopic subscore; MH: mucosal healing; M-MES: maximum score of Mayo endoscopic subscore; S-MES: sum of Mayo endoscopic subscore; UC: Ulcerative colitis.

Competing interests

The authors declare that they have no competing interest in connection with the publication of this manuscript.

Authors' contributions

Study concept and design: KK, SI and YK. Manuscript preparation: KK, SI and YM. Acquisition of data: KK, SI, TY, NF, NO, HK, YT, HS, RK, AO and IM. Statistical analysis: NF and KK. All authors read and approved the final manuscript.

Acknowledgements

The authors thank SRL Inc. for measurements of FC as well as shipping.

Author details

[1]Department of Internal Medicine II, Shimane University Faculty of Medicine, 89-1, Enya-cho, Izumo, Shimane 693-8501, Japan. [2]Division of Internal Medicine, Matsue Seikyo General Hospital, 8-8-8, Nishitsuda, Matsue 690-8522, Japan. [3]Cancer center, Shimane University Hospital, 89-1, Enya-cho, Izumo, Shimane 693-8501, Japan.

References

1. Rutgeerts P, Sandborn WJ, Feagan BG, Reinisch W, Olson A, Johanns J, et al. Infliximab for induction and maintenance therapy for ulcerative colitis. N Engl J Med. 2005;353:2462–76.
2. Armuzzi A, Pugliese D, Danese S, Rizzo G, Felice C, Marzo M, et al. Long-term combination therapy with infliximab plus azathioprine predicts sustained steroid-free clinical benefit in steroid-dependent ulcerative colitis. Inflamm Bowel Dis. 2014;20:1368–74.
3. Sandborn WJ, van Assche G, Reinisch W, Colombel JF, D'Haens G, Wolf DC, et al. Adalimumab induces and maintains clinical remission in patients with moderate-to-severe ulcerative colitis. Gastroenterology. 2012;142:257–65.
4. Reinisch W, Sandborn WJ, Panaccione R, Huang B, Pollack PF, Lazar A, et al. 52-week efficacy of adalimumab in patients with moderately to severely active ulcerative colitis who failed corticosteroids and/or immunosuppressants. Inflamm Bowel Dis. 2013;19:1700–09.
5. Danese S, Fiorino G, Peyrin-Biroulet L, Lucenteforte E, Virgili G, Moja L, et al. Biological agents for moderately to severely active ulcerative colitis: a systematic review and network meta-analysis. Ann Intern Med. 2014;160:704–11.
6. Ogata H, Kato J, Hirai F, Hida N, Matsui T, Matsumoto T, et al. Double-blind, placebo-controlled trial of oral tacrolimus (FK506) in the management of hospitalized patients with steroid-refractory ulcerative colitis. Inflamm Bowel Dis. 2012;18:803–8.
7. Feagan BG, Rutgeerts P, Sands BE, Hanauer S, Colombel JF, Sandborn WJ, et al. Vedolizumab as induction and maintenance therapy for ulcerative colitis. N Engl J Med. 2013;369:699–710.
8. Shelton E, Allegretti JR, Stevens B, Lucci M, Khalili H, Nguyen DD, et al. Efficacy of Vedolizumab as Induction Therapy in Refractory IBD Patients: A Multicenter Cohort. Inflamm Bowel Dis. 2015;21:2879–85.
9. Peyrin-Biroulet L, Ferrante M, Magro F, Campbell S, Franchimont D, Fidder H, et al. Scientific Committee of the European Crohn's and Colitis Organization. Results from the 2nd Scientific Workshop of the ECCO. I: Impact of mucosal healing on the course of inflammatory bowel disease. J Crohns Colitis. 2011;5:477–83.
10. Meucci G, Fasoli R, Saibeni S, Valpiani D, Gullotta R, Colombo E, et al. IG-IBD. Prognostic significance of endoscopic remission in patients with active ulcerative colitis treated with oral and topical mesalazine: a prospective, multicenter study. Inflamm Bowel Dis. 2012;18:1006–10.
11. Frøslie KF, Jahnsen J, Moum BA. Vatn MH. IBSEN Group Mucosal Heal inflamm Bowel Dis. 2007;133:412–22.
12. Menees S, Higgins P, Korsnes S, Elta G. Does colonoscopy cause increased ulcerative colitis symptoms? Inflamm Bowel Dis. 2007;13:12–8.
13. Vermeire S, Van Assche G, Rutgeerts P. Laboratory markers in IBD: useful, magic, or unnecessary toys? Gut. 2006;55:426–31.
14. Lasson A, Stotzer PO, Öhman L, Isaksson S, Sapnara M, Strid H. The intra-individual variability of faecal calprotectin: a prospective study in patients with active ulcerative colitis. J Crohns Colitis. 2015;9:26–32.
15. Røseth AG, Aadland E, Jahnsen J, Raknerud N. Assessment of disease activity in ulcerative colitis by faecal calprotectin, a novel granulocyte marker protein. Digestion. 1997;58:176–80.
16. Hanai H, Takeuchi K, Iida T, Kashiwagi N, Saniabadi AR, Matsushita I, et al. Relationship between fecal calprotectin, intestinal inflammation, and peripheral blood neutrophils in patients with active ulcerative colitis. Dig Dis Sci. 2004;49:1438–43.
17. D'Incà R, Dal Pont E, Di Leo V, Ferronato A, Fries W, Vettorato MG, et al. Calprotectin and lactoferrin in the assessment of intestinal inflammation and organic disease. Int J Colorectal Dis. 2007;22:429–37.
18. Langhorst J, Elsenbruch S, Koelzer J, Rueffer A, Michalsen A, Dobos GJ. Noninvasive markers in the assessment of intestinal inflammation in inflammatory bowel diseases: performance of fecal lactoferrin, calprotectin, and PMN-elastase, CRP, and clinical indices. Am J Gastroenterol. 2008;103:162–9.
19. Schoepfer AM, Beglinger C, Straumann A, Trummler M, Renzulli P, Seibold F. Ulcerative colitis: correlation of the Rachmilewitz endoscopic activity index with fecal calprotectin, clinical activity, C-reactive protein, and blood leukocytes. Inflamm Bowel Dis. 2009;15:1851–8.
20. Schoepfer AM, Beglinger C, Straumann A, Safroneeva E, Romero Y, Armstrong D, et al. Fecal calprotectin more accurately reflects endoscopic activity of ulcerative colitis than the Lichtiger Index, C-reactive protein, platelets, hemoglobin, and blood leukocytes. Inflamm Bowel Dis. 2013;19:332–41.
21. D'Haens G, Ferrante M, Vermeire S, Baert F, Noman M, Moortgat L, et al. Fecal calprotectin is a surrogate marker for endoscopic lesions in inflammatory bowel disease. Inflamm Bowel Dis. 2012;18:2218–24.
22. Daperno M, Castiglione F, de Ridder L, Dotan I, Färkkilä M, Florholmen J, et al. Scientific Committee of the European Crohn's and Colitis Organization. Results of the 2nd part Scientific Workshop of the ECCO. II: Measures and markers of prediction to achieve, detect, and monitor intestinal healing in inflammatory bowel disease. J Crohns Colitis. 2011;5:484–98.
23. Schroeder KW, Tremaine WJ, Ilstrup DM. Coated oral 5-aminosalicylic acid therapy for mildly to moderately active ulcerative colitis. A randomized study. N Engl J Med. 1987;317:1625–9.
24. Baron JH, Connell AM, Lennard-Jones JE. Variation between observers in describing mucosal appearances in proctocolitis. Br Med J. 1964;1:89–92.
25. Powell-Tuck J, Bown RL, Lennard-Jones JE. A comparison of oral prednisolone given as single or multiple daily doses for active proctocolitis. Scand J Gastroenterol. 1978;13:833–7.
26. Sutherland LR, Martin F, Greer S, Robinson M, Greenberger N, Saibil F, et al. 5-Aminosalicylic acid enema in the treatment of distal ulcerative colitis, proctosigmoiditis, and proctitis. Gastroenterology. 1987;92:1894–8.
27. Rachmilewitz D. Coated mesalazine (5-aminosalicylic acid) versus sulphasalazine in the treatment of active ulcerative colitis: a randomised trial. BMJ. 1989;298:82–6.
28. Silverberg MS, Satsangi J, Ahmad T, Arnott ID, Bernstein CN, Brant SR, et al. Toward an integrated clinical, molecular and serological classification of inflammatory bowel disease: report of a Working Party of the 2005 Montreal World Congress of Gastroenterology. Can J Gastroenterol. 2005;19 Suppl A:5A–36A.
29. Satsangi J, Silverberg MS, Vermeire S, Colombel JF. The Montreal classification of inflammatory bowel disease: controversies, consensus, and implications. Gut. 2006;55:749–53.
30. Kato J, Kuriyama M, Hiraoka S, Yamamoto K. Is sigmoidoscopy sufficient for evaluating inflammatory status of ulcerative colitis patients? J Gastroenterol Hepatol. 2011;26:683–7.
31. D'Haens G, Sandborn WJ, Feagan BG, Colombel JF. A review of activity indices and efficacy end points for clinical trials of medical therapy in adults with ulcerative colitis. Gastroenterology. 2007;132:763–86.
32. Samuel S, Bruining DH, Loftus Jr EV, Thia KT, Schroeder KW, Tremaine WJ, et al. Validation of the ulcerative colitis colonoscopic index of severity and its correlation with disease activity measures. Clin Gastroenterol Hepatol. 2013; 11:49–54.
33. Lobatón T, Bessissow T, De Hertogh G, Lemmens B, Maedler C, Van Assche G, et al. The Modified Mayo Endoscopic Score (MMES): A New Index for the Assessment of Extension and Severity of Endoscopic Activity in Ulcerative Colitis Patients. J Crohns Colitis. 2015;9:846–52.

17

Gastrointestinal tuberculosis following renal transplantation accompanied with septic shock and acute respiratory distress syndrome

Andrea Cikova[1], Diana Vavrincova-Yaghi[2*], Peter Vavrinec[2], Anna Dobisova[1], Andrea Gebhardtova[1], Zora Flassikova[1], Mark A. Seelen[3], Robert H. Henning[4] and Aktham Yaghi[1]

Abstract

Background: Post-transplant tuberculosis (PTTB) is a serious opportunistic infection in renal graft recipients with a 30-70 fold higher incidence compared to the general population. PTTB occurs most frequently within the first years after transplantation, manifesting as pulmonary or disseminated TB. Gastrointestinal TB (GITB) is a rare and potentially lethal manifestation of PTTB and may show delayed onset in renal transplant recipients due to the use of lower doses of immunosuppressants. Further, non-specificity of symptoms and the common occurrence of GI disorders in transplant recipients may delay diagnosis of GITB.

Case presentation: Here we report a rare survival case of isolated GITB in a renal transplant recipient, occurring seven years after transplantation. The patient's condition was complicated by severe sepsis with positive blood culture *Staphylococcus haemolyticus*, septic shock, multiple organ failure including acute respiratory distress syndrome (ARDS) and acute renal failure, requiring mechanical ventilation, vasopressor circulatory support and intermittent hemodialysis. Furthermore, nosocomial infections such as invasive aspergillosis and *Pseudomonas aeruginosa* occurred during hospitalization. Antituberculosis therapy (rifampicin, isoniazid, ethambutol and pyrazinamide) was initiated upon *Mycobacterium* confirmation. Moreover, treatment with voriconazole due to the *Aspergillus flavus* and meropenem due to the *Pseudomonas aeruginosa* was initiated, the former necessitating discontinuation of rifampicin. After 34 days, the patient was weaned from mechanical ventilation and was discharged to the pulmonary ward, followed by complete recovery.

Conclusion: This case offers a guideline for the clinical management towards survival of GITB in transplant patients, complicated by septic shock and multiple organ failure, including acute renal injury and ARDS.

Keywords: Gastrointestinal tuberculosis, Renal transplantation, Multiple organ failure, Acute respiratory distress syndrome, Septic shock

* Correspondence: vavrincova@fpharm.uniba.sk
[2]Department of Pharmacology and Toxicology, Faculty of Pharmacy, Comenius University in Bratislava, Bratislava, Odbojarov 10, 832 32 Bratislava, Slovakia
Full list of author information is available at the end of the article

Background

Post-transplant tuberculosis (PTTB) is a serious opportunistic infection in renal graft recipients significantly increasing mortality and morbidity [1]. The incidence of PTTB among transplant recipients is 30-70 fold higher compared to the general population, with a significant risk of graft loss and a mortality rate up-to 30% [2]. PTTB is usually the result of reactivation of latent tuberculosis infection, although primary infection or transmission of *Mycobacterium tuberculosis* via the renal graft has been occasionally reported [3]. PTTB occurs most frequently within the first 2 years after transplantation, with a median interval of 8 months [4]. The overall prevalence of PTTB is reported to be 0.3-1.7% in the United States and Western Europe. In developing countries, PTTB prevalence is much higher, ranging between 3.1-15.2% due to the higher prevalence of tuberculosis in those areas [1]. The most common manifestation of PTTB in renal transplant patients is pulmonary TB [5]. One third of all cases of PTTB involve disseminated and extra-pulmonary TB [6]. Amongst the very rare manifestations of PTTB is gastrointestinal TB (GITB) [1]. GITB is potentially lethal [7] and because of its nonspecific symptoms and laboratory findings, diagnosis is often challenging [8]. Moreover, limited data are available regarding the prevalence of GITB among renal transplant recipients [1]. Further, although uncommon, extensive TB of the pulmonary parenchyma, as observed in the course of miliary TB, may cause acute respiratory distress syndrome (ARDS) [9], which is associated with a 60% in-hospital mortality [10]. Mortality increases to 100% when acute kidney injury ensues [11]. So far, a case of post-transplant GITB complicated by ARDS has not been reported.

Here we report a case of isolated GITB in a renal transplant recipient, occurring seven years after transplantation. Moreover, the patient's condition was complicated by severe sepsis with positive blood culture for *Staphylococcus haemolyticus*, septic shock and multiple organ failure including ARDS and acute renal failure, requiring mechanical ventilation, vasopressor circulatory support and intermittent hemodialysis. Furthermore, nosocomial infections including invasive aspergillosis and *Pseudomonas aeruginosa* occurred during hospitalization.

Case presentation

A 53-year-old female renal allograft recipient with a history of hypertension presented to the intensive care unit (ICU) with a septic shock and multi-organ failure. In the past, left nephrectomy had been performed due to kidney dysfunction. Seven years before admission, she underwent deceased-donor renal transplantation due to pyelonephritis of the right kidney. The immunosuppressive regimen included methylprednisolone, mycophenolate mofetil (1000 mg-0-1000 mg) and cyclosporine (25 mg-0-50 mg).

Since 7 months, the patient had been re-admitted repeatedly to other hospitals because of recurrent fever, however without demonstration of an infectious agent. One month earlier she had been admitted to the hospital because of dyspnoea and dry cough. Atypical right bronchopneumonia was suspected based on computed tomography (CT) of the lungs and treated empirically with antibiotic therapy including piperacillin/tazobactam, metronidazole, and fluconazole. Since the patient was deteriorating, she was admitted to the pulmonary ICU of our hospital.

Post-surgery (PO) admission day 1

Because of a history of weight loss and the patient starting to complain of abdominal pain at the pulmonary ICU, and the presence of anemia and intestinal hemorrhage, an abdominal CT was performed. The CT revealed ascites, enlarged uterus with wall thickening, enlarged left ovarium, as well as enlarged mesenteric and retroperitoneal lymph nodes. Further, the low thoracic area showed bilateral pleural effusion and hydropericardium.

Because of the massive intestinal hemorrhage, surgery was needed four days after admission to the pulmonary ICU, during which a right-sided hemicolectomy with side-to-side ileotransverse anastomosis was performed. Additionally, left adnexectomy was performed, because inflammatory tumor lesions were found. As her condition deteriorated post-operatively, the patient was intubated, analgo-sedated to Glasgow Coma Scale 3 (GCS 3) and artificially ventilated with inspired FiO2 0.65-1. Norepinephrine was administered for hypotension. The patient was transferred to our ICU after 24 h of mechanical ventilation in the pulmonary ICU, because of progression of multiple organ failure, including acute renal failure.

On admission at 9:15 a.m., under norepinephrine administration (0.4 μg/kg/min), blood pressure was 110/50 mmHg, HR was 117/min, temperature 37.2 °C, and the patient was anuric. Laboratory analyses revealed combined metabolic and respiratory acidosis (pH 7.136, pCO2 7.8 kPa, BE −11 mmol/l, pO_2 12.65 kPa, HCO_3 16.1 mmol/l, O_2 saturation 93.4%, paO2/FiO2 94, arterial lactate 2.13 mmol/l), and hyperkalemia (6.29 mmol/l), hyperchloremia (121.7 mmol/l), elevated blood urea and creatinine (13.11 mmol/l and 179.5 μmol/l, respectively), AST 346.4 U/l and elevated C-reactive protein (196.2 mg/l) and procalcitonin (2.14 μg/l). Blood analyses corroborated massive blood loss (Hb 82 g/l, Ht 0.24, RBC 2.77×10^{12}/l) and showed WBC 14.2×10^9/l and PLT 147×10^9/l. After the admission, cannulation of left subclavian vein and the left radial artery was performed. Left thoracic drainage was performed due to an iatrogenic left anterior pneumothorax, confirmed by CT, which also showed extensive diffuse bilateral infiltrates (Fig. 1a, b). At 12 a.m., blood culture from a blood sample taken upon admission was found positive for *Staphylococcus haemolyticus.* Moreover, *Staphyloccocus aureus* was cultured from the abdominal cavity. Subsequently, linezolid was added to the therapeutical regimen.

Histology tissue specimens obtained from the abdominal cavity revealed granuloma, indicative of tuberculous enteritis, peritonitis, adnexitis and lymphadenitis. Ziehl-Neelsen staining revealed an abundance of gram positive bacterial pathogens type *Mycobacterium.* A final diagnose of systemic mycobacteriosis, with superinfection due to the chronic immunosuppressive therapy was made. Antimycobacterial therapy was initiated with rifampicin, isoniazid, ethambutol and pyrazinamide. Intravenous administration of ciprofloxacin, piperacillin/tazobactam and linezolid was continued. Following the advice of the nephrologist, mycophenolate mofetil was discontinued and immunosuppressive therapy was continued with hydrocortisone. Later that day, the patient was turned to the prone position because of severe ARDS (Fig. 1a, b), for seven hours without improvement in oxygenation (Fig. 2 – timeline with interventions and medications).

PO day 2 and further

On day 2 of admission to the ICU, oxygenation improved (paO2/FiO2 185), while norepinephrine was continued (up to 0.5 μg/kg/min.). As oliguria persisted, intermittent hemodialysis was indicated (4 h/day). Prior to dialysis, laboratory analyses showed urea 21 mmol/l, creatinine 261.9 μmol/l, potassium 6.22 mmol/l and metabolic acidosis.

Day 3. Intermittent hemodialysis was maintained (4 h/day) and spontaneous diuresis increased to 760 ml/24 h. Norepinephrine infusion rate was gradually lowered.

Day 4. Final intermittent hemodialysis was indicated (4 h/day).

Day 5. Norepinephrine was discontinued.

Day 6. Tracheostomy was performed. *Mycobacterium tuberculosis* in sputum was confirmed by polymerase chain reaction (PCR).

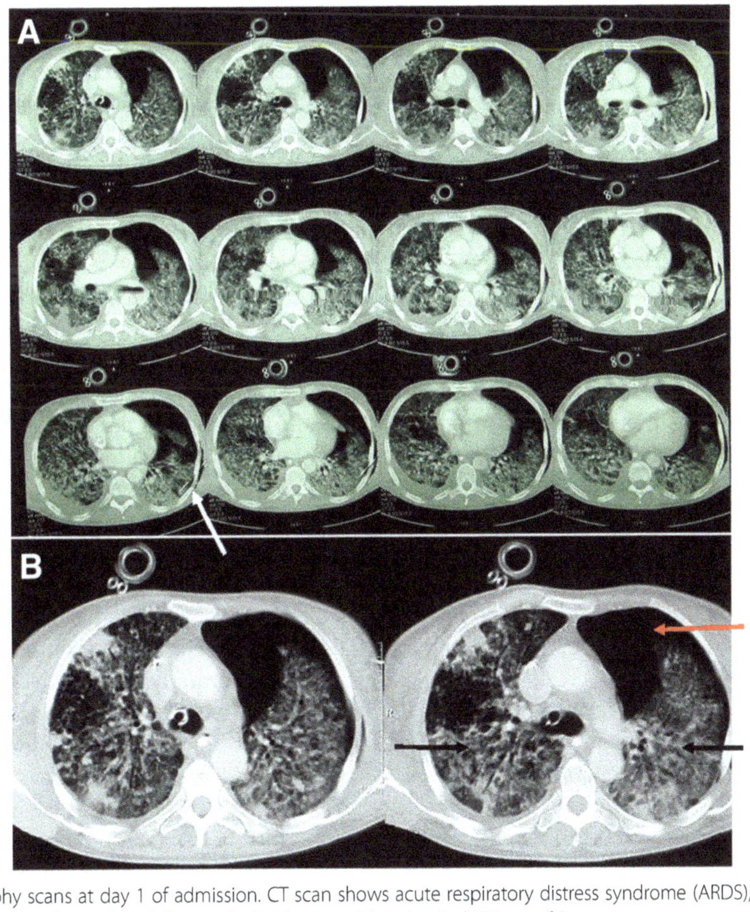

Fig. 1 Computer tomography scans at day 1 of admission. CT scan shows acute respiratory distress syndrome (ARDS), diffuse bilateral infiltrates (black arrows), pneumothorax (red arrow) and chest tube (white arrow) (**a**), detailed CT scan (**b**)

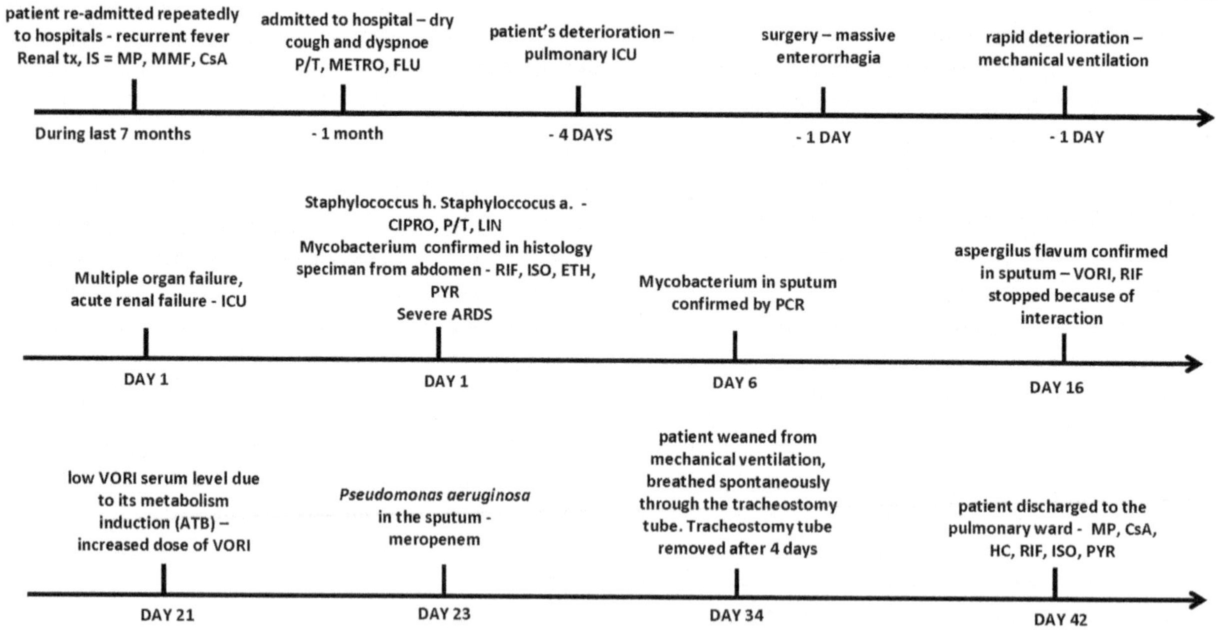

Fig. 2 Timeline with essential interventions and medications. tx, transplantation; IS, immunosuppressive regimen; MP, methylprednisolone; MMF, mycophenolate mofetil; CsA, cyclosporine; P/T, piperacillin/tazobactam; METRO, metronidazole; FLU, fluconazole; LIN, linezolid; CIPRO, ciprofloxacin; RIF, rifampicin; ISO, isoniazid; ETH, ethambutol; PYR, pyrazinamide; ARDS, acute respiratory distress syndrome; PCR, polymerase chain reaction; VORI, voriconazole; HC, hydrocortisone; ATB, antituberculosis therapy

Day 11. Mycophenolate mofetil was re-added to the immunosuppressive regimen.

Day 15. The analyses of sputum revealed filamentous fungi without further specification – the clinical pharmacologist prescribed anidulafungin for yeast superinfection following sensitivity testing (initial dose 200 mg i.v., then 100 mg i.v. every 24 h).

Day 16. Anidulafungin resistant *Aspergillus flavus* was confirmed in sputum, prompting addition of voriconazole to the current treatment (initial dose 300 mg i.v. every 12 h, then 200 mg i.v. every 12 h). The pulmonologist was consulted because of interaction between antimycotic agents and rifampicin. Because of the invasive aspergillosis, rifampicin was stopped.

Day 21. Because of low voriconazole serum level, the dose was increased to 400 mg i.v. every 12 h.

Day 23. Due to the *Pseudomonas aeruginosa* in the sputum, meropenem i.v. was added to the antimicrobial regimen.

Day 34. The patient was weaned from mechanical ventilation and breathed spontaneously through the tracheostomy tube with O_2. The tracheostomy tube was removed four days later.

Day 42. The patient was discharged to the pulmonary ward, with the following medication: methylprednisolone, cyclosporine, hydrocortisone, rifampicin, isoniazid and pyrazinamide.

Discussion and conclusions

This case demonstrates both typical and non-typical features associated with GITB in renal transplant patients. First, reactivation of latent TB infection was only observed 7 years after transplantation, which is unusually late, as most cases occur in the first 2 years after transplantation [1]. However, several reports show that the median time of onset of GITB may be longer in renal transplant recipients, possibly due to the lower doses of immunosuppressants in those recipients compared to other transplant recipients [1, 3]. This might have been also the case of our patient, as her immunosuppressive regimen consisted of lower doses of mycophenolate mofetil (1000 mg two times daily) compared to e.g. heart or liver transplant patients (1500 mg two times daily). Moreover, the dose of cyclosporine was decreased several weeks after renal transplantation.

GITB occurs usually due to the reactivation of latent TB infection because of immunosuppressive therapy, or (but less commonly) it is transmitted by the allograft itself; alternatively, it may result from primary infection [3]. Immunosuppressive therapy affecting the function of cell-mediated immunity such as cyclosporine, mycophenolate mofetil and monoclonal and polyclonal antibodies during the first years after transplantation have been associated with TB reactivation [3, 12–14]. Our patient's immunosuppressive therapy included both cyclosporine and mycophenolate mofetil, however, other risk factors of reactivation (such as pretransplant diabetes, the number of acute rejections of transplanted graft resulting in higher dosing of immunosuppression, opportunistic infections, chronic liver diseases and duration of pretransplant hemodialysis) were unknown. Interestingly, the receipt of a graft from a deceased donor rather than other sources of donors was recently identified as important risk factor for developing TB in liver or kidney transplant recipients [15], which is in accordance with our case.

Although GITB in our patient occurred most likely due to the latent reactivation, primary infection or transmission via the renal graft cannot be explicitly excluded. However, no recent TB exposure, or significant travel history was reported.

On readmission to the hospital, and subsequent admission to pulmonary ICU, the patient displayed several symptoms commonly found in GITB, including recurrent fever, weight loss, abdominal pain and anemia. The symptoms of GITB in non-transplant patients constitute abdominal pain, weight loss - even anorexia, fever, anemia and bowel habit change [8, 16]. However, in renal transplant recipients, the most common symptoms of decreased inflammatory response due to the immunosuppressive therapy [1, 8] are GI bleeding accompanied by fever and abdominal pain [1]. Furthermore, the symptoms in renal transplant recipients are also often very vague and sometimes plain unusual. Moreover, GI disorders in transplant recipients are relatively common, and are also associated with immunosuppressive therapy or bacterial, viral or parasitic infection [2, 3]. One of the main adverse effects of mycophenolate mofetil is GI irritation [17]. Together, these are causing an important delay in the diagnosis, contributing to the extremely high mortality of renal transplant recipients with GITB. Some authors reported that the late manifestation of GITB in renal transplant recipients is related mainly to this diagnostic delay because of lack of specific symptoms [18]. Therefore, all GI symptoms in renal transplant recipients, although vague, require diagnostic follow up for GITB, albeit confirming the diagnosis may be challenging. CT may often reveal inflammation, ascites (our patient) and lymphadenopathy (our patient). These unspecific features may lead to alternative diagnoses (neoplasms, inflammation or nontuberculosis bacterial or other viral infections or parasites). The microbiological confirmation is often tricky because of difficulties in obtaining the suitable tissue, low sensitivity of microbiological examination and the protracted time needed for culture [19]. Moreover, in immunosuppressed patients skin anergy is frequent; resulting in negative skin tuberculin tests [20] and endoscopic distinction between GITB and other GI diseases (e.g. Crohn's disease) is difficult. In our patient, tissue specimens obtained from abdominal cavity revealed granulomas with *Mycobacterium*. Six days later, *Mycobacterium tuberculosis* was confirmed by PCR in the sputum. However, CT scan of the lungs revealed no specific lesions, except for atypical right bronchopneumonia. Although we advocate that PCR may be the first line tool in GITB diagnosis, it does not differentiate between an active and latent infection [21]. GITB can coexist with pulmonary involvement; however reports have shown that less than 50% of patients infected with GITB have radiographic evidence of pulmonary disease. A case report of Yilmaz et al. demonstrated renal transplant recipient with GITB, however without X-ray abnormalities [22]. Swallowing of infected sputum in patients with active pulmonary TB belongs to the most common mechanism of GITB origin [23].

In addition, massive intestinal bleeding occurred in line with previous reports showing GI bleeding present in most renal transplant recipients with GITB [1]. As mentioned above, GI bleeding is the most common symptom of posttransplant GITB (in contrast with GITB in a non-transplant population). This could be again due to the decreased inflammatory response because of the immunosuppression; hence the ulcerative disease component is predominant rather than obstructive bowel wall inflammation [1]. Moreover, tissue specimens obtained from the abdominal cavity revealed granuloma, the indicative of tuberculous enteritis, peritonitis, adnexitis and lymphadenitis, which is in line with a previous report [7]. Except for its very late onset, likely due to the low doses of immunosuppressive therapy, and further complications, this case thus represents a typical example of reactivation of latent tuberculosis infection, resulting in GITB with vague abdominal complaints and intestinal bleeding.

Upon observing *Mycobacterium* in tissue obtained from the abdominal cavity, antituberculosis therapy was initiated, consisting of rifampicin, isoniazid, ethambutol and pyrazinamide. However, antituberculosis therapy increases the risk of interactions and toxic hepatitis. Rifampicin is a strong inducer of microsomal enzyme P450 3A4, which leads to increased metabolism of calcineurin-inhibitors, rapamycin and steroids [24]. Rifampicin reduces plasma levels of cyclosporine 2-5 fold and tacrolimus 4-10 fold [1], which increases the risk of rejection [13]. Moreover, common TB medications may lead to interactions with other required drugs, as documented with our case. Therefore, it is strongly recommended to closely monitor and adjust plasma concentrations of drugs, particularly those of the calcineurin-inhibitors, to avoid both toxicity and graft rejection. Therefore mycophenolate mofetil was discontinued for 11 days due to the septic shock (severe infection), while cyclosporine dosage was increased from

25 mg-0-50 mg to 100 mg-0-100 mg. Moreover, our patient's condition was complicated with aspergillosis and *Pseudomonas aeruginosa* infection. Therefore, voriconazole and meropenem was added to the therapeutic regimen. However, low plasma level of voriconazole was found in the plasma of our patient, likely because of the interaction with rifampicin. Thus, the voriconazole doses also had to be adjusted, while rifampicin was discontinued for one day.

During hospitalization, nosocomial infections including anidulafungin resistant *Aspergillus flavus* and *Pseudomonas aeruginosa* occurred. Immunocompromised patients are more vulnerable for nosocomial infections, especially early after transplantation. On day 1 PO mycophenolate mofetil was discontinued, however on day 11 PO was again re-added to the therapeutic regimen. Subsequently, both *Aspergillus flavus* and *Pseudomonas aeruginosa* was confirmed from the sputum on day 16 and 23 PO. *Aspergillus* infection occurs almost exclusively in immunosuppressed hosts [25], and is associated with increased morbidity and mortality among transplant recipients [26]. *Pseudomonas aeruginosa*, a major nosocomial pathogen, belongs to the life-threatening complication after abdominal organ transplantation. The survival rates are significantly lower for patients with hypotension and on mechanical ventilation, and the predictor of mortality related to *Pseudomonas* bacteremia is the onset of bacteremia in the ICU [27]. Furthermore, the multiple nosocomial infections could be related to previous repeated admission to the hospital or to the prolonged ICU stay (>3 days). In order to reduce risk of nosocomial infection in immunocompromised patients, it is necessary to take preventive measures, such as thorough decontamination and hand hygiene, aseptic procedures, or prophylactic antibiotic therapy. Moreover it is important to reduce the infection risk from use of catheters, cannulas, or tubes. Transplant recipients should receive an empirical antibiotic treatment as well as directed therapy adjusted according to the severity of the infection [28].

Our patient's condition was furthermore complicated with severe sepsis with *Staphylococcus haemolyticus* blood culture, septic shock, multiple organ failure including ARDS and acute renal failure requiring mechanical ventilation, vasopressor circulatory support and intermittent hemodialysis. Reports of ARDS associated with TB are not scarce; most studies report ARDS to be caused by pulmonary TB, which is associated with in-hospital mortality rates higher than from non-TB causes (e.g. pneumonia) [10, 29]. ARDS may be very rarely caused by miliary TB [10]. To our best knowledge however, there is no case study investigated posttransplant GITB complicated with ARDS.

Although treatable and very rare, GITB is a potentially lethal complication after solid organ transplantation. Onset of GITB is most commonly about 2 years after transplantation, however in renal transplant recipients, with modest immunosuppressive therapy time to manifestation can be longer (our patient). Diagnosis of GITB is challenging, because symptoms are often vague and atypical and renal graft recipients often display GI symptoms. However, early diagnosis is crucial for successful treatment. Therefore, both GI symptoms and fever at any time after transplantation should trigger active diagnostic workup for GITB, especially in the absence of another confirmed infection. Furthermore, (GI)TB treatment in transplant patients poses specific problems because of interactions between antituberculosis drugs and immunosuppressive therapy, especially when other comorbidities such as aspergillosis need to be treated (our patient). Thus, plasma drug levels need to be closely monitored. In case septic shock occurs (our patient), the immunosuppressive therapy may be discontinued. Moreover, GITB could be complicated with multiple organ failure including ARDS and acute renal failure, which may necessitate mechanical ventilation, vasopressor circulatory support and hemodialysis. Nevertheless, the case currently presented demonstrates that by implementing the above recommendations, survival from GITB complicated by septic shock and multiple organ failure including acute renal injury and ARDS may be accomplished.

Abbreviations

ARDS: Acute respiratory distress syndrome; AST: Aspartate aminotransferase; ATB: Antituberculosis therapy; CIPRO: Ciprofloxacin; CsA: Cyclosporine; CT: Computed tomography; ETH: Ethambutol; FLU: Fluconazole; GCS 3: Glasgow Coma Scale; GITB: Gastrointestinal tuberculosis; Hb: Hemoglobin; HC: Hydrocortisone; HR: Heart rate; Ht: Hematocrit; ICU: Intensive care unit; IS: Immunosuppressive regimen; ISO: Isoniazid; LIN: Linezolid; METRO: Metronidazole; MMF: Mycophenolate mofetil; MP: Methylprednisolone; P/T: Piperacillin/tazobactam; PCR: Polymerase chain reaction; PLT: Platelets; PO: Post-surgery; PTTB: Post-transplant tuberculosis; PYR: Pyrazinamide; RBC: Red blood cells; RIF: Rifampicin; TB: Tuberculosis; TX: Transplantation; VORI: Voriconazole; WBC: White blood cells

Acknowledgements

Not applicable.

Funding

This work was supported by Science Grant Agency (VEGA 1/0223/15 and 1/0247/17), Slovak Republic.

Authors' contributions

AC performed the research. DVY wrote the manuscript and performed analyses. PV wrote the initial draft manuscript. AD performed the research. AG performed the research. ZF performed the research. MAS reviewed and edited the manuscript. RHH reviewed and edited the manuscript. AY reviewed the manuscript and conducted the research. All authors read and approved the final manuscript.

Competing interests
The authors declare that they have no competing interests.

Author details
[1]University Hospital Bratislava, Nemocnica Ruzinov, ICU, KAIM, Clinic of Anesthesiology and Intensive Care Medicine, Faculty of Medicine, Comenius University in Bratislava, Bratislava, Slovakia. [2]Department of Pharmacology and Toxicology, Faculty of Pharmacy, Comenius University in Bratislava, Bratislava, Odbojarov 10, 832 32 Bratislava, Slovakia. [3]Department of Internal Medicine, University of Groningen, University Medical Center Groningen, Groningen, the Netherlands. [4]Department of Clinical Pharmacy and Pharmacology, University of Groningen, University Medical Center Groningen, Groningen, the Netherlands.

References
1. Jarrett O, Grim SA, Benedetti E, Clark NM. Gastrointestinal tuberculosis in renal transplant recipients: case report and review of the literature. Transpl Infect Dis. 2011;13:52–7.
2. Munoz P, Rodriguez C, Bouza E. Mycobacterium tuberculosis infection in recipients of solid organ transplants. Clin Infect Dis. 2005;40:581–7.
3. Singh N, Paterson DL. Mycobacterium tuberculosis infection in solid-organ transplant recipients: impact and implications for management. Clin Infect Dis. 1998;27:1266–77.
4. Chen SY, Wang CX, Chen LZ, Fei JG, Deng SX, Qiu J, Li J, Chen GO, Fu HM, Xie CM. Tuberculosis in southern Chinese renal-transplant recipients. Clin Transpl. 2008;22:780–4.
5. Sundaram M, Adhikary SD, John GT, Kekre NS. Tuberculosis in renal transplant recipients. Indian J Urol. 2008;24:396–400.
6. Karuthu S, Blumberg EA. Common infections in kidney transplant recipients. Clin J Am Soc Nephrol. 2012;7:2058–70.
7. Chan HW, Cheung CY, Chan YH, Chu YY, Lee KC, Chau KF, Li CS. Intestinal tuberculosis as a cause of gastrointestinal bleeding in a renal transplant recipient. Transpl Int. 2010;23:657–60.
8. Horvath KD, Whelan RL. Intestinal tuberculosis: return of an old disease. Am J Gastroenterol. 1998;93:692–6.
9. Nam SJ, Cho YJ. The successful treatment of refractory respiratory failure due to miliary tuberculosis: survival after prolonged extracorporeal membrane oxygenation support. Clin Respir J. 2016;10:393–9.
10. Lee K, Kim JH, Lee JH, Lee WY, Park MS, Kim JY, Kim KC, Lee MG, Jung KS, Kim YS, Shin YM, Koh Y. Acute respiratory distress syndrome caused by miliary tuberculosis: a multicentre survey in South Korea. Int J Tuberc Lung Dis. 2011;15:1099–103.
11. Strunk AK, Ciesek S, Schmidt JJ, Kuhn C, Hoeper MM, Welte T, Kielstein JT. Single- and multiple-dose pharmacokinetics of ethambutol and rifampicin in a tuberculosis patient with acute respiratory distress syndrome undergoing extended daily dialysis and ECMO treatment. Int J Infect Dis. 2016;42:1–3.
12. John GT, Shankar V, Abraham AM, Mukundan U, Thomas PP, Jacob CK. Risk factors for post-transplant tuberculosis. Kidney Int. 2001;60:1148–53.
13. Azevedo P, Freitas C, Silva H, Aguiar P, Farrajota P, Almeida M, Pedroso S, Martins LS, Dias L, Vizcaino JR, Castro HA, Cabrita A. A case series of gastrointestinal tuberculosis in renal transplant patients. Case Rep Nephrol. 2013;2013:213273.
14. Atasever A, Bacakoglu F, Toz H, Basoglu OK, Duman S, Basak K, Guzelant A, Sayiner A. Tuberculosis in renal transplant recipients on various immunosuppressive regimens. Nephrol Dial Transplant. 2005;20:797–802.
15. Liu J, Yan J, Wan Q, Ye Q, Huang Y. The risk factors for tuberculosis in liver or kidney transplant recipients. BMC Infect Dis. 2014;14:387.
16. Zedtwitz-Liebenstein K, Podesser B, Peck-Radosavljevic M, Graninger W. Intestinal tuberculosis presenting as fever of unknown origin in a heart transplant patient. Infection. 1999;27:289–90.
17. Parfitt JR, Jayakumar S, Driman DK. Mycophenolate mofetil-related gastrointestinal mucosal injury: variable injury patterns, including graft-versus-host disease-like changes. Am J Surg Pathol. 2008;32:1367–72.
18. Sikalias N, Alexiou K, Mountzalia L, Triantafyllis V, Efstathiou G, Antsaklis G. Acute adomen in a transplant patient with tuberculous colitis: a case report. Cases J. 2009;2:9305.
19. Niewczas M, Ziolkowski J, Rancewicz Z, Szymanska K, Kwiatkowski A, Galazka T, Senatorski G, Paczek L. Tuberculosis in patients after renal transplantation remains still a clinical problem. Transplant Proc. 2002;34:677–9.
20. Woeltje KF, Mathew A, Rothstein M, Seiler S, Fraser VJ. Tuberculosis infection and anergy in hemodialysis patients. Am J Kidney Dis. 1998;31:848–52.
21. Honore-Bouakline S, Vincensini JP, Giacuzzo V, Lagrange PH, Herrmann JL. Rapid diagnosis of extrapulmonary tuberculosis by PCR: impact of sample preparation and DNA extraction. J Clin Microbiol. 2003;41:2323–9.
22. Yilmaz E, Balci A, Sal S, Cakmakci H. Tuberculous ileitis in a renal transplant recipient with familial Mediterranean fever: gray-scale and power Doppler sonographic findings. J Clin Ultrasound. 2003;31:51–4.
23. Tulczynska JM, Fleischman JK. Abdominal tuberculosis: an unusual cause of abdominal pain. Respir Care. 2010;55:346–9.
24. Finch CK, Chrisman CR, Baciewicz AM, Self TH. Rifampin and rifabutin drug interactions: an update. Arch Intern Med. 2002;162:985–92.
25. Linden E, Restrepo D, Dikman S, Murphy B, Huprikar S. Aspergillus infection limited to renal allograft: case report and review of literature. Transpl Infect Dis. 2006;8:177–81.
26. Atılgan A, Özdemir BH, Kırnap M, Akdur A, Yılmaz Akçay E, Akar Özkan E, Haberal M. Invasive fungal infections in liver transplant recipients. Exp Clin Transplant. 2014;12(Suppl 1):110–6.
27. Su H, Ye Q, Wan Q, Zhou J. Predictors of mortality in abdominal organ transplant recipients with pseudomonas aeruginosa infections. Ann Transplant. 2016;21:86–93.
28. Aguado JM, Silva JT, Fernández-Ruiz M, Cordero E, Fortún J, Gudiol C, Martínez-Martínez L, Vidal E, Almenar L, Almirante B, Cantón R, Carratalá J, Caston JJ, Cercenado E, Cervera C, Cisneros JM, Crespo-Leiro MG, Cuervas-Mons V, Elizalde-Fernández J, Fariñas MC, Gavaldà J, Goyanes MJ, Gutiérrez-Gutiérrez B, Hernández D, Len O, López-Andujar R, López-Medrano F, Martín-Dávila P, Montejo M, Moreno A, Oliver A, Pascual A, Pérez-Nadales E, Román-Broto A, San-Juan R, Serón D, Solé-Jover A, Valerio M, Muñoz P, Torre-Cisneros J. Spanish Society of Transplantation (SET); Group for Study of infection in transplantation of the Spanish Society of Infectious Diseases and Clinical Microbiology (GESITRA-SEIMC); Spanish network for research in infectious diseases (REIPI) (RD16/0016): management of multidrug resistant gram-negative bacilli infections in solid organ transplant recipients: SET/GESITRA-SEIMC/REIPI recommendations. Transplant Rev (Orlando). 2017 Jul 26; doi:10.1016/j.trre.2017.07.001. [Epub ahead of print].
29. Lee PL, Jerng JS, Chang YL, Chen CF, Hsueh PR, Yu CJ, Yang PC, Luh KT. Patient mortality of active pulmonary tuberculosis requiring mechanical ventilation. Eur Respir J. 2003;22:141–7.

18

Case report on pathogenetic link between gluten and IgA nephropathy

Stefano Costa[1], Giovanni Currò[1], Salvatore Pellegrino[1*], Maria Cristina Lucanto[1], Giovanni Tuccari[2], Antonio Ieni[2], Giuseppina Visalli[3], Giuseppe Magazzù[1] and Domenico Santoro[4]

Abstract

Background: A relationship between IgA nephropathy (IgAN) and celiac disease (CD) has been reported. We show the pathogenetic link for the first time.

Case presentation: A 39-year-old man with cystic fibrosis (CF) and CF-related diabetes started to present gross hematuria, back pain and headache. At admission, laboratory analysis showed increase in serum creatinine of 1. 5 mg/dl, together with hematuria and mild proteinuria (1 g/24 h). He underwent a renal biopsy to investigate the cause of hematuria and renal failure. Biopsy was consistent with IgAN. In view of patient reported dyspepsia, an upper gastrointestinal endoscopy with duodenal biopsies was undertaken and was normal. We looked for mucosal deposits of tTG-2 in the duodenum and the renal mesangium. tTG-2 deposits were found both in the duodenum and in renal biopsies, where they topographically replicated mesangial IgA deposits. After one year on a continued gluten containing diet, the patient developed a Marsh 2 type duodenal pathology.

Conclusions: Our findings suggest a connection between CD and IgAN in terms of an immune-mediated gluten-induced pathogenesis even in the absence of villous atrophy and serum celiac autoantibodies.

Keywords: IGA nephropathy, Celiac disease, Tissue transglutaminase, Immunofluorescence technique, Pathogenesis

Background

A relationship between celiac disease and other autoimmune inflammatory disorders is known [1]. With regardto IgA nephropathy (IgAN), some studies report an increased incidence of celiac disease [2] and postulate a role of gluten in the pathogenesis of this disorder [3, 4]. A double immunofluorescence technique to detect intestinal deposits of anti-tissue transglutaminase IgA was successfully performed in patients with dermatitis herpetiformis (DH) [5] and gluten ataxia (GA) [6] showing a link between gluten and these diseases even in absence of duodenal atrophy or positive celiac serology.

We used this technique to detect anti-TG2 in the mesangium and duodenum of a patient with IgAN.

Case presentation

A 39-year-old man with CF and CF-related diabetes came to our Unit due to symptoms of pulmonary exacerbation. At the same time, he started to present gross hematuria, back pain and headache. At admission, laboratory analysis showed increase in serum creatinine of 1.5 mg/dl together with hematuria and mild proteinuria (1 g/24 h). Intravenous antibiotics for pulmonary exacerbation (piperacillin/tazobacatam and colimycin) were started and a renal biopsy performed to investigate the cause of hematuria and renal failure. Biopsy was consistent with IgAN (see Fig. 1d), with morphological features of mesangial and endocapillary hypercellularity (Oxford classification M1, E1, S0, T0) [7] As the patient presented dyspepsia, he was offered upper gastrointestinal endoscopy with duodenal biopsies (one from duodenal bulb and three from descending duodenum). Duodenal mucosa was reported as normal on hematoxylin/eosin stain. While compatible HLA alleles for celiac disease (DQ2) were identified, both serum anti-endomysium (EMA) and anti-tissue transglutaminase antibodies (anti-tTG) were negative. It has been demonstrated that coeliac IgA targets intestinal TG2 early in disease development even when serum celiac autoantibodies are not present. Extraintestinal deposits of coeliac IgA further indicate that

* Correspondence: salvatorepellegrino2014@gmail.com
[1]Celiac Regional Centre, Pediatric Gastroenterology and Cystic Fibrosis Unit, University of Messina, Via Consolare Valeria 1, 98125 Messina, Italy
Full list of author information is available at the end of the article

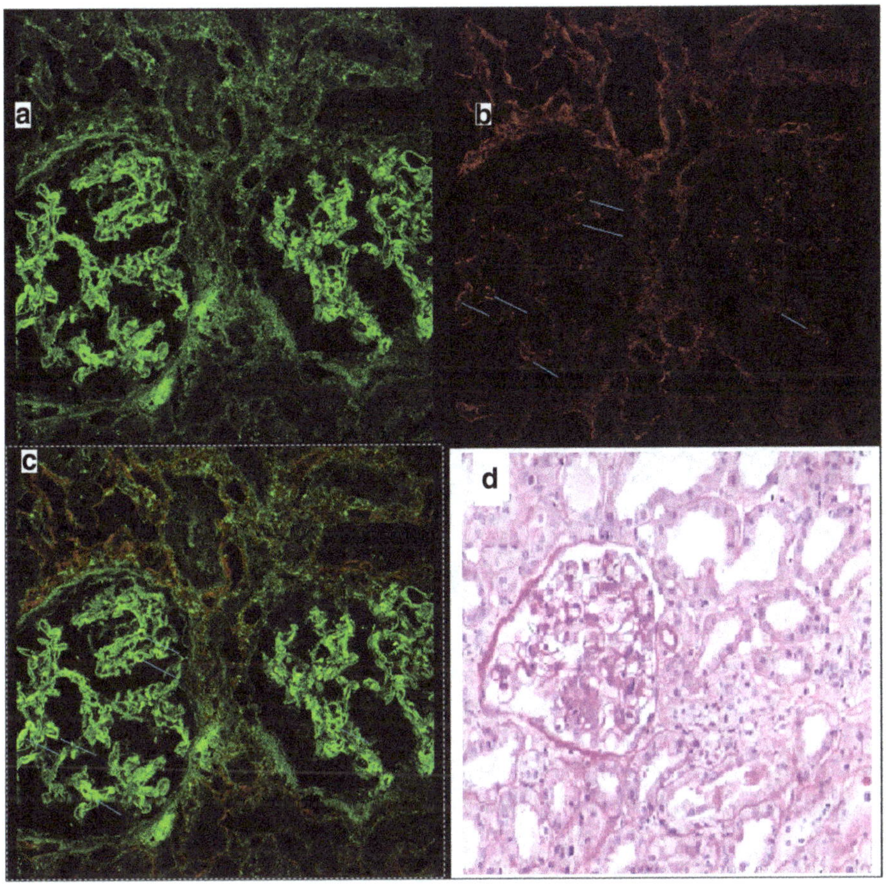

Fig. 1 Renal biopsy. Immunofluorescence (**a**) showing mesangial deposition of IgA in green. In **b**, in red, deposition of TG2. In **c**, the overlap of red and green, in yellow, showing deposition of a-tTG2. The blue lines show the more intense deposition of IgA and TG2. In **d**, hematoxylin/eosin stain of renal biopsy

humoral immunity may have a pathogenetic role [8]. Therefore, double immunofluorescence on duodenal mucosa was performed to detect mucosal deposits of anti-tissue transglutaminase type 2 using the technique described by Karponay-Szabo et al., with some modification [8]. Briefly, 5 μm sections from the duodenal specimen included in optimal cutting temperature (OCT) compound were obtained and stored at – 80° in liquid nitrogen. Sections were fixed in acetone and incubated with Normal Rabbit Serum (Calbiochem Germany) for 20 min to block nonspecific sites. Sections were then incubated with anti-tissue transglutaminase type 2 (anti-tTG-2) from mouse (CUB7402 from Neomarker, Fremont CA) for one hour, and then with secondary antibodies conjugated with fluorochromes to detect total IgA (in green using Polyclonal Rabbit anti-Human IgA/FICT from Dako, Denmark) and anti-tTG-2 (in red using Polyconal Rabbit anti-Mouse RPE F (ab') 2 from Dako, Denmark) for 30 min. The overlap of green and red (yellow) indicates the deposits of anti-tTG2. Analysis was performed on confocal microscopy. The same technique was performed on 5 μm renal sections. In both cases, an overlap of green and red in yellow was seen, thus demonstrating deposits of tTG-2 (Fig. 2a, b and c). In particular, in renal biopsies, deposits of tTG-2 that topographically replicated mesangial deposits of IgA (Fig. 1) were detected.

Given the morphological features of IgAN, and the presence of proteinuria, steroid therapy was started according to a standardized six month's protocol [9]. After one month, proteinuria decreased to 100 mg/24 h and hematuria resolved. Steroids were stopped after six months of treatment. The patient continued on a gluten containing diet.

Considering that intestinal deposits of anti-tissue transglutaminase IgA are predictive of forthcoming enteropathy [10] after one year arepeat upper endoscopy was performed even though anti-tTG were still negative. At this time, a Marsh 2 type duodenal pathology was detected (Fig. 3a, b). A gluten free diet was started (for a complete timeline history see Additional file 1: Table S1).

Discussion and conclusions

To our knowledge, this is the first demonstration of the pathogenetic role of gluten in IgAN. IgAN is a rare complication of CF [11]. In these cases, it is supposed that

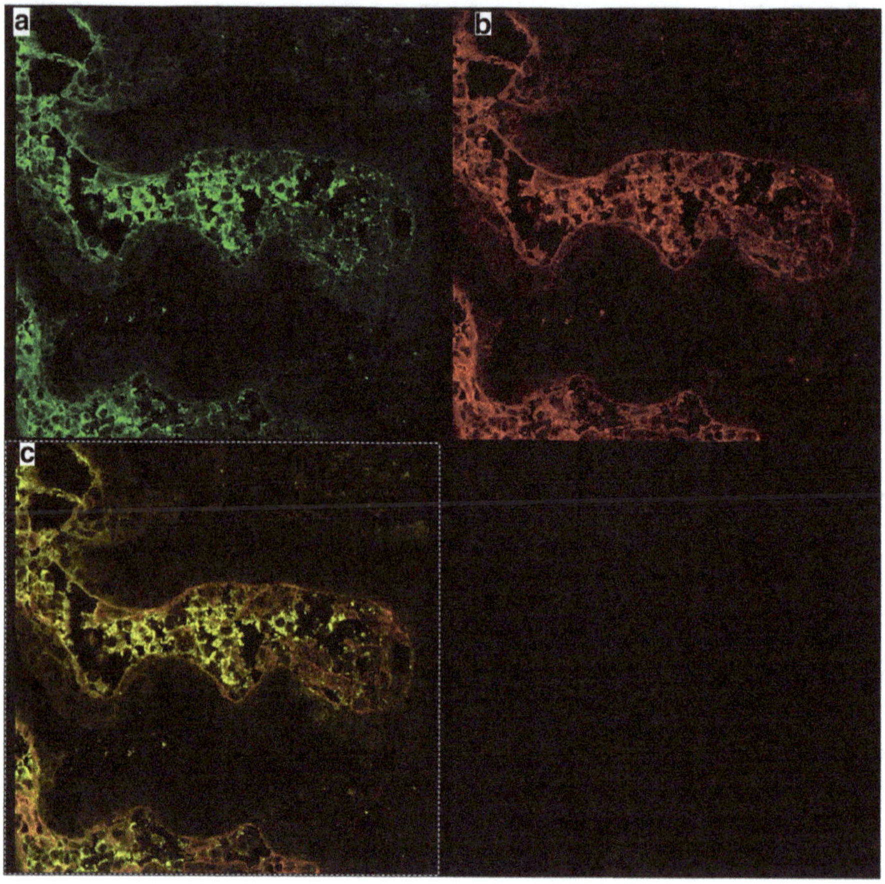

Fig. 2 Duodenal biopsy. In **a**, deposition of IgA is showed in green. In **b**, deposition of TG2 is shown in red. In **c**, in yellow, the overlap of green and red demonstrating the presence of a-tTG2

aninfectious stimulus acts as a trigger. On the other hand, a relationship between CD and IgAN has previously been suggested. In 2002, Collin et al. demonstrated an incidence of 3.6% of biopsy proven CD in IgAN [2]. On the other hand, a recent study demonstrated an increased risk of biopsy-verified IgAN among individuals with CD [12]. Another link between these two diseases is represented by the ability of gliadin to act as a lectin and to form immunocomplexes with IgA1N (oligosaccharide-containing IgA). Coppo et al. were able to induce experimental IgAN in mice immunized with gliadin [3]. The same authors showed a positive effect of a gluten free diet on proteinuria and on progression of renal failure in patients with IgAN. Berthelot et al. showed how activation of transglutaminase 2 is crucial for the deposition of immune-complexes in the mesangium of patients with IgAN [13]. Lechner et al. showed that the removal of IgA deposits by a proteases led to a decrease of TG2 staining thus confirming the presence of the enzyme in mesangial immunocomplexes [14].

In several case reports, an improvement of IgAN is described following a gluten free diet [15–17]. All these cases are characterized by the presence of a biopsy proven CD and in no caseis a contemporary immune activation in intestine and kidney reported before the development of duodenal atrophy.

Our finding can explain how CD and IgAN are related. As we found deposits of IgA anti-tissue transglutaminase both in the duodenum and glomerular mesangium we can argue that an autoimmune activation, triggered by gluten in intestinal mucosa and involving tissue transglutaminase, mayoccur in extraintestinal target sites. This kind of association has been demonstrated in other diseases such as GA and in DH, where the role of gluten is well recognized, and a gluten free diet is beneficial [5, 6]. Duodenal atrophy can be absentalso in these diseases, as auto-antibodies production is directed against specific transglutaminase isotypes represented, in dermis, by isotype 3, and in myelin by isotype 6, in DH and GA, respectively, In particular, in GA a contemporary presence of anti-tTG2 deposits was found in jejunal mucosa and within the muscular layer of brain vessels and brain parenchyma particularly of the cerebellum, regardless of the presence of duodenal atrophy or positive celiac serology.

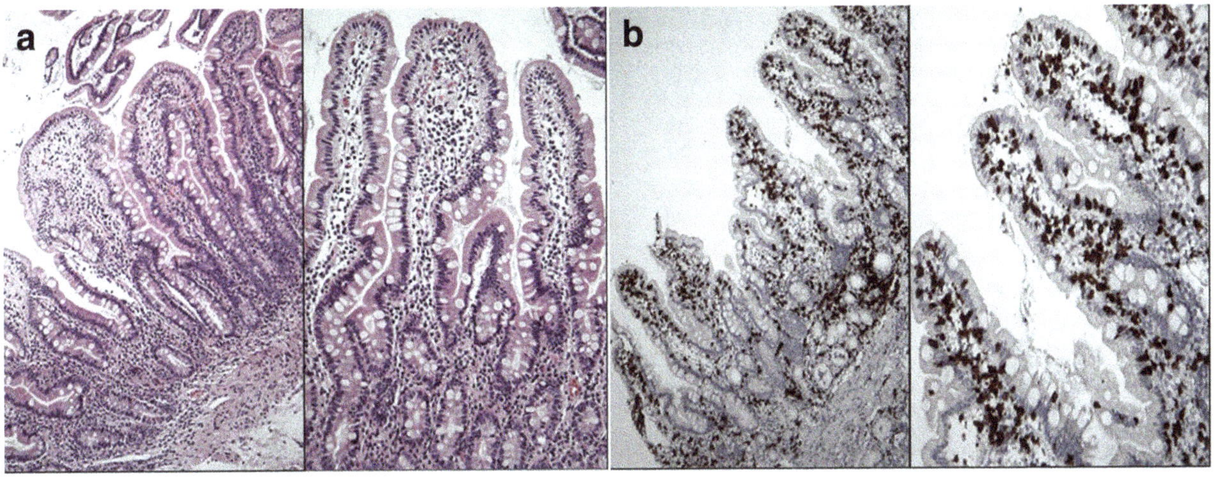

Fig. 3 Duodenal biopsy after one year. In **a**, hematoxylin/eosin stain showing cryptic hyperplasia. In **b**, the CD3 immunostained section for the count of intraepithelial lymphocytes

In our case the strength of pathogeneticassociation between CD and IgAN depends on the diagnostic power of the technique we adopted to detect a gluten dependent immune activation. Duodenal deposits oftTG2 are very sensitive and specific for diagnosis of celiac disease, even in the absence of duodenal atrophy and positive celiac serology [18]. Moreover, Salmi et al. [10] showed how mucosal anti-tTG2 deposits strongly predict forthcoming duodenal atrophy.

Actually, after one year, the patient developed a duodenal pathology, thus confirming that intestinal deposits of anti-tTG2 were the initial manifestation of a gluten driven inflammation. As transglutaminase 2 is the most represented isoform in the mesangium, we suggest that mesangial deposition of anti-tTG-2 may play a determinant role in pathogenesis of the disease even in the absence of other signs suggesting celiac disease.

Our findings suggest an immune-mediated gluten-induced pathogenetic link between CD and IgAN even in the absence of villous atrophy and serum celiac autoantibodies. Searching for mesangial deposits of anti-tTG2 in a large series of new cases of IgAN will allow to define how many cases are caused by this autoimmune mechanism and if a gluten free diet can really improve renal outcome of these patients.

Abbreviations

CD: Celiac disease; CF: Cystic fibrosis; DH: Dermatitis herpetiformis; EMA: Anti-endomysium; GA: Gluten ataxia; IgAN: IgA nephropathy; IgA-tTG: IgA-tissue antitransglutaminase antibodies

Acknowledgements

The authors thank Trays Macdonnell for the English language revision of the article.

Authors' contributions

SC, GC, SP, DS and GM planned the study, analyzed data and drafted the article. MCL, AI, GT and GV gave substantial contributions to conception and design, acquisition and interpretation of data, revising the article critically for important intellectual content. All authors read and approved the final manuscript.

Competing interests

The authors declare that they have no competing interests.

Author details

[1]Celiac Regional Centre, Pediatric Gastroenterology and Cystic Fibrosis Unit, University of Messina, Via Consolare Valeria 1, 98125 Messina, Italy. [2]Department of Human Pathology of Adult and Evolutive Age 'Gaetano Barresi', University of Messina, Messina, Italy. [3]Department of Biomedical and Dental Sciences and Morphofunctional Imaging, University of Messina, Messina, Italy. [4]Department of Clinical and Experimental Medicine, Unit of Nephrology and Dialysis, University of Messina, Messina, Italy

References

1. Ventura A, Magazzù G, Greco L. Duration of exposure to gluten and risk for autoimmune disorders in patients with celiac disease. SIGEP Study Group for Autoimmune Disorders in Celiac Disease. Gastroenterology. 1999;117(2):297–303.
2. Collin P, Syrjänen J, Partanen J, Pasternack A, Kaukinen K, Mustonen J. Celiac disease and HLA DQ in patients with IgA nephropathy. Am J Gastroenterol. 2002;97:2572–6.
3. Coppo R, Amore A, Roccatello D. Dietary antigens and primary immunoglobulin A nephropathy. J Am Soc Nephrol. 1992;2(Suppl 10): S173–80.
4. Papista C, Lechner S, Ben Mkaddem S, LeStang MB, Abbad L, Bex-Coudrat J, Pillebout E, Chemouny JM, Jablonski M, Flamant M, Daugas E, Vrtovsnik F, Yiangou M, Berthelot L, Monteiro RC. Gluten exacerbates IgA nephropathy in humanized micethrough gliadin-CD89 interaction. Kidney Int. 2015;88(2): 276–85.
5. Donaldson MR, Zone JJ, Schmidt LA, Taylor TB, Neuhausen SL, Hull CM, Meyer LJ. Epidermal transglutaminase deposits in perilesional and uninvolved skin in patients with dermatitis herpetiformis. J Invest Dermatol. 2007;127:1268–71.
6. Hadjivassiliou M, Mäki M, Sanders DS, Williamson CA, Grünewald RA, Woodroofe NM, Korponay-Szabó IR. Autoantibody targeting of brain and intestinal transglutaminase in gluten ataxia. Neurology. 2006;66:373–7.
7. Eitner F, Floege J. Glomerular disease: the Oxford classification–predicting progression of IgAN. Nat Rev Nephrol. 2009;5:557–9.
8. Korponay-Szabo IR, Halttunen T, Szalai Z, Laurila K, Kirly R, Kovács JB, Fésüs L, Mäki M. In vivo targeting of intestinal and extraintestinal transglutaminase 2 by coeliac autoantibodies. Gut. 2004;53:641–8.

9. Pozzi C, Andrulli S, Del Vecchio L, Melis P, Fogazzi GB, Altieri P, Ponticelli C, Locatelli F. Corticosteroid effectiveness in IgA nephropathy: long-term results of a randomized, controlled trial. J Am Soc Nephrol. 2004;15:157–63.
10. Salmi TT, Collin P, Järvinen O, Haimila K, Partanen J, Laurila K, Korponay-Szabo IR, Huhtala H, Reunala T, Mäki M, Kaukinen K. Immunoglobulin Aautoantibodies against transglutaminase 2 in the small intestinal mucosa predict forthcoming coeliac disease. Aliment Pharmacol Ther. 2006;24(3):541–52.
11. Yahiaoui Y, Jablonski M, Hubert D, Mosnier-Pudar H, Noël L, Stern M, Grenet D, Grűnfeld JP, Chauveau D, Fakhouri F. Renal involvement in cystic fibrosis: diseases spectrum and clinical relevance. Clin J Am Soc Nephrol. 2009;4:921–8.
12. Welander A, Sundelin B, Fored M, Ludvigsson JF. Increased risk of IgA nephropathy among individuals with celiac disease. J Clin Gastroenterol. 2013;47:678–83.
13. Berthelot L, Papista C, Maciel TT, Biarnes-Pelicot M, Tissandie E, Wang PH, Tamouza H, Jamin A, Bex-Coudrat J, Gestin A, Boumediene A, Arcos-Fajardo M, England P, Pillebout E, Walker F, Daugas E, Vrtosvnik F, Flamant M, Benhamou M, Cogné M, Moura IC, Monteiro RC. Transglutaminase is essential for IgA nephropathydevelopment acting through IgA receptors. J Exp Med. 2012;209(4):793–806.
14. Lechner SM, Abbad L, Boedec E, Papista C, Le Stang MB, Moal C, Maillard J, Jamin A, Bex-Coudrat J, Wang Y, Li A, Martini PG, Monteiro RC, Berthelot L. IgA1 protease treatment reverses mesangial deposits and hematuria in a model of IgA Nephropathy. J Am Soc Nephrol. 2016;27(9):2622–9.
15. Koivuviita N, Tertti R, Heiro M, Metsärinne K. A case report: a patient withIgA nephropathy and coeliac disease. Complete clinical remission followinggluten-free diet. NDT Plus. 2009;2(2):161–3.
16. La Villa G, Pantaleo P, Tarquini R, Cirami L, Perfetto F, Mancuso F, Laffi G. Multiple immune disorders in unrecognized celiac disease: a case report. World J Gastroenterol. 2003;9(6):1377–80.
17. Woodrow G, Innes A, Boyd SM, Burden RP. A case of IgA nephropathy with celiac disease responding to a gluten-free diet. Nephrol Dial Transplant. 1993;8(12):1382–3.
18. Kaukinen K, Peräaho M, Collin P, Partanen J, Woolley N, Kaartinen T, Nuutinen T, Halttunen T, Mäki M, Korponay-Szabo I. Small-bowel mucosal transglutaminase2-specific IgA deposits in coeliac disease without villous atrophy: a prospectiveand randomized clinical study. Scand J Gastroenterol. 2005;40(5):564–72.

Rate and determinants of non-adherence to a gluten-free diet and nutritional status assessment in children and adolescents with celiac disease in a tertiary Brazilian referral center

Maraci Rodrigues[1*], Glauce Hiromi Yonamine[2] and Carla Aline Fernandes Satiro[2]

Abstract

Background: Compliance with a gluten-free diet (GFD) is difficult at all ages but particularly for teenagers due to social, cultural, economic, and practical pressures. The multidisciplinary team responsible for the treatment of patients with celiac disease and give support to their parents plays a special role on strengthening GFD and assessing the nutritional and physical health.

Methods: A cross-sectional and retrospective study including patients under 20 years of age, with biopsy-confirmed CD, followed regularly at the Department of Pediatrics, Division of Gastroenterology, *Hospital das Clínicas*, University of Sao Paulo, School of Medicine, Sao Paulo, Brazil, were surveyed using a questionnaire and serologic test applied between November 2011 and February 2012. A retrospective chart review of these patients was performed to collect the anthropometric data along with the results of the serologic test performed at the time of diagnosis and after at least 1 year of treatment with a GFD.

Results: We evaluated 35 patients aged between 2.4 and 19.9 years. Of these 68.6% were female, 88.6% had the typical form of the disease and 51.4% had other comorbidities. The mean age at diagnosis was 5.4 years. Despite dietary guidance, 20% reported non-adherence to the diet. Most children recovered the weight and height deficit after 5 years of treatment, and in some children, excessive weight gain became a concern.

Conclusion: The majority of transgressions occurred intentionally at home or at parties. There was a risk of excessive weight gain, especially in the first two years of treatment. More alternatives and easier access to low cost gluten-free foods, increasing the discussion about the benefits of adhering to a GFD among patients, families, and the general population, besides the acquisition of self-management skills, are crucial to fostering independent children and adolescents who have the knowledge and tools to manage life with CD.

Keywords: Celiac disease, Nutritional status, Gluten-free diet

* Correspondence: maraci@uol.com.br
[1]Department of Gastroenterology, Hospital das Clínicas, School of Medicine, University of Sao Paulo (SMUSP), Av. Dr Eneas de Carvalho Aguiar, 255, 05403-000, Sao Paulo, Brazil
Full list of author information is available at the end of the article

Background

Celiac disease is now defined as a genetically predisposed systemic autoimmune condition characterized by the presence of a variable combination of gluten-dependent enteropathy, other clinical manifestations, and CD-specific antibodies such as anti-tissue transglutaminase antibodies 2 (TG2-IgA and TG2-IgG) and anti-endomysial antibodies (EMAs) [1] . The disease occurs in individuals carrying the HLA class II DQ2 or DQ8 allelic variants haplotype and is characterized by an inflammatory enteropathy with various degrees of severity, and a wide range of gastrointestinal and extraintestinal symptoms and signs [1]. CD can reach far beyond the intestine and has been associated with many non-gastrointestinal signs and symptoms such as dermatitis herpetiformis, short stature, osteoporosis, iron deficiency anemia, arthritis, headaches, fatigue, liver function abnormalities, myalgias, adverse pregnancy outcomes, tooth enamel defects, and others [2]. A strong association with autoimmune conditions such as type 1 diabetes mellitus has been observed, and it has been linked with some congenital disorders, such as IgA deficiency and Down syndrome [2] . This pathology is considered a major public health problem because of its high prevalence worldwide. Studies from the United States and Europe estimated that the mean prevalence of CD in the general population is approximately 1%, with some regional differences. A similar disease prevalence has been found in other countries mostly populated by European descendants [3].

In Brazil, the prevalence of biopsy-confirmed CD in apparently healthy volunteer blood donors ranged from 1:214 to 1:286 in Sao Paulo city [4, 5] 1:273 in Sao Paulo countryside [6], 1:417 in southern Brazil [7] and 1:681 in Brasilia [8] . These preliminary results support the view that CD is not a rare disease in Brazil.

Currently, the treatment of CD is based on lifelong exclusion of wheat, rye and barley [9], oats (because in Brazil oats may be contaminated with gluten), and other gluten-containing food products from the diet.

Adherence to a GFD is crucial not only for intestinal mucosal recovery and alleviation of symptoms, but also for the prevention of complications such as anemia, osteoporosis fractures and small-bowel lymphoma [9].

Compliance with a GFD is difficult at all ages but particularly for teenagers due to social, cultural, economic, and practical pressures. At this age group, the diet may be a psychological and social challenge. Occasions such as birthday parties, sleepovers, eating out, and even snack time at school can be difficult to be managed. A survey among college students with CD revealed that they were motivated to adhere to the diet but they experienced challenges related to dining services and social meetings [10].

The strategies required for a GFD to be successful must include education for the patient, family and all those involved with the patient (e.g. healthcare team and school) regarding product ingredients, labeling all gluten-free flours, having snacks on hand at school or work, and bringing gluten-free foods to social events [11]. With regard to parental knowledge, there is the need for clinicians and healthcare professionals to provide better education and more efficient counseling about gluten-free products for parents [12].

Although evidence-based recommendations for follow-up of pediatric patients with CD have not yet been established, some experts advise a yearly follow-up visit and monitoring of dietary compliance, with evaluation of the improvement in symptoms and signs, and analysis for biochemical and serologic markers of CD and screening for associated autoimmune thyroiditis [13].

Therefore, the aims of this study were to examine the rate and determinants of non-adherence to a GFD, as well as the dietary habits and nutritional status of children and adolescents diagnosed with CD at a tertiary referral center.

Methods

This was a cross-sectional and retrospective study, and included 35 patients with CD who attended a medical consultation, conducted in the Pediatric Gastroenterology Outpatient Clinic of the Department of Pediatrics, SMUSP, Sao Paulo, Brazil, between November 2011 and February 2012. These patients were children and adolescents with confirmed diagnosis according to the CD consensus of 2012 [14]:

1.Typical or atypical manifestations or belonging to a group at risk for CD;

2.Positive serology (TG2 IgA, EMAs, or TG2 IgG if hypogammaglobulinemia IgA was diagnosed) or presence of human histocompatibility antigen genes (HLA) class II DQ2 or DQ8 allelic variants;

3. Confirmation of the diagnosis by duodenal biopsy, from the bulb (at least one biopsy) and from the second and third portion of the duodenum (at least four biopsies), and grading according to marsh-Oberhuber [15].

The celiac follow-up visits were defined as attending a medical appointment that addressed CD and documented symptoms associated with CD, GFD compliance, and/or CD serologies.

The medical team included pediatric gastroenterologists, nutritionists and social assistants to assess each child and teenage carrier of CD, and their parents, in relation to symptoms, nutritional status, education, adherence and social difficulties associated with adhering to a GFD.

Patients younger than 1 year or older than 20 years and those who did not attend the consultation and/or with whom contact was not possible because of obsolete phone numbers were excluded. Two patients did not agree to participate in the study.

Data were collected using a questionnaire constructed for this study comprising two open questions on social events and difficulties with the GFD, and closed questions about food routine (home, school, parties, travel), awareness, adherence and difficulties regarding the GFD.

This questionnaire was applied by trained professionals. Parents of patients younger than 13 years of age were instructed to complete the survey with their child. Adolescents older than 13 years of age were asked to complete the survey themselves, during the appointment. The questionnaire are presented in Additional file 1.

Additional information was obtained from medical records, including associated diseases, laboratory tests and anthropometric assessment at the time of diagnosis, 1, 2 and 5 years after diagnosis.

The anthropometric data of weight and height were measured during the medical consultation, on the day of application of the questionnaire. Weight was measured on digital scales, with accuracy to 100 g, while the patient was barefoot and in his underwear. Height was measured using a horizontal stadiometer in children under 2 years of age and a vertical stadiometer in children above this age.

The anthropometric data of weight, height and body mass index (BMI) were expressed as Z scores using the World Health Organization (WHO) multicentre growth reference study group [16].

The laboratory tests were performed according to the reference laboratory of SMUSP.

Ethics approval and consent to participate

This project was approved by the Research Ethics Committee (REC) and the Ethics Committee for review of research projects (CAPPesq) under the number 829/11.

Patients (above 16 years of age), parents or legal guardians (in the case of children under 16) only participated in the study after signing the informed consent, which provided information on the goals of the study and other relevant information.

Permission to conduct the study was sought from relevant ethical committees at Department of Pediatric, Instituto da Criança, Hospital das Clinicas, São Paulo, Brazil. All patients were entered into the study after a written informed consent, either given by the patients themselves or their guardians in the case where patients were not able to.

Statistics

All data were coded in numerical form. The data tabulation and analysis were performed using Microsoft Excel, Epi Info, version 6.04, and the Statistical Package for the Social Sciences, version 13.0 (SPSS Inc. Chicago, IL, USA).

Fisher's exact test was the statistical test used to determine if there were nonrandom associations between two categorical variables, and McNemar's test was used to compare paired proportions. Significance was defined as $P < 0.05$.

Results

Characterization of the population

Were included a total of 35 patients, aged from 2.4 to 19.9 years (mean: 10.77, standard deviation: 4.16 and median: 11 years); 68.6% were female. In most cases (51.35%), the questionnaires were answered by the patient's mother (Table 1).

Patients or their family considered their health to be good, very good or great (91.4%) when compared to other people of the same age without the disease.

About 51.4% of respondents had another disease besides CD, the most cited were: diabetes mellitus type 1 23% (n = 8), asthma 14% (n = 5), and rhinitis and epilepsy 11.5% (both with four cases).

The majority of patients (91.4%) did not have knowledge about CD before diagnosis, and 93.8% reported that they had been suffering from symptoms characteristic of the disease (mainly diarrhea) for about 23.6 months before diagnosis (DP: 24 months).

Dietary treatment

Most patients consumed meat, milk, fruit and vegetables on a daily basis, as per Table 2.

When at school, 48% (n = 24) of the patients brought a snack from home, 18% (n = 9) bought lunch. When the option was to purchase food at school, the favorites were: cheese bread (25.7%),wich is very popular in Brazil and it is made with cassava flour and cheese, snacks (22.9%), soda (14.3%); and 69.2% did not receive GFD at school.

All patients were instructed to follow a restricted diet, but 20% (n = 7) reported that they did not avoid gluten at all times. The latter presented a positive EMAs result.

Factors cited as justifications for transgressions were the high cost of a GFD (n = 2; 15.4%), the low acceptance of these foods (n = 2; 15.4%), lack of choice (n = 1; 7.7%), visiting friends (n = 1; 7.7%), and voluntary choice (n = 7; 53.8%).

Transgressions occurred at parties (n = 12; 23.5%), home (n = 11; 21.6%), school (n = 10; 19.6%), while shopping (n = 8; 15.7%), with friends (n = 7; 13.7%), and while traveling (n = 3; 5.9%). A total of 51.9% claimed that the transgressions were intentional and 63.3% reported having symptoms after the transgressions, primarily diarrhea (41.4%) and abdominal pain (41.4%).

Table 1 Characteristics of the population

Features	N	%
Gender		
Boys	24	68.6
Girls	11	31.4
Age group		
2–5 years	5	14.3
5–12 years	15	42.9
> 12 < 19.9 years	15	42.9
Manifestation of the disease		
Typical	31	88.6
Atypical	4	11.4
Age at diagnosis		
0–2 years	8	22.9
2–5 years	9	25.7
5–12 years	14	40
> 12 years	0	0
No response	4	11.4
Time of disease		
0–2 years	8	22.9
2–4 years	5	14.3
4–6 years	4	11.4
6–8 years	4	11.4
8–10 years	3	8.6
> 10 years	6	17.1
No response	5	14.3
Monthly income		
Up to 1 minimum wage	9	25.7
Up to 2 minimum wage	13	37.1
Up to 3 minimum wage	7	20
> 3 minimum wage	6	17.1
Number of residents in the house		
1–3	8	22.9
4–6	25	71.4
> 7	1	2.9
No response	1	2.9

Table 2 Food profile of patients with celiac disease

	Meat	Milk	Fruit	Greens and vegetables
Daily	62.9%	91.4%	62.9%	54.3%
2 to 4 times a week	37.1%	8.6%	31.4%	37.1%
Does not consume	–		5.7%	8.6%

The frequency of flatulence was higher in the group that did not strictly adhere to the diet ($p = 0.083$).

When asked about their behavior at parties and social events, the majority reported taking food from home to avoid eating food containing gluten, while 62.8% of patients stated that they never attended events due to their disease. See Table 3.

Gluten-free recipes were prepared by 88.6% of the patients and/or their guardians, and 41.9% prepared special recipes three times a week. The main recipes with satisfactory sensory characteristics, according to the patients, were: cakes (80%) and pies (20%). Bread (20%) and pancakes (8.57%) were considered to have less satisfactory sensory characteristics. The flours mostly used as a substitute for gluten were: corn starch, corn flour and potato starch. All patients reported buying gluten-free foods in conventional supermarkets ($n = 30$) and specialist shops ($n = 26$).

Meals outside the home were eaten a few times per month by 45.7% of the patients, mainly in restaurants and coffee shops.

When asked about difficulties related to adhering to the treatment of celiac disease, 37.1% had no difficulty, 25.7% little difficulty, and 20% average difficulty, while 17.1% found it very difficult. The majority of patients (74.3%) were able to talk with ease about celiac disease, but a significant percentage, either disliked or were ashamed of talking about it, 17.1% and 14.3% respectively. All claimed to know about the risks of non-adherence to the diet and to know that dietary treatment would be lifelong.

There was no association between diet transgression and gender form of presentation of the disease, eating habits, behaviors in relation to food in school and social events or knowledge about the disease.

Nutritional evaluation

Out of the 35 patients, 27 had anthropometric data of diagnosis, enabling an assessment of nutritional evolution. The remaining patients were diagnosed in another service or did not have this data in their chart.

At the time of diagnosis 4 children were classified as having a nutritional deficit according to their BMI/age, either being underweight or extremely underweight but

Table 3 Behavior of patients with celiac disease at parties and social events

Behavior at parties	%
Takes food from home	65.7%
Ashamed and does not attend	11.4%
Only eats permitted foods	5.7%
Does not eat	8.6%
Infringes the GFD	5.7%

this index improved considerably during treatment; no child had a weight deficit at the end of the study.

In the same way, when the children were evaluated in accordance with their stature/age i.e. the number of children with a height deficit decreased during treatment.

The number of children who were overweight or obese increased throughout the follow-up of these patients. See Tables 4 and 5.

There was no difference in the nutritional parameters (BMI/age and stature/age) between patients who reported transgression of the diet and those who demonstrated adherence to treatment.

It was also assessed the laboratory tests of these patients, and the main change was the EMAs, with about 28 patients with a positive result. The results of this blood tests were not statistically different over time.

Discussion

This study demonstrated that 20% of evaluated patients did not adhere completely to the GFD. The reasons for transgressions were related to the GF products (high cost, low palatability and lack of availability), social events with friends and voluntary choice. Surprisingly, the nutritional parameters were not influenced by the adherence to the diet. Probably, the transgression of the GFD was not high enough to compromise the weight gain and growth of the patients.

Our sample was small compared with some previous studies [12, 17–23], but larger than in others [24, 25], because our study was conducted in a single center and included only patients with regular outpatient gastroenterologist visits in the period between November 2011 and February 2012.

The majority of our patients were women (68.6%), which was consistent with other studies, in which a slight predominance of females was observed [12, 17–20, 22, 24, 26].

The mean age of the 35 children included in this study was 10.77 years and the median was 11 years; they were older than in some studies [17, 22, 25] and younger than in other studies [12, 19, 20, 24].

In our study, the genre and clinical presentation of celiac disease at diagnosis had no effect on adherence. This is consistent with several other studies [12, 18, 22], but contrasts with others [27], in which adherence was better in girls than in boys.

In our study, the adherence of adolescents (older than 13 years of age) to a GFD was particularly low while dining at restaurants, maybe due to lack of easy availability of GF foods outside the home or peer pressure when dining out, as in other studies [12, 18, 19, 21]. In the Ljungman and Myrdal study [27], they stratified the adolescents' ages and observed that the adherence was better in younger adolescents aged 12 to 14 years old than in older adolescents aged 15 to 17 years old, probably because the latter group had greater social exposure than the former.

In our study the majority (93.8%) of patients reported that they had suffered from symptoms of the disease for about 23.6 months before diagnosis (DP: 24 months), similar to the time span reported in another study [12], and longer than in others [17, 18, 22, 26].

In our series, most of the children had typical symptoms of CD (88.6%), which was consistent with the study by Charalampopoulos et al. [12] but higher than in other studies [17, 18, 22, 26]. Our findings also contrast with those of Munoz et al. [24], who reported that children with atypical symptoms before diagnosis and patients with screening diagnosis by serologic testing had a higher rate of transgression than children with typical symptoms.

Other studies reported similar reasons, regarding to the availability of GF foods and costs as the most significant barriers to adherence to a GFD [24, 28].

In contrast as described previously [18], in our study there was not an association between non-adherence and environment. Our study also agree with others studies [19, 29] that most CD patients on a GFD, specially teenagers, found it easier to adhere to the diet at home and school than when out in social situations. Our study found that the most transgressions did not occur only at friends′ house and birthday parties, but also at home and school, as reported by Munoz et al. [24].

In our patients, as well as in other study [30], when asked about the behavior at parties and social events,

Table 4 Nutritional status of patients with celiac disease according to the body mass index for age (BMI/age)

	At time of diagnosis	1 year	2 years	5 years	Current
Extremely underweight	2	0	0	0	0
Underweight	2	0	1	0	0
Eutrophy	18	16	8	9	19
Risk of overweight	2	4	3	0	2
Overweight	2	3	2	0	4
Obesity	1	2	2	2	2
Total	27	25	16	11	27

Table 5 Stature for age of patients with celiac disease at diagnosis and over time

	At time of diagnosis	1 year	2 years	5 years	Current
Very short stature for age	4	3	2	1	1
Short stature for age	5	4	2	1	3
Appropriate stature for age	18	18	12	9	22
Total	27	25	16	11	26

the majority reported that successful diet adherence strategies included planning ahead and taking their own food to social events to avoid meals containing gluten.

Most patients in our study found the GFD relatively easy to follow, were comfortable talking about their disease and realized that they would need to follow a GFD for entire life. This results differs from that reported by Bravo & Munoz [24] reported that 70% found the diet hard to follow, 55% had difficulty following the diet, 42.8% were not sure what they could eat, and 51.5% reported that the GFD was causing financial distress in the family.

In respect of involuntary transgression, it is worth mentioning the possibility of occurring with the acquisition of cheese bread outside the home (cited by nine patients) as this may be contaminated with other gluten foods produced and served alongside the bread. In addition, despite reporting adherence to the diet, the positive EMAs results in 28/35 patients indicate unintentional transgression.

Error or mistake was also cited in the literature as a reason for transgressions. In Brazil the law requires that all processed products show the information "contains" or "does not contain gluten", and even with disbelief in some information on the label, it facilitates the purchase of industrial products. However, errors or mistakes often happen with ready-to-eat products, consumed in cafes, restaurants and while traveling, so it is important that patients and families are able to cope with these situations. In this study, 48.1% of patients report that the transgression was not intentional, but rather due to the lack of adequate information about the preparation of food.

Similar to our results, several studies have found that patients found it particularly difficult to adhere to a GFD when dining out or at social events, due to variability in the availability of GFD foods or cross-contamination with gluten.

As our study, the higher price of gluten free products is a point of great concern, and several studies from North America and Europe have demonstrated that the cost of GFD food products is significantly higher than that of gluten-containing foods [31–33].

Similar to our results, Tapsas et al. [20] reported different symptoms after incidental intake of gluten, including abdominal pain (64.8%), vomiting (33.3%), and diarrhea (24.1%). They found that in two-thirds of the children in their study, symptoms were noticed soon after consumption, that is, during the first 3 h. No correlation was found between the amount of accidental gluten intake and the time of symptom onset. Some patients, however, experienced symptoms later, that is, after more than 24 h.

Dietary adherence has been the subject of several investigations in pediatric CD and these studies have varied with respect to sample size and method of assessment of adherence. Measures used to assess adherence included self-report, interview, dietary record, and biossay methods, and each measure has its strengths and limitations. Available methods are insufficiently accurate to identify occasional gluten exposure that may cause intestinal mucosal damage. Serological tests are highly sensitive and specific for diagnosis, but do not predict recovery and are not useful for follow-up. Serial endoscopy is invasive and impractical for frequent monitoring, and dietary interview can be subjective [10]. The detection of gluten immunogenic peptides in feces and urine as new non-invasive biomarkers of gluten intake has been suggested, but requires further investigation [34].

In our study, the overall rate of adherence was 80%, as measured by questionnaire and serologic testing. Another Brazilian study conducted by ACELBRA (Brazilian Celiac Association) [35] found that 29.5% of patients reported transgressions in their diet, a higher percentage than the present study. The rates of adherence to GFD in the literature vary from 39% to 79%, depending on factors including self-reporting, laboratory testing and prediagnosis symptoms [12, 18, 19, 36–39]. Some of the studies, despite the small sample, illustrated that non-adherence to GFD is related to poorer bone health [36, 37], shorter stature [37]. Parent report adherence via interview was higher than bioassay data [38] tTG antibodies were significantly more sensitive at identifying occasional non-adherence than EMAs data [39]. Younger age at diagnosis, currently being a teenager, and current symptoms were associated with non-adherence [18]. There was a relationship between compliance, children's age and perceived parental knowledge [12]. Younger age at diagnosis and shorter duration since the diagnosis were associated with a better adherence rate [22].

Our study did not compare the potential difference in diet adherence when questionnaires were filled in by adolescents or by their parents, or if the CD education program for parents and caregivers of celiac patients improved adherence to GFD rate. In our service all the family and responsible for celiac patients receive education about CD routinely.

It has been reported that parents could give us a false picture of the children's compliance with the GFD [12, 40] On the other hand, other authors reported that the perceived parental knowledge was also independently and significantly associated with dietary compliance [12].

We would like to strengthen the importance of the education on CD and the adherence of a GFD not only to the pediatric patients but also to the family and all those involved with the patient to achieve the adherence to a strict lifelong gluten-free diet (GFD).

In our study, children and adolescents recovered their nutritional status after starting treatment, with a significant increase in the proportion of overweight patients over the years. There was no statistical relationship between adherence to treatment and nutritional status, which result was in agreement with other study [41]. They also reported that children who did not adhere to the GFD had lower values of the Z-score of stature/age in comparison with children who adhered to the GFD; 5.9% of children were overweight, which was lower than found in our study.

Other study which reported nutritional status [26], found that almost 19% of patients had an elevated BMI at diagnosis (12.6% overweight, 6% obese) and 74.5% presented with a normal BMI. Seventy-five percent of patients with an elevated BMI at diagnosis decreased their BMI Z-score significantly after adherence to a GFD, normalizing it in 44% of cases. Of patients with a normal BMI at diagnosis, weight Z-scores increased significantly after treatment, and 13% became overweight. In this study, a GFD may have a beneficial effect upon the BMI of overweight and obese children with CD. Other aspect about nutrition and CD was observed in other study [25] which reported that children with CD had high intakes of fiber, and foods with a high glycemic index, and glycemic load, and lower folate content than controls. This has implications for dietary counseling in this population.

The limitations of our study were the sample size and the lack of complete data regarding nutritional evolution, which may have interfered in the absence of association between transgression and other variables, including nutritional status. The retrospective analysis of medical records and questionnaires may involve registration and memory bias, respectively, which may influence the accuracy of the results.

Conclusion

In this study, a fifth of the patients was voluntarily transgressing the GFD, mainly because of the high cost, lack of availability and poor palatability related to the diet. Possibly, part of the children in sample is also involuntarily eating gluten, as observed by the positivity of the serologic tests. There was a catch-up growth in patients with nutritional deficit and a risk of excessive weight gain during follow-up. The early diagnosis and continuous education, with a multidisciplinary clinical care model, is essential to promote adherence to the diet.

Abbreviations

ACELBRA: Brazilian Celiac Association; BMI: Body mass index; CAPPesq: Ethics Committee for review of research projects; CD: Celiac disease; EMAs: Anti-endomysial antibodies; GFD: Gluten-free diet; HLA: Human histocompatibility antigen genes; REC: Research Ethics Committee; SMUSP: School of Medicine, University of Sao Paulo; SPSS: Statistical Package for the Social Sciences; TG2-IgA: Transglutaminase antibodies 2; WHO: World Health Organization

Acknowledgements

We are grateful to all the patients who participated in this study.

All the authors have read this manuscript and approved the submission for publication. All authors fulfill the criteria given in the authorship defined by your journal. All author concor with the submittion and none of the data have been previously reported or are under consideration for publication elsewhere.

No conflict of interest exists for any of the authors.

Funding

No funding was recieved.

Authors´ contributions

MR: coordinated and designed the study, participated in analysis and interpretation of data, wrote and finalized the manuscript. CAS: participated in the collection, writing and interpretation of data. GHY: participated in the collection, writing and interpretation of data. All authors read and approved the final version of the manuscript.

Competing interests

The authors declare that they have no competing interests.

Author details

[1]Department of Gastroenterology, Hospital das Clínicas, School of Medicine, University of Sao Paulo (SMUSP), Av. Dr Eneas de Carvalho Aguiar, 255, 05403-000, Sao Paulo, Brazil. [2]Department of Pediatric, Instituto da Criança, Division of Nutrition, Hospital das Clínicas, School of Medicine, University of Sao Paulo (SMUSP), Sao Paulo, Brazil.

References

1. Fasano A, Araya M, Bhatnagar S, Cameron D, Catassi C, Dirks M, Mearin ML, Ortigosa L, Phillips A; Celiac Disease Working Group, FISPGHAN. Federation Of international societies of pediatric gastroenterology, hepatology, and nutrition consensus report on celiac disease. J Pediatr Gastroenterol Nutr 2008;47(2):214–219.

2. Leffler DA, Green PHR, Fasano A. Extraintestinal manifestations of coeliac disease. Nat Rev Gastroenterol Hepatol. 2015;12:561–71.
3. Catassi C, Gatti S, Lionetti E. World perspective and celiac disease epidemiology. Dig Dis. 2015;33(2):141–6.
4. Oliveira RP, Sdepanian VL, Barreto JA, Cortez AJ, Carvalho FO, Bordin JO, de Camargo Soares MA, da Silva Patrício FR, Kawakami E, de Morais MB, Fagundes-Neto U. High prevalence of celiac disease in Brazilian blood donor volunteers based on screening by IgA antitissue transglutaminase antibody. Eur J Gastroenterol Hepatol. 2007;19(1):43–9.
5. Alencar ML, Ortiz-Agostinho CL, Nishitokukado L, Damião AO, Abrantes-Lemos CP, Leite AZ, Td B, Chamone Dde A, Silva ME, Giannella-Neto D, Sipahi AM. Prevalence of celiac disease among blood donors in São Paulo: the most populated city in Brazil. Clinics (Sao Paulo). 2012;67(9):1013–8.
6. Melo SB, Fernandes MI, Peres LC, Troncon LE, Galvão LC. Prevalence and demographic characteristics of celiac disease among blood donors in Ribeirão Preto, state of São Paulo, Brazil. Dig Dis Sci. 2006;51(5):1020–5.
7. Pereira MA, Ortiz-Agostinho CL, Nishitokukado I, Sato MN, Damião AO, Alencar ML, Abrantes-Lemos CP, Cançado EL, de Brito T, Ioshii SO, Valarini SB, Sipahi AM. Prevalence of celiac disease in an urban area of Brazil with predominantly European ancestry. World J Gastroenterol. 2006, 28;12(40):6546–50.
8. Gandolfi L, Pratesi R, Cordoba JC, Tauil PL, Gasparin M, Catassi C. Prevalence of celiac disease among blood donors in Brazil. Am J Gastroenterol. 2000; 95(3):689–92.
9. Garnier-Lengliné H, Cerf-Bensussan N, Ruemmele FM. Celiac disease in children. Clin Res Hepatol Gastroenterol. 2015;39(5):544–51.
10. Hommel KA, Mackner LM, Denson LA, Crandall WV. Treatment regimen adherence in pediatric gastroenterology. J Pediatr Gastroenterol Nutr. 2008; 47(5):526–43.
11. Zarkadas M, Dubois S, MacIsaac K, Cantin I, Rashid M, Roberts KC, La Vieille S, Godefroy S, Pulido OM. Living with coeliac disease and a gluten-free diet: a Canadian perspective. J Hum Nutr Diet. 2013;26(1):10–23.
12. Charalampopoulos D, Panayiotou J, Chouliaras G, Zellos A, Kyritsi E, Roma E. Determinants of adherence to gluten-free diet in Greek children with coeliac disease: a cross-sectional study. Eur J Clin Nutr. 2013;67(6):615–9.
13. Valitutti F, Trovato CM, Montuori M, Cucchiara S. Pediatric Celiac Disease: Follow-Up in the Spotlight. Adv Nutr. 2017, 15;8(2):356–361.
14. Husby S, Koletzko S, Korponay-Szabó IR, Mearin ML, Phillips A, Shamir R, Troncone R, Giersiepen K, Branski D, Catassi C, Lelgeman M, Mäki M, Ribes-Koninckx C, Ventura A, Zimmer KP; ESPGHAN working group on coeliac disease diagnosis.; ESPGHAN gastroenterology committee.; European Society for Pediatric Gastroenterology, hepatology, and nutrition. European Society for Pediatric Gastroenterology, Hepatology, and Nutrition guidelines for the diagnosis of coeliac diseaseJ Pediatr Gastroenterol Nutr 2012;54(1):136–160.
15. Oberhuber G, Granditsch G, Vogelsang H. The histopathology of coelic disease: time for a standardized report scheme for pathologists. Eur J Gastroenterol Hepatol. 1999;11:1185–94.
16. WHO Multicentre Growth Reference Study Group. WHO child growth standards: length/height-for-age, weight-for-age, weight-for-length, weight-for-height and body mass index-for-age: methods and development. Geneva: World Health Organization; 2006.
17. Mozer-Glassberg Y, Zevit N, Rosenbach Y, Hartman C, Morgenstern S, Shamir R. Follow-up of children with celiac disease - lost in translation? Digestion. 2011;83(4):283–7.
18. Kurppa K, Lauronen O, Collin P, Ukkola A, Laurila K, Huhtala H, Mäki M, Kaukinen K. Factors associated with dietary adherence in celiac disease: a nationwide study. Digestion. 2012;86(4):309–14.
19. MacCulloch K, Rashid M. Factors affecting adherence to a gluten-free diet in children with celiac disease. Paediatr Child Health. 2014;19(6):305–9.
20. Tapsas D, Fälth-Magnusson K, Högberg L, Hammersjö JÅ, Hollén E. Swedish children with celiac disease comply well with a gluten-free diet, and most include oats without reporting any adverse effects: a long-term follow-up study. Nutr Res. 2014;34(5):436–41.
21. Barnea L, Mozer-Glassberg Y, Hojsak I, Hartman C, Shamir R. Pediatric celiac disease patients who are lost to follow-up have a poorly controlled disease. Digestion. 2014;90(4):248–53.
22. Sarkhy AA, El Mouzan MI, Saeed E, Alanazi A, Alghamdi S, Anil S, Assiri A. Clinical Characteristics of Celiac Disease and Dietary Adherence to Gluten-Free Diet among Saudi Children. Pediatr Gastroenterol Hepatol Nutr. 2015;18(1):23–9.
23. Webb C, Myléus A, Norström F, Hammarroth S, Högberg L, Lagerqvist C, Rosén A, Sandström O, Stenhammar L, Ivarsson A, Carlsson A. High adherence to a gluten-free diet in adolescents with screening-detected celiac disease. J Pediatr Gastroenterol Nutr. 2015;60(1):54–9.
24. Bravo MF, Munõz FMP. Adherence and impact of gluten free diet in children with celiac disease. Rev Chil Pediatr. 2011;82(3):191–7.
25. Alzaben AS, Turner J, Shirton L, Samuel TM, Persad R, Mager D. Assessing nutritional quality and adherence to the gluten-free diet in children and adolescents with celiac disease. Can J Diet Pract Res. 2015;76(2):56–63.
26. Reilly NR, Aguilar K, Hassid BG, Cheng J, Defelice AR, Kazlow P, Bhagat G, Green PH. Celiac disease in normal-weight and overweight children: clinical features and growth outcomes following a gluten-free diet. J Pediatr Gastroenterol Nutr. 2011;53(5):528–31.
27. Ljungman G, Myrdal U. Compliance in teenagers with coeliac disease-a Swedish follow-up study. Acta Paediatr. 1993;82(3):235–8.
28. Rashid M, Cranney A, Zarkadas M, Graham ID, Switzer C, Case S, Molloy M, Warren RE, Burrows V, Butzner JD. Celiac disease: evaluation of the diagnosis and dietary compliance in Canadian children. Pediatrics. 2005;116(6):e754–9.
29. Olsson C, Lyon P, Hörnell A, Ivarsson A, Sydner YM. Food that makes you different: the stigma experienced by adolescents with celiac disease. Qual Health Res. 2009;19(7):976–84.
30. Bacigalupe G, Plocha A. Celiac is a social disease: family challenges and strategies. Fam Syst Health. 2015;33(1):46–54.
31. Stevens L, Rashid M. Gluten-free and regular foods: a cost comparison. Can J Diet Pract Res. 2008 Fall;69(3):147–50.
32. Lee AR, Ng DL, Zivin J, Green PH. Economic burden of a gluten-free diet. J Hum Nutr Diet. 2007;20(5):423–30.
33. Singh J, Whelan K. Limited availability and higher cost of gluten-free foods. J Hum Nutr Diet. 2011;24(5):479–86.
34. Moreno ML, Rodríguez-Herrera A, Sousa C, Comino I. Biomarkers to Monitor Gluten-Free Diet Compliance in Celiac Patients. Nutrients. 2017, 6;9(1), pii: E46..
35. Sdepanian VL, de Morais MB, Fagundes-Neto U. [Celiac disease: evaluation of compliance to gluten-free diet and knowledge of disease in patients registered at the Brazilian Celiac Association (ACA)]. Arq Gastroenterol 2001; 38(4):232–239.
36. Mora S, Barera G, Beccio S, et al. A prospective, longitudinal study of long – term effect of treatment on bone density in children with celiac disease. J Pediatr. 2001;139:516–21.
37. Hartman C, Hino B, Lerner A, et al. Bone quantitative ultrasound and boné mineral density in children with celiac disease. JPediatr Gastroenteorl Nutr. 2004;39:504–10.
38. Tommasini A, Not T, Kiren V, et al. Mass screening for coelic disease using antihuman transglutaminase antibody assay. Arch Dis Child. 2004;89:512–5.
39. Bazzigaluppi E, Roggero P, Parma B, et al. Antibodies to recombinant human tissue-transglutaminase in coeliac disease: diagnostic effectiveness and decline pattern after gluten-free diet. Dig Liver Dis. 2006;38:98–102.
40. Byströn IM, Hollen E, Fälth-Magnusson K, Johansson A. Health-related quality of life in children and adolescents with celiac disease: from the perspectives of children and parents. Gastroenterol Res Pract. 2012;2012(986475)
41. Andreoli CS, Cortez APB, Sdepanian VL, Morais MB. Nutritional evaluation and food intake of celiac disease patients compliant or not with a gluten-free diet. Rev Nutr. Campinas. 2013;26(3):301–11.

20

Expression profiling and intracellular localization studies of the novel Proline-, Histidine-, and Glycine-rich protein 1 suggest an essential role in gastro-intestinal epithelium and a potential clinical application in colorectal cancer diagnostics

Satu Oltedal[1], Ivar Skaland[2], Jodi Maple-Grødem[3,4], Kjersti Tjensvoll[1], Emiel A. M. Janssen[2], Bjørnar Gilje[1], Rune Smaaland[1], Reino Heikkilä[5] and Oddmund Nordgård[1*]

Abstract

Background: The primary function of the intestines is the absorption of water and nutrients. Although our knowledge about these processes on the cellular level is extensive, a number of important intracellular elements remain unknown. Here, we characterize the novel proline-, histidine-, glycine-rich 1 (PHGR1) mRNA and protein on the molecular level and propose a functional role of the PHGR1 protein in the intestinal and gastric epithelium.

Methods: PHGR1 mRNA and protein expression in human tissues and cell lines were characterized by quantitative RT-PCR, in situ hybridization, Northern blotting, Western blotting, and immunohistochemistry. Glycosylation was assessed by a chemical deglycosylation assay, whereas intracellular localization was studied by immunofluorescent staining of cell line cells. PHGR1 mRNA levels in HT29 cells was reduced by RNA interference and the resulting global changes in gene expression assessed by microarray hybridization.

Results: PHGR1 mRNA and protein were found to be expressed specifically in epithelial cells of intestinal mucosa, with the highest expression in the most mature and differentiated cells. PHGR1 protein was found to be glycosylated and to localize to both the cytoplasm and nucleus. Transcript profiling and gene ontology analysis of HT29 cells subjected to PHGR1 knockdown suggested a functional relationship with transport and metabolic processes. Examination of PHGR1 mRNA and protein levels in lymph nodes with known colorectal cancer metastases indicated that they may serve as biomarkers for detection of such metastases.

Conclusions: Functional analyses of the novel PHGR1 mRNA and protein suggest an essential role in gastrointestinal epithelium and a clinical application in detection of colorectal cancer lymph node metastases.

Keywords: Colon, Mucosa, Glycoprotein, Transport, Metastasis, Cancer

* Correspondence: nood@sus.no
[1]Department of Hematology and Oncology, Stavanger University Hospital, 4068 Stavanger, Norway
Full list of author information is available at the end of the article

Background

The intestinal mucosa forms an important barrier against nutrients and microorganisms within the intestines. Other primary functions of the mucosa are absorption, secretion, and maintaining symbiosis with the intestinal microbiota [1].

The intestinal mucosa is covered by a single cell layer consisting primarily of four cell types [1, 2]. The most abundant cells are the absorptive *enterocytes*; *goblet* cells and *enteroendocrine* cells secrete mucus and various hormones; and *Paneth* cells secrete bactericidal proteins, such as lysozyme and defensins. The mucosal cell layer forms crypts, and in the small intestine protrusions called villi are formed, maximizing the surface area. Mature enterocytes, goblet cells, and enteroendocrine cells cover the villi of the small intestine and the luminal surface of the large intestine. Paneth cells and immature enterocytes, goblet, and enteroendocrine cells reside in the basal parts of the crypts, which is a niche of proliferation and cell differentiation. The bottom of each crypt also harbors stem cells that give rise to all of the cell types described above [2].

The enterocytes are highly polarized columnar cells with an apical surface facing the lumen and a basolateral surface connecting the mucosa to the other cell layers of the intestinal wall [3]. The apical surface is covered by numerous membrane protrusions, called the brush-border, further maximizing the surface area and absorptive capacity of the cell. The brush-border is covered by layers of mucus and glycocalyx, which provides protection and contains digestive enzymes [1]. Substantial membrane and cytoplasmic asymmetry is required to maintain the brush-border structure and facilitate the transport of nutrients and water from the intestinal lumen to the basolateral surface. Membrane asymmetry is generated and maintained primarily by vesicular transport, including both specific transport of newly synthesized proteins from the trans-Golgi network and recycling of existing membrane proteins via recycling endosomes [3, 4].

Vesicular transport is also responsible for the direct transport of some nutrients across the mucosal cell layer in a process called transcytosis [4]. However, the gross absorption of nutrients, electrolytes, and water from the lumen is performed by specific membrane-spanning transporter proteins [5]. Specific transporters also secrete water and electrolytes, maintaining an intricate chemical homeostasis both inside the cells and in the neighboring compartments.

Enterocytes also play a role in the immunological defense system of the gut [1], as they contribute to the activation of the immune system against disease-causing microorganisms and to the suppression of immune reactions against the beneficial inhabitants of the gut. These activities include uptake and presentation of antigens, interaction with immune cells and secretion of immunoglobulin A and antimicrobial peptides [1].

Even if many aspects of intestinal biology are well-described, important details are still lacking regarding the level of molecular mechanisms, signaling, and integration of processes. Through bioinformatic searches for colorectal cancer biomarkers, we identified the novel gastrointestinal-specific proline-, histidine-, glycine-rich protein 1 (PHGR1). Here, we describe the first molecular characterization of PHGR1 and suggest a clinical utility in colorectal cancer diagnostics.

Methods

PHGR1 5′ end cDNA cloning and sequencing

The complete 5′ end of *PHGR1* cDNA was cloned by RNA ligase-mediated rapid amplification of 5' cDNA ends (RLM-RACE), using the GeneRacer kit (Invitrogen) according to the kit protocol. The 5′ end of *PHGR1* cDNA was then PCR amplified, using one adapter-specific primer and a *PHGR1*-specific primer with the following sequence: 5′- TTC TCT CAG GCT TGC CAT CTT GT -3′. The PCR products were cloned using the Zero Blunt TOPO PCR Cloning Kit for Sequencing (Invitrogen). DNA sequencing was performed using the BigDye Terminator v3.1 Cycle sequencing Kit (Applied Biosystems) and capillary electrophoresis at the sequencing facility of the SARS center in Bergen. We sequenced four clones, from two different individuals, and they were identical. Our *PHGR1* mRNA sequence (5′ end) was uploaded to Genbank (Genbank: KT007223).

Cell culture

Caco-2, LS174T, HT29, and HCT116 cells were cultured according to the recommendations of the provider (ECACC).

For the differentiation experiments, non-confluent Caco-2 cells were plated in each well of 12-well culture plates, corresponding to a density 2.9 x 10^4 cells/cm^2 and approximately 50% confluence. The culture medium was exchanged every second day until the last cultures were harvested after 14 days. The cells reached confluence at day 2. After 0, 1, 2, 4, 6, 8, 10, and 14 days of growth, three cultures were washed with phosphate-buffered saline (PBS) (37 °C) and lysed in 350 μl of RLT buffer (from the Allprep DNA/RNA/Protein Mini kit, Qiagen).

For the intracellular localization studies Caco-2 cells were seeded at a density of 2.9 x 10^4 cells/cm^2 in 12-well transparent polyethylene terephthalate (PET) hanging cell culture filter inserts (Millipore) with 1.0 μm pores. The cells reached confluence at day 2 and the medium was exchanged every second day until harvesting. Parallel cultures were stained according to the protocol in the "Immunofluorescent staining" section or lysed in RLT buffer for RNA isolation.

Northern blotting

RNA (5 µg) from the LS174T cell line, a colorectal adenocarcinoma sample and a normal colonic mucosa sample were subjected to agarose gel (1.2%) electrophoresis using MOPS electrophoresis buffer and 2% formaldehyde in the gel, according to the "DIG Application Manual for Filter Hybridization" (Roche). A digoxigenin (DIG)-labeled RNA size standard was analyzed in parallel. RNA was blotted onto a positively charged nylon membrane by capillary transfer and hybridized to 2.5 pmol of four PHGR1-specific DIG-labeled DNA hybridization probes, according to the same DIG application manual. The sequences of the hybridization probes were: 5′-GGA GTA AGA GCA GGG AAT ACC TGA GAG TGC AGA GCA GGG GCA GGA AGT C-3′, 5'-GCC CGC AGT GAC CTG GAG GAT GGC CAT GCC CCC CAC AGT G-3′, 5'-GGC CCT GGA CCA TGG TGG GGG GGT GGC CCG CAG G-3′ and 5'-GGC CTC ATT CCA GGT CAG CTG GGC AAT TCT CTC AGG CTT GCC-3′. The hybridization signals were detected by an alkaline phosphatase-conjugated DIG antibody according to the application manual.

In situ hybridization

In situ hybridization was performed essentially as described in the DIG Application Manual for Nonradioactive In Situ Hybridization (3rd edition, Roche). DIG-labeled cRNA probes were prepared using a DIG-RNA-labeling kit (Roche). The antisense and probe mixture consisted of the same four probes as described in the Northern blotting section, 20 ng of each probe per slide. The sense probe mixture (negative control) consisted of four probes, 20 ng of each probe per slide. Unbound RNA probe was not digested, but removed by washing at 37 °C five times for 15 min each in decreasing concentrations of SSC buffer. The hybridization signals were detected by an alkaline phosphatase-conjugated DIG antibody according to the DIG Application Manual.

RNA and protein purification

RNA and protein were isolated from cell cultures and tissue samples using the Allprep DNA/RNA/Protein Mini kit according to the manufacturer's protocol (Qiagen). Protein pellets from mucosa tissue samples required 8 M urea/2% SDS and incubation at 70 °C for 2–3 h to dissolve.

DNAse-treatment and reverse transcription

RNA was treated with DNAse by mixing 500 ng total RNA from each sample with 1 unit RQ1 RNAse-free DNAse (Promega) in a total volume of 20 µl First Strand Synthesis buffer (Invitrogen) containing 10 units RNAse-OUT RNAse inhibitor (Invitrogen). The reaction mixture was incubated at 37 °C for 30 min and the DNAse inactivated by adding 1 µl RQ1 stop solution and incubating for 10 min at 65 °C. Complementary DNA was synthesized by M-MLV reverse transcriptase in a total volume of 40 µl according to the manufacturer's protocol (Life Technologies).

Quantitative PCR

PCR amplification of *PHGR1, HPRT1,* and *BCR* cDNA was performed with the qPCR SYBR Green Core kit (Eurogentec) according to the manufacturer's recommendations. Thermocycling and real-time fluorescence measurements were performed in an Mx3000P real-time PCR instrument (Stratagene). The DNA sequences of the PCR primers were: PHGR1-F: 5'-CCCTGCTCTGCACTCT-CAG-3′, PHGR1-R: 5'-CGCAGTGACCTGGAGGAT-3′, HPRT1-F: 5'-TTCCTTGGTCAGGCAGTA-3′, HPR T1-R: 5′- TATCCAACACTTCGTGGG-3′, BCR-F: 5'-GCTCTATGGGTTTCTGAATG-3′, BCR-R: 5'-AAAT ACCCAAAGGAATCCAC-3′.

Relative levels of *PHGR1* mRNA were determined by normalization against a reference transcript *(HPRT1* or *BCR*) and a calibrator sample according to the $2^{\Delta\Delta Cq}$ method [6]. All analyses were performed in duplicates or triplicates.

PHGR1 mRNA expression profiling was done by measuring the relative *PHGR1* mRNA levels in 2 µl of cDNA from Multiple Tissue cDNA Panels I and II (BD Bioscences), cDNA from normal colon mucosa biopsies and lymph nodes from healthy controls described below. The means from three independent experiments were presented.

ALPL, MAPK3, MAPK13, SLC2A1, SLC44A2, S100A3, SPRR1A, DDIT4, RASD1, and *SLC4A* mRNA levels were measured relative to *HPRT1* mRNA using TaqMan assays (Thermo Fischer), according to the manufacturer's protocol.

Antibody synthesis

A polyclonal rabbit antibody against a synthetic subpeptide of the PHGR1 protein was raised in two rabbits through a custom antibody production service (Eurogentec). The peptide sequence of the synthetic subpeptide was N-CGPPPGHGPGHPPPGP-C, which is part of the repeated region of PHGR1. The antibody was affinity purified from antiserum after the final bleed.

Western blotting

Proteins were separated according to size by SDS-PAGE using 15% polyacrylamide gels and a Tris-glycine buffer system in a Mini-Protean electrophoresis unit (Bio-Rad).

Separated proteins were blotted onto PVDF membranes (Bio-Rad Immunoblot) by semi-dry electro-blotting for 20 min at 15 V using a Transblot SD unit (Bio-Rad). The anode filter paper (Extra thick blot paper, Bio-Rad) and membrane were soaked in 25 mM Tris base/20% methanol, whereas the cathode filter paper was soaked in 25 mM Tris base/20 mM 6-Aminocaproic acid/20% methanol. Proteins were fixed to the membranes by incubation in methanol for 2 min and reversibly stained with Ponceau stain to validate blotting quality. The membranes were blocked by incubation for 30 min with shaking in TBS-T (10 mM Tris-HCl pH 8.0, 0.15 M NaCl, 0.05% Tween-20) buffer added 5% skimmed milk powder, then shaken for two hours at room temperature with primary antibodies (rabbit anti-PHGR1 1:2000 and rabbit anti-GAPDH (Abcam) 1:1000) in TBS-T/milk buffer. Subsequently, the membranes were washed 3 × 20 min in TBS-T/milk buffer and incubated for one hour of shaking with an alkaline phosphatase-conjugated goat antibody against rabbit immunoglobulin G (Sigma-Aldrich), diluted 1:10,000 (PHGR1) or 1:5000 (GAPDH) with TBS-T/milk. Finally, the membranes were rinsed 6 times with TBS-T, washed for 20 minutes with TBS-T, incubated for one minute in 0,1 M Tris-HCl pH 9.5/0,1 M NaCl and overlaid with BCIP/NBT purple liquid substrate system for membranes (Sigma Aldrich) in darkness. Color reactions were stopped after sufficient signal development (5–15 min) by rinsing with distilled water.

Chemical deglycosylation

The protein fraction was extracted from 5 to 10 million LS174T cells by the Allprep DNA/RNA/protein Mini kit according to the manufacturer's protocol (Qiagen) and dissolved in 5% SDS. The SDS was subsequently removed by purification on PD Spintrap G-25 gel filtration spin columns (GE Healthcare) using milli-Q water as the equilibration buffer in accordance with the manufacturer's protocol. The water was removed by vacuum centrifugation. Protein extracts were chemically deglycosylated using the GlycoProfile IV chemical deglycosylation kit (Sigma-Aldrich) according to the manufacturer's protocol. In short, 75 µl pre-cooled (2-8 °C) Trifluoromethanesulfonic (TFMS) acid was added to pre-cooled dried protein extracts. The reaction tubes were immediately sealed and proteins dissolved by gentle shaking for 2–5 min. The samples were incubated on ice for 25 min and added pre-cooled (methanol-dry ice bath) pyridine solution dropwise until the pH reached approximately 6 (bromophenol blue turned blue). The reaction vessel was cooled on methanol-dry ice water bath during the first phase of pyridine addition to avoid freezing. Finally, deglycosylated proteins were dialyzed using the PlusOne Mini Dialysis kit (GE Healthcare), concentrated by vacuum centrifugation, and analyzed by Western blotting as described above. The volume of deglycosylated protein extract loaded on the acrylamide gel for SDS-PAGE corresponded to the volume of undeglycosylated protein extract loaded, corrected for dilutions and up-concentration during deglycosylation. The experiment was repeated four times, two times according to kit protocol A and two times according to protocol B (using anisole scavenger), producing the same results in all replicates.

Immunofluorescent staining

Caco-2 cells grown on PET hanging cell culture filter inserts (Millipore) were washed in PBS, fixed in 4% paraformaldehyde, permeabilized, blocked and incubated for 1 h at room temperature in a 1:500 dilution of our rabbit polyclonal PHGR1 antibody in blocking solution or an isotype-specific control antibody for polyclonal rabbit antibodies (Life Technologies 08–6199). The cells were washed and incubated for 30 min in a 1:2000 dilution of the secondary antibody (goat polyclonal FITC-conjugated antibody against rabbit IgG, Sigma-Aldrich). The cells were subsequently washed and incubated for 30 min with a 1:500 dilution of a mouse monoclonal Alexa Fluor 594-conjugated antibody against occludin (Life Technologies). The cells were then washed and incubated for 10 min in a 0.2 µg/ml dilution of 4′,6-diamidino-2-phenylindole dihydrochloride (DAPI, Sigma-Aldrich). The filters were removed from the inserts using a scalpel and mounted on glass slides with fluorescent mounting medium (Dako). Pictures were obtained at room temperature with an Axioplan 2 fluorescence microscope (Carl Zeiss) and a JAI M4+ HiRes Digital CCD camera, using fixed exposure times (1 s.) for the green and red channels and automatic exposure times for the blue channel. The objectives were Carl Zeiss 10× Plan-APOCHROMAT /0.45 NA and 100× Plan-NEOFLUAR/1.3 NA oil. The software ISIS version 5.2.23 was utilized for capture and image processing. Lower signal thresholds were the same for all images obtained with the same magnification. The images shown in Fig. 4 and Additional file 3 are representative of the majority of the investigated Caco-2 cells.

Images were also taken using an inverted Nikon A1R confocal laser scanning microscope with a 60X Plan-Apo/1.20 NA oil objective. Excitations used laser lines at 408 nm, 488 nm, or 561 nm, and images were recorded at 450/50 nm, 525/50 nm, or 595/50 nm, respectively. Stacks of images were acquired with a 0.2 µm confocal slice. NIS-Elements imaging software 4.0 (Nikon, Japan) was used for image capture, and the brightness of the resulting pictures was increased by adjusting the signal threshold.

Immunohistochemistry

Paraffin-embedded tissue sections were mounted onto Superfrost Plus slides (Menzel, Braunschweig, Germany) and dried overnight at 37 °C followed by 1 h at 60 °C. The sections were deparaffinized in xylene and rehydrated in decreasing concentrations of alcohol. Antigen was retrieved using a highly stabilized retrieval system (ImmunoPrep, Instrumec, Oslo, Norway) at high temperature and pressure. The sections were incubated for 30 min with a 1:20,000 dilution of our rabbit polyclonal PHGR1 antibody in Dako antibody diluent. The EnVisionTMFlex detection system (Dako) was used for visualization. After washing the sections, they were incubated for 5 min with peroxidase-blocking reagent, 20 min with the EnVision™ FLEX/HRP Detection Reagent, 10 min with EnVision™ FLEX DAB+ Chromogen/EnVision™ FLEX Substrate Buffer mix and 5 min with EnVision™ FLEX Hematoxylin. The slides were dehydrated and mounted. All immunohistochemical stainings were performed using a Dako Autostainer Link 48 instrument and EnVision™ FLEX Wash Buffer. Micrographs were obtained with an Olympus IX81 microscope and a MMI CellCamera 1.4 camera, using Olympus 20× LUCPlanFLN/0.45 NA and 100× UPlanSApo/1.4 NA oil objectives. The MMI CellTools-4-4 software was used.

PHGR1 knockdown in HT29 cells

Proliferating HT29 cells were plated in 12-well culture plates at a density of 30,000 cells per well and cultured overnight without antibiotics. These cells were then transfected separately with three different small interfering RNAs (siRNAs) in quadruplicates using Dharmafect 4 transfection reagent (Dharmacon/GE healthcare), according to the manufacturer's protocol. Two siRNAs (A and B) were targeted against PHGR1, whereas the third was a negative control (C). The siRNA sequences were siPHGR1-A: 5′-GAUGGCAAGCCUGAGAGAA(dTdT)-3′ (MWG Biotech siMAX), siPHGR1-B: 5′-AGAUGGACCCAGGUC CGAA(dTdT)-3′, and a negative control siRNA: AGGUAG UGUAAUCGCCUUG(dTdT)-3′ (scramble). Untransfected control wells were also included. Subsequently, the cells were cultured for 48 h and lysed in RLT buffer containing β-mercaptoethanol. RNA was isolated with the RNeasy Mini kit according to the kit protocol, using the optional on-column DNAse digestion step. The RNA quality was verified on the Bioanalyzer 2100 (Agilent).

PHGR1 mRNA knockdown was confirmed by quantitative RT-PCR as described above. A separate, identical transfection experiment was performed to verify the reduced PHGR1 protein level upon siRNA transfection. The cells were then lysed and analyzed by Western blot according to the protocol described above.

Global mRNA profiling and data analysis

One microgram of RNA from each transfected HT29 culture was amplified and labeled using the Illumina RNA Amplification kit and hybridized to Illumina Human-6 Expression BeadChips (48,000 different probes and 1.6×10^6 beads). Fluorescence was measured in a BeadArray Reader (Illumina). Amplification, hybridization and fluorescence measurements were performed by the Norwegian Microarray Consortium (NMC) in Oslo.

Data extraction and initial quality control were performed using BeadStudio version 3.1.3.0 from Illumina (http://www.illumina.com) and Gene Expression module 3.2.6. Additional quality control and statistical and gene ontology analysis were performed using the R (version 3.0.2, http://www.r-project.org) and Bioconductor (version 2.22.0, http://www.bioconductor.org) software packages [7, 8]. Raw fluorescence values were quantile normalized, log-transformed and submitted to the Gene Expression Omnibus (GEO) database (GEO: GSE70053). Differential gene expression between samples was assessed with the limma package in Bioconductor. *P*-values were adjusted for multiple testing by the Benjamini and Hochberg method [9]. Transcripts with significantly different levels (adjusted $P < 0.001$) in both comparison groups (A vs. control and B vs. control) were considered to be significantly upregulated and downregulated.

Gene ontology analysis was performed using the Database for Annotation, Visualization and Integrated Discovery (DAVID) [10] web service version 6.7 and GOstat [11] version 2.28.0 for Bioconductor. Similar results were obtained with both methods, but only the DAVID results are shown in the article. The gene ontology annotations of significantly upregulated or downregulated genes were compared with the annotations for all genes analyzed in the mRNA profiling, in order to identify over- or underrepresented gene ontology categories. *P*-values were adjusted for multiple testing by the Benjamini-Hochberg method. Under-represented categories were only assessed by the GOstats package (not shown), but were complementary to the over-represented categories.

Other bioinformatics

Expressed sequence tag (EST) databases at the Cancer Gene Anatomy Project (CGAP; US National Cancer Institute) were searched for potential colorectal cancer biomarkers using the cDNA digital gene expression displayer (DGED) tool in June 2004. Libraries from normal colon and colon cancers (including cell lines) were compared to all other available libraries.

Multiple sequence alignments were analyzed using MUSCLE 3.51 software. The alignment was colored by JalView version 2.7. Homology searches were performed with the blastn, blastp, tblastn, Phi-blast, PSI-blast, Delta-blast and HMMER3 software programs in the Genbank nr and Swissprot databases. The subcellular localization of PHGR1 was predicted by PSORT II. No clear predictions were possible from the primary sequence of PHGR1 (data not shown).

Patients and control samples

Colon and lung tumor biopsies, normal mucosa, and lymph node biopsies were obtained from patients and controls recruited into two prospective clinical studies previously approved by the Norwegian Regional Ethical Committee West (approval 197.04) and the Norwegian Regional Ethical Commmittee South (approval S-05307) [12–14]. Written informed consents from the donors were obtained for the use of their tissue samples in research. The colon cancer study included operable colon cancer patients, and the lung cancer study included operable non-small cell lung cancer patients. The samples analyzed in Fig. 6a and b were selected from the existing biobanks by randomization. Clinicopathological data for the 209 colon cancer patients analyzed in Fig. 6b and c are shown in Additional file 8. RNA from other human tissues was purchased from BD Bioscences and Asterand Bioscience.

Results

In Silico identification and characterization of PHGR1

EST libraries at the Cancer Gene Anatomy project (CGAP) were searched for potential colorectal cancer biomarkers using the cDNA digital gene expression displayer tool, by comparing libraries for normal colon and colon cancers to all other available libraries. Among the mRNAs apparently only expressed in normal and neoplastic colon tissues were several well-known colonic differentiation markers and a novel mRNA later denoted as proline-, histidine-, glycine-rich protein 1 (PHGR1).

The gene and mRNA sequences of *PHGR1* from several species were available in Genbank and equivalent sequence databases. We verified experimentally that the human *PHGR1* mRNA sequence in Genbank had a complete 5′ end (Genbank: KT007223). The human RefSeq *PHGR1* mRNA has 434 bases (without the polyA tail) and consists of four exons (Genbank: NM_001145643). The human *PHGR1* gene is located on chromosome 15 band q15.1.

Two alternative open reading frames (ORFs) have been suggested in the publicly available sequence databases, encoding either an 82 amino acid (aa) or a 93 aa polypeptide (human). Therefore, we performed multiple sequence alignments for both groups of predicted polypeptides and found the 82-aa ORF to be best conserved and probably also the one that is translated. The predicted PHGR1 peptide sequence has extraordinarily high proline (29%), histidine (18%) and glycine (31%) content. Fig. 1 shows a multiple sequence alignment of the predicted PHGR1 protein orthologs, revealing that many of the glycine, proline, and histidine residues were well conserved. In addition, three cysteines and a lysine residue were present in all orthologs. Sequence analysis also revealed five repeats of approximately 11 aa in the N-terminal part of the peptide (Additional file 1). The predicted molecular weight of the PHGR1 polypeptide was 7.7 kDa.

Homology searches were performed with both the peptide sequence alone and the multiple sequence alignment (Fig. 1) as a query. When using compositional adjustment, only weak similarities were found, probably because very few amino acids in PHGR1 are not proline, histidine, or glycine. However, without compositional adjustment we found several proteins with significant similarity to the repeat region of PHGR1, mostly histidine and proline-rich proteins of various classes. The most significant hits with functional annotations were histidine-rich glycoproteins from animals, proline-rich cell wall glycoproteins from plants, and salivary proline-rich proteins and proline-rich proteoglycans from mammals. Several of these proteins had sequence repeats in their proline-rich regions and many of them were secretory and had signaling peptides. However, no conventional signaling peptide was present in PHGR1.

PHGR1 mRNA characterization

Northern blotting revealed a single *PHGR1* mRNA variant of approximately 490 bases in normal colonic

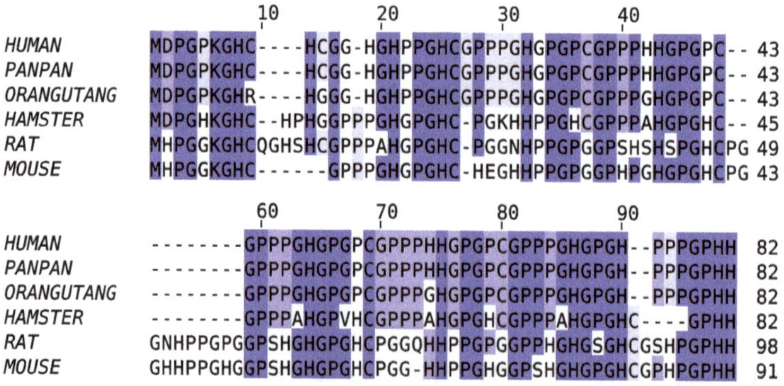

Fig. 1 Multiple sequence alignment of PHGR1 orthologs. Predicted PHGR1 polypeptides from *Homo sapiens* (human), *Pan paniscus* (PanPan), *Pongo abelii* (orangutan), *Cricetulus griseus* (hamster), *Rattus norvegicus* (rat) and *Mus musculus* (mouse) were aligned by the MUSCLE multiple sequence alignment software. Identical residues across all peptides are shown in dark blue and conserved residues (positive BLOSUM62 score) in light blue

mucosa, a colorectal tumor biopsy, and the colorectal cancer cell line LS174T (data not shown). This corresponded well to the RefSeq mRNA sequence of 434 bases without the polyA tail. The *PHGR1* mRNA expression profile in various normal tissues was determined by quantitative reverse transcription PCR (Fig. 2a). Very high levels of *PHGR1* mRNA were present in the intestines and stomach, but low levels were present in most other tissues. However, the prostate and pancreas had moderate levels of *PHGR1* mRNA.

To identify the colonic cell types with high levels of *PHGR1* mRNA, we performed *PHGR1* mRNA in situ hybridization in colon tissue biopsies (Fig. 2b). *PHGR1* mRNA was predominantly expressed in the upper parts of the crypts, where the more mature epithelial cells reside. Both the mucus-producing goblet cells and the absorptive enterocytes expressed high levels of *PHGR1* mRNA, whereas the mature epithelial cells facing the lumen of the colon had somewhat lower levels.

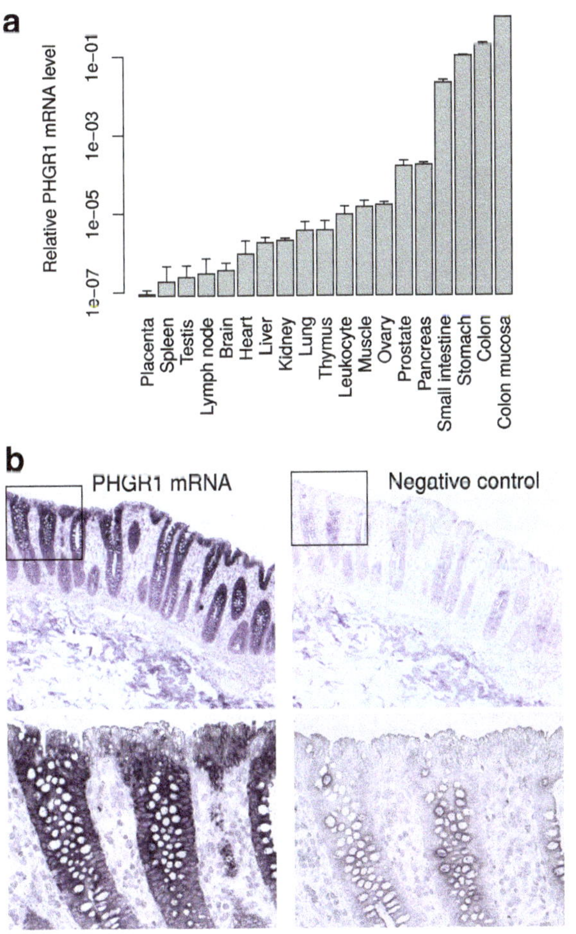

Fig. 2 *PHGR1* mRNA characterization. **a** *PHGR1* mRNA levels in various tissues presented relative to a reference mRNA and the pooled colon mucosa samples. The error bars represent the standard deviation from three independent experiments. **b** In situ hybridization of *PHGR1* mRNA in the colon wall. The left panels show 10× and 40× (insert) microscopy images of a tissue section hybridized to *PHGR1*-specific probes. The right panels show corresponding images of an adjacent tissue section hybridized to a negative control probe. Nuclear counterstaining (blue) was achieved with hematoxylin

PHGR1 protein characterization

On Western blots using a polyclonal antibody against PHGR1 the LS174T, HT29, and HCT116 colorectal cancer cell lines and normal mucosa samples did not have a protein band around the expected molecular weight for PHGR1 (7.7 kDa). Instead, a strong band was observed near 40 kDa, in addition to a number of weaker bands with a larger size interval (Fig. 3a). PHGR1 mRNA levels were measured in the same samples, showing a remarkably good correlation with the protein levels (Additional file 2). PHGR1 protein levels were highest in the mucosa samples and the mucin-producing, goblet cell-like LS174T cell line [15] and almost absent in the low-differentiated and more aggressive HCT116 cell line. The HT29 cell line, which can differentiate into both enterocyte-like and mucin-producing lineages [16], had intermediate levels of PHGR1 protein.

Covalent modification of the PHGR1 peptide could explain its unexpectedly slow migration in SDS-PAGE. Further analyses showed that the PHGR1 peptides were resistant to trypsin digestion, but not proteinase K digestion. This finding was consistent with the presence of only one trypsin site at the very beginning (6th amino acid residue) of the predicted PHGR1 polypeptide (data not shown), which would probably not result in detectable changes in migration. This observation indicated that a covalently conjugated heterotypic protein complex was not a probable explanation for the apparently large size. The PHGR1 peptides seemed generally very stable, resisting incubation for several hours in a crude protein extract containing endogenous proteases without protease inhibitors (data not shown).

Variable protein glycosylation may be an alternative explanation for the numerous weaker bands observed in SDS-PAGE. Thus, we tried to remove the potential glycosylation of PHGR1 both enzymatically and chemically. However, the enzymatic deglycosylation did not result in any shift in electrophoretic mobility for the observed protein bands (data not shown). On the other hand, the chemical deglycosylation revealed a protein band at 10 kDa (Fig. 3b), supporting the hypothesis that PHGR1 is glycosylated.

Some proteins without a signaling peptide have been reported to be directed to secretion based on specific glycosylation [17]. However, we did not detect any PHGR1 in the growth medium of LS174T cells after 2 days of culture (data not shown).

Immunohistochemical expression pattern of the PHGR1 protein

To investigate the pattern of PHGR1 protein expression, we performed immunohistochemical (IHC) staining of PHGR1 in normal colon, breast, liver, kidney, thyroid, pancreas, and placenta (Fig. 3c and Additional file 2). PHGR1 protein levels were high in colonic mucosa, but very low or undetectable in the other normal tissues tested. The PHGR1 protein levels were also highest in the upper parts of the colonic crypts, where the most mature epithelial cells reside, corresponding well with the expression pattern we observed for *PHGR1* mRNA.

Interestingly, IHC staining also revealed that the PHGR1 protein was present in both the cytoplasm and nucleus, with nuclear levels increasing more than cytoplasmic levels during differentiation. Accordingly, we analyzed several colorectal cancers and observed both cytoplasmic and nuclear localization in highly differentiated tumors. Tumors with a lower differentiation grade primarily had cytoplasmic localization of

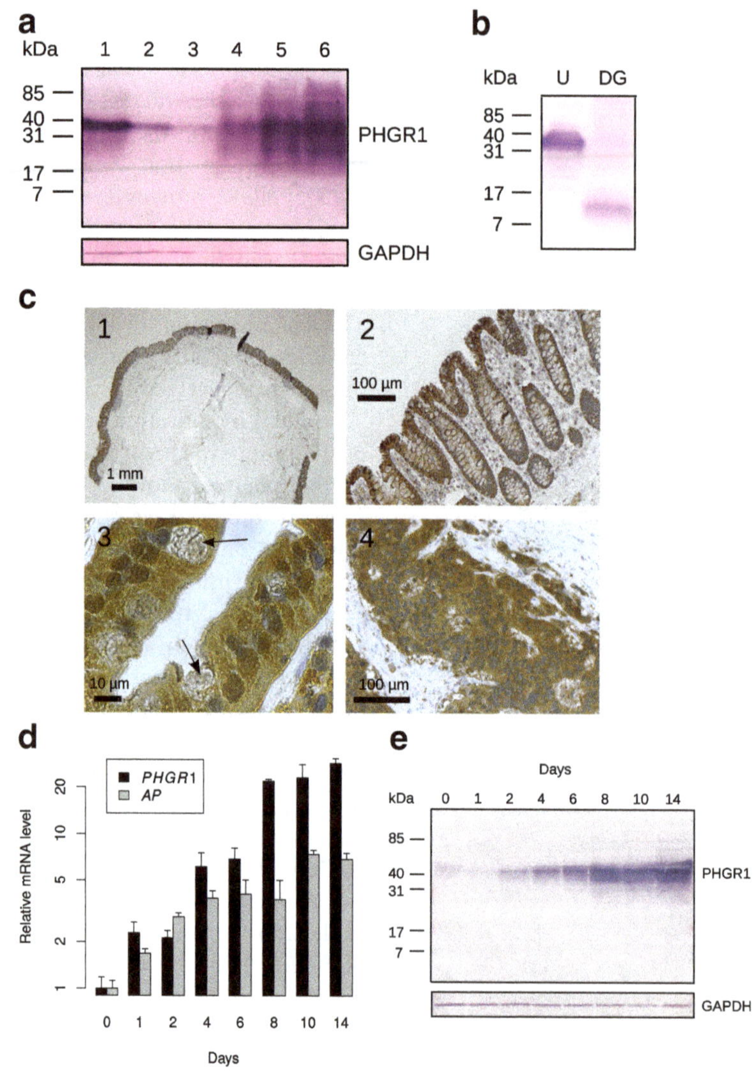

Fig. 3 PHGR1 protein characterization. **a** Western blot of PHGR1 protein in the colorectal cancer cell lines LS174T (lane 1), HT29 (lane 2), and HCT116 (lane 3) and normal mucosa samples (lanes 4–6). GAPDH was included as a loading control. **b** Western blot of untreated (U) and chemically deglycosylated (DG) protein extracts from the LS174T cell line, stained with a polyclonal antibody against PHGR1. The volumes loaded corresponded to the same volume of original protein extract. **c** Immunohistochemical staining of PHGR1 in colon and colorectal cancer. 1) PHGR1-stained (brown) normal colon (2.5× microscope objective). 2) PHGR1-stained normal colon mucosa (20× objective). 3) PHGR1-stained normal mucosa (100× objective), upper part of a crypt. The arrows indicate goblet cells. 4) PHGR1-stained colorectal carcinoma (20× objective). Nuclear counterstaining was achieved with hematoxylin (blue). **d** Relative *PHGR1* and alkaline phosphatase (*AP*) mRNA levels during Caco-2 cell differentiation. mRNA levels were normalized both against the reference mRNA *HPRT1* and the day 0 sample. Data are represented as mean values from three biological replicates. The error bars represent standard deviation. **e** Western blot of Caco-2 cells cultured to confluence and beyond (0–14 days) using antibodies against PHGR1 (upper panel) and GAPDH (lower panel)

PHGR1 (Fig. 3c and data not shown). In general, both secretory goblet cells and absorptive enterocytes had high levels of PHGR1 protein. However, a few mature goblet cells with lower nuclear PHGR1 levels were also observed in normal mucosa (arrows in Fig. 3c).

PHGR1 levels during enterocyte differentiation

When cultured beyond confluency, the Caco-2 human adenocarcinoma cell line expresses characteristics of enterocytic differentiation [18]. Therefore, to investigate *PHGR1* mRNA levels in a model of enterocytic differentiation, we measured *PHGR1* mRNA levels in differentiating Caco-2 cells by quantitative RT-PCR (Fig. 3d). We observed a strong increase in *PHGR1* mRNA levels during Caco-2 cell differentiation. The differentiation process was verified by measuring alkaline phosphatase mRNA levels in parallel. Moreover, Western blotting of protein lysates from the same Caco-2 cultures demonstrated a similar increase in the PHGR1 protein levels during differentiation (Fig. 3e).

Intracellular localization of PHGR1 during enterocyte differentiation

To determine the intracellular localization of PHGR1 protein during differentiation we cultured Caco-2 cells beyond confluence on optically transparent permeable filter inserts. The previously observed upregulation of *PHGR1* expression during Caco-2 cell differentiation was verified in the filter-grown cells by quantitative RT-PCR (Additional file 3). Immunofluorescent staining of PHGR1 protein revealed a primarily cytoplasmic localization in these differentiating cells (Fig. 4). Interestingly, immunofluorescent analyses revealed a striking heterogeneity in PHGR1 protein levels among the Caco-2 cells, especially in the early phase of differentiation. Some cells had high PHGR1 levels, but the majority had very low levels. The overall increase in PHGR1 protein levels during differentiation seemed to be caused by an increase in the fraction of Caco-2 cells expressing the PHGR1 protein, rather than by an increase in PHGR1 protein levels in cells already expressing the protein.

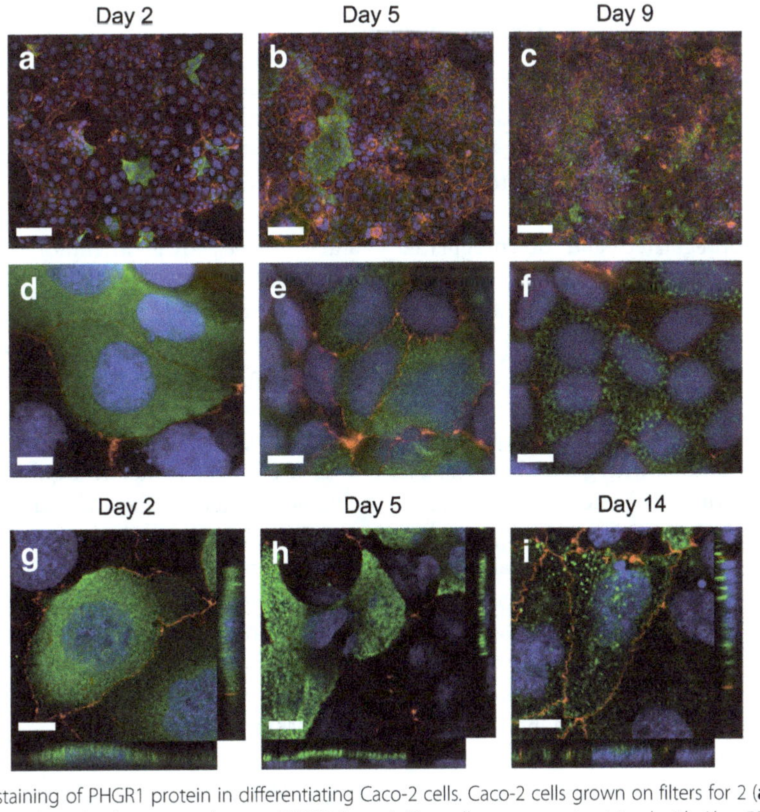

Fig. 4 Immunofluorescent staining of PHGR1 protein in differentiating Caco-2 cells. Caco-2 cells grown on filters for 2 (**a, d, g**), 5 (**b, e, h**), 9 (**c, f**) and 14 (**i**) days were stained with antibodies against human PHGR1 (green). The cells were counterstained with Alexa594-conjugated antibodies against the tight-junction protein occludin (red) and the DNA dye DAPI (blue). See Additional file 3 for negative isotype control staining of the Caco-2 cells. **a-c** Images taken with a 10× objective. Scale bars = 100 μm. **d-f** Images taken with a 100× objective. Scale bars = 10 μm. **g-i** Images taken with a confocal laser scanning microscope at 60× magnification. Scale bars = 10 μm. Z-X and Z-Y views are shown in the side panels

The cytosolic distribution of PHGR1 protein in Caco-2 cells at day 2 revealed an almost homogeneous distribution of tiny spots (Fig. 4d). Interestingly, the distribution shifted towards larger speckles of PHGR1 (Fig. 4f) inside the cytoplasm at day 9. From the focal plan we also judged the large speckles in later stages to be located on the apical side of the cells. Examination of the slides with a confocal laser scanning microscope confirmed this distribution (Fig. 4h and i). The speckles were reminiscent of intracellular vesicles.

Transcript profile in response to PHGR1 downregulation

To elucidate the functional pathways related to PHGR1 expression, we investigated the global transcriptional effects of PHGR1 knockdown in HT29 colon cancer cells. The HT29 cancer cell line was chosen because of its moderately high *PHGR1* mRNA levels in growing cultures. To eliminate non-specific side effects of siRNA transfection, two different PHGR1-targeted siRNAs were used in addition to a negative control siRNA (scramble). Knockdown of *PHGR1* mRNA (70% reduction) and protein levels in transfected HT29 cells was verified by quantitative RT-PCR and Western blotting (Additional file 4).

Global mRNA profiling by microarray analysis of HT29 cells transfected separately with two different PHGR1-targeted siRNAs (siRNA A and B) revealed 406 genes that were significantly upregulated and 369 genes significantly downregulated in response to PHGR1 knockdown (Additional files 5 and 6). Clustering and heatmap analysis of significantly upregulated or downregulated genes unveiled substantial changes in the mRNA profiles due to PHGR1 knockdown (Fig. 5a). The biological replicates clustered together as expected. Upregulated and downregulated transcripts with high fold changes or well-known functions were verified by quantitative RT-PCR in a separate transfection experiment (Additional file 4).

To further characterize the functional relationships of PHGR1, we performed gene ontology analysis, searching for ontologies over- and under-represented among the upregulated and downregulated genes. As shown in Fig. 5b and Additional file 7, genes associated with localization and transport were over-represented among the upregulated genes. On the other hand, genes associated with metabolic processes were over-represented among the downregulated genes, whereas metabolic and biosynthetic biological processes were under-represented among the upregulated genes and catabolic processes were under-represented among the downregulated genes (results not shown).

PHGR1 is a potential marker for detection of lymph node metastasis in colorectal cancer

We hypothesized that PHGR1 may serve as a clinically useful biomarker for detection of lymph node metastasis in colorectal cancer patients because of our observation that *PHGR1* mRNA levels are high in normal colon mucosa and very low in normal lymph nodes and several other tissues (Fig. 2a). To investigate this hypothesis, we measured the levels of *PHGR1* mRNA in parallel with the mRNA levels of the established lymph node metastasis marker *KRT20* in tumors from colon, pancreas, breast, prostate and lung (non-small cell) cancer patients, as well as normal lymph nodes and lymph nodes with known colon cancer metastases (Fig. 6a and b). On average, *PHGR1* mRNA levels were 3.4×10^5 times higher in colon tumors than normal lymph nodes, whereas *KRT20* mRNA levels were 1.3×10^5 times higher ($P = 0.02$). Median *PHGR1* mRNA level were 1.4×10^5 times higher in lymph nodes with known metastases compared with normal lymph nodes ($P < 0.001$), whereas the corresponding number was 2.5×10^4 for *KRT20* ($P < 0.001$). This finding suggested that PHGR1 may be a promising alternative to KRT20 for detecting lymph node metastases. The mean *PHGR1* and *KRT20* mRNA levels in examined colon cancers were 620- and 90-times higher than the mean level in the other tumor types tested ($P < 0.001$), respectively, indicating that PHGR1 is also more colon cancer-specific than KRT20.

Downregulation during tumorigenesis is a recognized weakness of using differentiation markers such as KRT20 as markers of tumor metastasis. To compare PHGR1 and KRT20 in this context, we measured *PHGR1* and *KRT20* mRNA levels in tumor biopsies from 209 patients with operable colon cancer and normal mucosa biopsies from 76 of the 209 patients (Fig. 6c and d). The mean *PHGR1* and *KRT20* mRNA levels were 6.2 and 6.7-times lower in tumors than in the mucosa, respectively. No significant association was found between primary tumor *PHGR1* mRNA levels and clinicopathological parameters or survival (Additional file 8 and data not shown). PHGR1 protein was also detected by IHC in all examined colorectal tumors ($n = 17$, Fig. 3c and data not shown).

As a proof-of-principle experiment, we immunohistochemically stained the PHGR1 protein in several lymph nodes with known CRC metastases (Fig. 6e). All examined lymph nodes ($n = 4$) were clearly positive for PHGR1 in the metastatic areas, suggesting that the PHGR1 protein is a potential marker of lymph node metastasis in colorectal cancer.

Discussion

Here, we report the first molecular characterization of the novel PHGR1 protein, which is specifically expressed in the gastrointestinal tract. PHGR1 is expressed primarily in the mature epithelial cells of the mucosal lining of the tract, is glycosylated and localizes in both the cytoplasm and nucleus. Transcript profiling

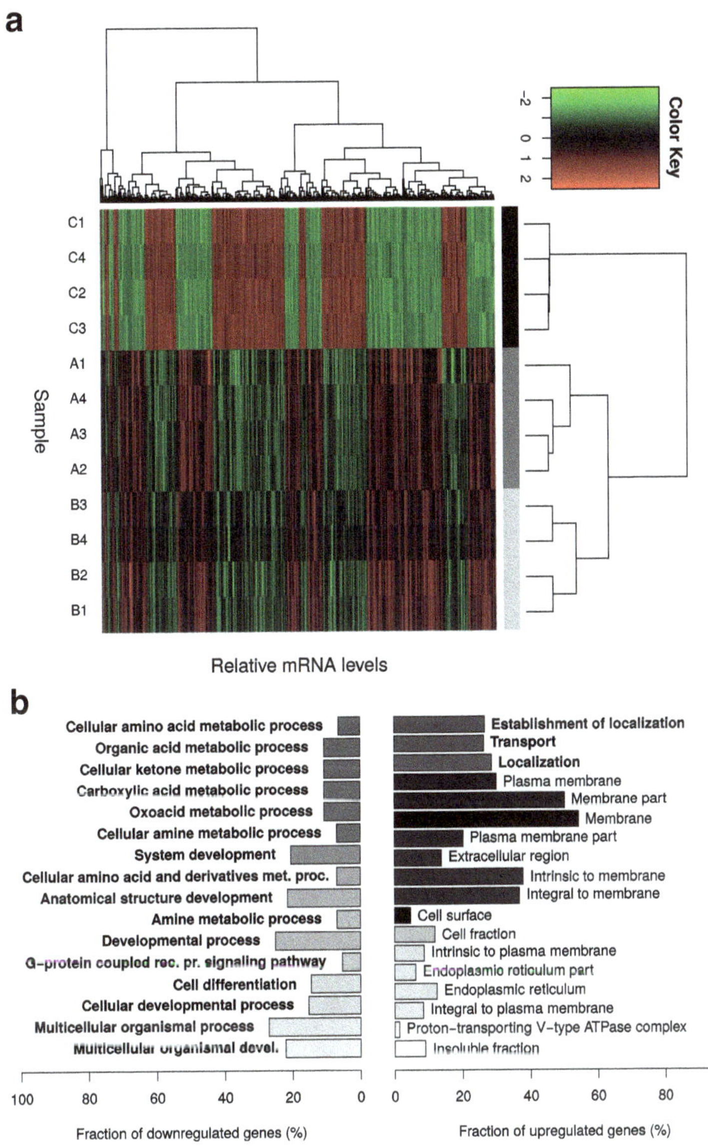

Fig. 5 Transcript profiling of HT29 cells subjected to PHGR1 downregulation. **a** Hierarchical clustering of samples (horizontal) and mRNAs (vertical) in the global mRNA profile of HT29 cells subjected to PHGR1 knockdown. Only the mRNAs with significant changes in response to PHGR1 knockdown are shown. The color key is scaled for each mRNA (row) to visualize differences. The sample names are shown on the left side of the heatmap; letters denote siRNA (C = negative control siRNA, A and B = PHGR1-targeting siRNA A and B) and numbers denote biological replicates. **b** Gene ontology analysis of genes down- and upregulated in response to PHGR1 knockdown. Gene ontology terms significantly enriched after correction for multiple testing are listed, biological processes (GO_BP) in bold fonts and cellular compartments (GO_CC) in plain fonts. Bar lengths show the fraction of downregulated (left panel) and upregulated (right panel) genes associated with the specific gene ontology terms, whereas the bar color reflects the adjusted *P*-value for each term (white: $P = 0.05$, black: $P \rightarrow 0$)

and gene ontology analysis of HT29 cells subjected to PHGR1 knockdown revealed a functional relationship with transport and metabolic processes. Finally, we demonstrated that PHGR1 mRNA and protein could be promising biomarkers for the detection of lymph node metastases in colorectal cancer patients.

Homology searches often reveal structurally similar proteins that may shed light on the function of a novel protein. However, the small size and extraordinarily high proline, histidine, and glycine content of PHGR1 represented a challenge for this approach. Nonetheless, we found several apparent homologs when performing the searches without compositional adjustment. Thus, the similarities were based more on similar amino acid composition than actual sequence homology. Some of the proteins also had other interesting similarities with PHGR1. The proline-rich salivary proteins PRB2 and PRB3 are also glycosylated and have tandem repeats [19].

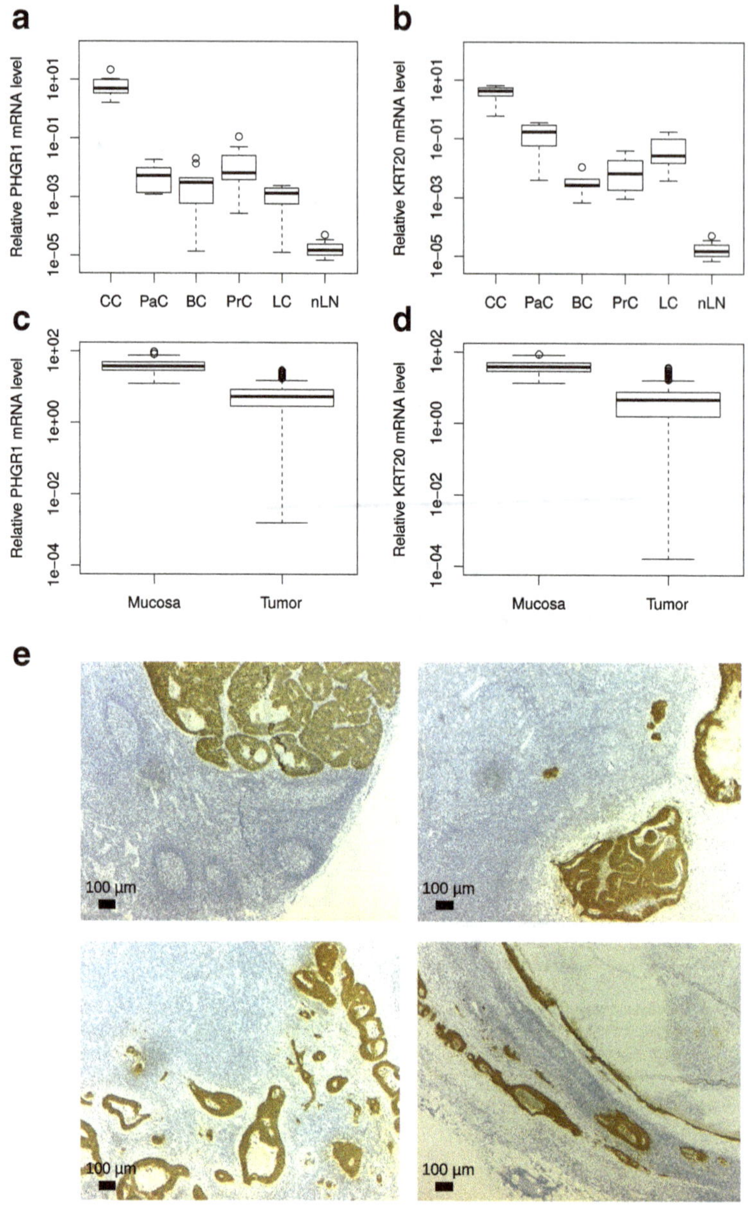

Fig. 6 PHGR1 is a potential marker of lymph node metastasis. **a** Relative *PHGR1* mRNA levels in colon cancers (CC, $n = 10$), pancreatic cancers (PaC, $n = 5$), breast cancers (BC, $n = 10$), prostate cancers (PC, $n = 10$), non-small cell lung cancers (LC, $n = 10$), normal lymph nodes (nLN, $n = 10$), and lymph nodes with known colon cancer metastases (mLN, $n = 10$). **b** Relative *KRT20* mRNA levels in the same tissue samples as in (**a**). **c** Relative *PHGR1* mRNA levels in mucosa ($n = 76$) and tumor ($n = 209$) tissue samples from patients with operable colon cancer. **d** Relative *PHGR1* and *KRT20* mRNA levels in the same samples as in (**c**). **e** Immunohistochemical staining of PHGR1 protein in CRC lymph node metastases. Tissue sections from four different lymph nodes with known metastases were stained with PHGR1 antibody (brown) and nuclear counterstain (blue). The images were obtained with a 2.5× microscope objective

Several collagens are also proline-rich, repetitive and glycosylated [20]. Another family of small proline-rich proteins, the SPRRs, are crosslinked in a multi-protein complex of stratified squamous epithelium, called the cornified envelope [21]. These proteins are small (8–18 kDa) and harbor internal repeats of 8–12 amino acids, similar to PHGR1. Interestingly, in our study the genes encoding SPRR1B and SPRR3 were both significantly upregulated in response to PHGR1 down-regulation (Additional file 5).

The multiple PHGR1 protein bands of unexpected size in our Western blot analysis encouraged us to affinity purify and validate our polyclonal PHGR1 antibody thoroughly. The strong correlation between protein and mRNA levels in multiple experiments (compare Figs. 2c and 3c, Fig. 3a and Additional file 2, and Fig. 3d and e) strengthened our perception that the PHGR1 antibody reaction was specific despite the unexpected results. Therefore, we searched other explanations for the unexpected band sizes, which were most likely due to some kind of post-translational modification of PHGR1. The modification had to be covalent because weaker bonds, such as disulfide bridges, are broken during SDS-PAGE. One alternative was isopeptide bonds generated by transglutaminases or ubiquitin/SUMO ligases [22, 23]. The single lysine residue of PHGR1 was the sole potential target for such modification. However, the resistance to trypsin digestion and the small differences in band sizes, corresponded to a modifier of flexible size and suggested glycosylation as a more likely explanation [24]. Intriguingly, the predicted PHGR1 peptide has very few potential glycosylation sites. The remaining alternative was hydroxylation and O-glycosylation of prolines or the single lysine residue. Glycosylation of hydroxyprolines has only been described for plants, whereas glycosylation of hydroxylysine occurs in collagens [20, 25]. The PHGR1 lysine being well conserved (Fig. 1) and having a glycine at the + 1 position, which is similar to the glycine required for collagen hydroxylation [20], supports O-glycosylation of this lysine residue in its potential hydroxylated form. TMFS acid treatment succeeded in removing the glycosylation, whereas enzymatic deglycosylation failed. This may be due to the complexity of O-glycosylation, which can block common enzymatic deglycosylation approaches [26].

The primary cytoplasmic distribution of PHGR1 protein in Caco-2 cells contrasted with the shift towards nuclear distribution observed in normal colonic mucosa cells (compare Figs. 4 and 3c). Interestingly, we also observed minor subclones of Caco-2 cells with PHGR1 present in both the nucleus and cytoplasm after 14 days of culture (Additional file 3). Full differentiation of all cells in a culture requires more time than full differentiation of minor clones [18], and the Caco-2 cells may therefore not have differentiated completely during our 14 day experiment. Varying culturing lengths have been reported for full differentiation of Caco-2 cells (from 14 to 30 days), possibly reflecting the heterogeneous nature of the cell line, which we also observed [18, 27, 28]. However, the biology of cancer cell lines is perturbed in various ways due to culturing, compared to the tissues from which they originate. Therefore, even if Caco-2 cells are generally accepted as a good model for intestinal enterocytes [18], our observations in this model should be interpreted with caution.

The speckled distribution of PHGR1 that we observed in differentiating Caco-2 cells (Fig. 4) suggested that PHGR1 may be associated with intracellular vesicles, such as endosomes [29, 30]. The resolution of the immunohistochemistry images in Fig. 3c was not sufficient to distinguish whether PHGR1 had a uniform or speckled distribution in the cytoplasm of normal enterocytes. Interestingly, the gene ontology analysis of genes significantly upregulated in response to PHGR1 knockdown revealed an over-representation of gene products localized to cellular membrane compartments (Fig. 5). Genes associated with transport were also significantly over-represented, suggesting that PHGR1 may be related to vesicle-mediated transport. We even found an over-representation of genes related to the proton–transporting vacuole-type ATPase complex found in the membrane of endosomes and other organelles [31]. The laser scanning microscope images indicated an apical, rather than basolateral, distribution of PHGR1 (Fig. 4g-i). Interestingly, evidence indicates that protein glycosylation plays a role in apical vesicle sorting, and that vesicle transport is important for maintenance of epithelial cell polarity [3, 32]. These observations encourage further research to elucidate the potential role of PHGR1 in vesicle-mediated transport.

The effects of knocking down a gene of interest on specific biological processes is difficult to interpret. The relationship between the gene of interest and the process may be indirect and the gene product may make a positive or a negative contribution to the process, neither of which can be unveiled by simple mRNA profiling.Therefore, the relationship between PHGR1 and metabolism and transport reported in our study is only hypothesis-generating. However, the transport aspect was supported by additional evidence (localization) and is also closely connected to the primary functions of intestinal epithelial cells: absorption and secretion [1].

Finally, we obtained evidence that both PHGR1 mRNA and protein may be promising biomarkers for the detection of metastases in colorectal cancer, as they have superior characteristics compared to the established metastasis marker KRT20. Differentiation markers (e.g. KRT20 and PHGR1) can be used to detect small deposits of tumor cells in clinical samples normally negative for such markers, such as lymph nodes from resection specimens [33]. This is valuable from a clinical point of view because metastases to regional lymph nodes is a well-known prognostic and predictive factor [34].

Conclusions

We have here unveiled important pieces of the functional puzzle for the novel protein PHGR1. Our present evidence suggests a functional role in mature intestinal epithelial cells that is specifically related to vesicle-mediated transport. However, further research is required to complete the picture. We also expect medical researchers to explore the biomarker potential of PHGR1 in clinical studies, notably with regard to colorectal cancer.

Additional files

Additional file 1: PHGR1 peptide sequence analysis.

Additional file 2: PHGR1 protein characterization. A) The barplot shows relative PHGR1 mRNA levels in the same samples that was analyzed in Fig. 3a, reproduced above. B) Immunohistochemical staining of PHGR1 in normal breast (1), liver (2), kidney (3), thyroid (4), pancreas (5) and placenta (6).

Additional file 3: Immunofluorescent staining of PHGR1 protein in differentiating Caco-2 cells.

Additional file 4: Verification experiments in relation to transcript profiling of HT29 cells subjected to PHGR1 downregulation.

Additional file 5: Upregulated genes.

Additional file 6: Downregulated genes.

Additional file 7: Gene ontology analysis.

Additional file 8: Clinicopathological data for the colorectal cancer patient cohort.

Abbreviations

AP: Alkaline phosphatase; CGAP: Cancer Gene Anatomy Project; DGED: Digital gene expression displayer; DIG: Digoxigenin; EST: Expressed sequence tag; ORF: Open reading frame; PBS: Phosphate-buffered saline; PET: Polyethylene terephthalate; PHGR1: Proline-histidine-glycine rich 1; RLM-RACE: RNA ligase-mediated rapid amplification of 5′ cDNA ends; siRNA: Small interfering RNA; TFMS: Trifluoromethanesulfonic

Acknowledgments

We are grateful to Dr. Åslaug Haga and Dr. Odd-Terje Brustugun for providing us with RNA from non-small cell lung tumors. None of the authors have any conflict of interest.

Funding

The study was financially supported by the Folke Hermansen fund and partly by the Western Norway Health Authorities. The funders had no role in study design, data collection and interpretation, or the decision to submit the work for publication.

Authors' contributions

SO did the PHGR1 cDNA cloning, mRNA expression profiling, mRNA in situ hybridization, some Western blotting, enzymatic deglycosylation and the mRNA quantification in general. IS did the immunohistochemistry. JG did the laser scanning microscopy. KT isolated and reverse transcribed RNA from cell cultures. EJ, BG, RS and RH provided technical and scientific advice, both regarding experimental design and interpretation of results. RH and ON initiated and planned the study. ON also led the study, did the bioinformatics, the Northern blotting, the majority of Western blotting, the Caco-2 differentiation, PHGR1 immunofluorescence, deglycosylation and PHGR1 knockdown by RNAi. ON drafted the manuscript and all authors contributed to the further manuscript preparation and approved the final manuscript.

Competing interests

The authors declare that they have no competing interests.

Author details

[1]Department of Hematology and Oncology, Stavanger University Hospital, 4068 Stavanger, Norway. [2]Department of Pathology, Stavanger University Hospital, 4068 Stavanger, Norway. [3]The Norwegian Centre for Movement Disorders, Stavanger University Hospital, 4068 Stavanger, Norway. [4]Centre for Organelle Research, University of Stavanger, 4036 Stavanger, Norway. [5]Oslo University Hospital, 0424 Oslo, Norway.

References

1. Henderson P, van Limbergen JE, Schwarze J, Wilson DC. Function of the intestinal epithelium and its dysregulation in inflammatory bowel disease. Inflamm Bowel Dis. 2011;17:382–95.
2. Clevers H. The intestinal crypt, a prototype stem cell compartment. Cell. 2013;154:274–84.
3. Apodaca G, Gallo LI, Bryant DM. Role of membrane traffic in the generation of epithelial cell asymmetry. Nat Cell Biol. 2012;14:1235–43.
4. Golachowska MR, Hoekstra D, van IJzendoorn SC. Recycling endosomes in apical plasma membrane domain formation and epithelial cell polarity. Trends Cell Biol. 2010;20:618–26.
5. Geibel JP. Secretion and absorption by colonic crypts. Annu Rev Physiol. 2005;67:471–90.
6. Livak KJ, Schmittgen TD. Analysis of relative gene expression data using real-time quantitative PCR and the 2(−Delta Delta C(T)) method. Methods. 2001;25:402–8.
7. R Development Core Team. R: a language and environment for statistical computing. Vienna: Foundation for Statistical Computing; 2007.
8. Gentleman RC, Carey VJ, Bates DM, et al. Bioconductor: open software development for computational biology and bioinformatics. Genome Biol. 2004;5:R80.
9. Benjamini Y. Discovering the false discovery rate. J R Stat Soc: Series B (Statistical Methodology). 2010;72:405–16.
10. Huang DW, Sherman BT, Lempicki RA. Systematic and integrative analysis of large gene lists using DAVID bioinformatics resources. Nat Protoc. 2009;4:44–57.
11. Falcon S, Gentleman R. Using GOstats to test gene lists for GO term association. Bioinformatics. 2007;23:257–8.
12. Nordgård O, Oltedal S, Kørner H, Aasprong OG, Tjensvoll K, Gilje B, et al. Quantitative RT-PCR detection of tumor cells in sentinel lymph nodes isolated from colon cancer patients with an ex vivo approach. Ann Surg. 2009;249:602–7.
13. Nordgård O, Singh G, Solberg S, Jørgensen L, Halvorsen AR, Smaaland R, et al. Novel molecular tumor cell markers in regional lymph nodes and blood samples from patients undergoing surgery for non-small cell lung cancer. PLoS One. 2013;8:e62153.
14. Nordgård O, Oltedal S, Aasprong OG, Søreide JA, Søreide K, Tjensvoll K, et al. Prognostic relevance of occult metastases detected by cytokeratin 20 and mucin 2 mRNA levels in sentinel lymph nodes from colon cancer patients. Ann Surg Oncol. 2012;19:3719–26.
15. van Klinken BJ, Oussoren E, Weenink JJ, Strous GJ, Büller HA, Dekker J, et al. The human intestinal cell lines Caco-2 and LS174T as models to study cell-type specific mucin expression. Glycoconj J. 1996;13:757–68.
16. Yeung TM, Gandhi SC, Wilding JL, Muschel R, Bodmer WF. Cancer stem cells from colorectal cancer-derived cell lines. Proc Natl Acad Sci U S A. 2010;107:3722–7.
17. Hönig E, Schneider K, Jacob R. Recycling of galectin-3 in epithelial cells. Eur J Cell Biol. 2015;94:309–15.
18. Sambuy Y, De Angelis I, Ranaldi G, Scarino ML, Stammati A, Zucco F. The Caco-2 cell line as a model of the intestinal barrier: influence of cell and culture-related factors on Caco-2 cell functional characteristics. Cell Biol Toxicol. 2005;21:1–26.
19. Kim HS, Lyons KM, Saitoh E, Azen EA, Smithies O, Maeda N. The structure and evolution of the human salivary proline-rich protein gene family. Mamm Genome. 1993;4:3–14.
20. Yamauchi M, Sricholpech M. Lysine post-translational modifications of collagen. Essays Biochem. 2012;52:113–33.
21. Kalinin AE, Kajava AV, Steinert PM. Epithelial barrier function: assembly and structural features of the cornified cell envelope. BioEssays. 2002;24:789–800.
22. Eckert RL, Kaartinen MT, Nurminskaya M, Belkin AM, Colak G, Johnson GVW, et al. Transglutaminase regulation of cell function. Physiol Rev. 2014;94:383–417.
23. Johnson ES. Protein modification by SUMO. Annu Rev Biochem. 2004; 73:355–82.
24. Moremen KW, Tiemeyer M, Nairn AV. Vertebrate protein glycosylation: diversity, synthesis and function. Nat Rev Mol Cell Biol. 2012;13:448–62.
25. Hijazi M, Velasquez SM, Jamet E, Estevez JM, Albenne C. An update on post-translational modifications of hydroxyproline-rich glycoproteins: toward a model highlighting their contribution to plant cell wall architecture. Front Plant Sci. 2014;5:395.

26. Marino K, Bones J, Kattla JJ, Rudd PM. A systematic approach to protein glycosylation analysis: a path through the maze. Nat Chem Biol. 2010;6:713–23.
27. Jumarie C, Malo C. Caco-2 cells cultured in serum-free medium as a model for the study of enterocytic differentiation in vitro. J Cell Physiol. 1991;149:24–33.
28. Esclatine A, Lemullois M, Servin AL, Quero AM, Geniteau-Legendre M. Human cytomegalovirus infects Caco-2 intestinal epithelial cells basolaterally regardless of the differentiation state. J Virol. 2000;74:513–7.
29. D'Souza RS, Semus R, Billings EA, Meyer CB, Conger K, Casanova JE. Rab4 orchestrates a small GTPase cascade for recruitment of adaptor proteins to early endosomes. Curr Biol. 2014;24:1187–98.
30. Gould GW, Lippincott-Schwartz J. New roles for endosomes: from vesicular carriers to multi-purpose platforms. Nat Rev Mol Cell Biol. 2009;10:287–92.
31. Marshansky V, Rubinstein JL, Grüber G. Eukaryotic V-ATPase: novel structural findings and functional insights. Biochim Biophys Acta. 1837;2014:857–79.
32. Kolset SO, Prydz K, Pejler G. Intracellular proteoglycans. Biochem J. 2004;379:217–27.
33. Nordgård O, Oltedal S, Korner H, Aasprong OG, Tjensvoll K, Gilje B, et al. The potential of cytokeratin 20 and mucin 2 mRNA as metastasis markers in regional lymph nodes of colon cancer patients investigated by quantitative RT-PCR. Int J Color Dis. 2009;24:261–8.
34. Edge S, Byrd D, Compton C, Fritz A, Greene F, Trotti A, editors. AJCC cancer staging manual. 7th ed. New York: Springer; 2010.

21

Celiac crisis, a rare and profound presentation of celiac disease

Elizabeth Ann Forrest*, Mark Wong, Srinivasa Nama and Siddharth Sharma

Abstract

Background: Celiac crisis is a life-threatening manifestation of celiac disease and is rare in adults, with only a handful of cases documented worldwide and mostly in children.

Case presentation: A profoundly emaciated 43-year-old female presented with profuse diarrhoea, shortness of breath, left leg swelling with ulceration and immobility (Body Mass Index (BMI) = 14.7 kg/m^2). The patient had normal anion-gap metabolic acidosis (pH = 7.16) with persisting hypokalemia, hyponatremia, hypomagnesemia and hypophosphatemia. In addition, severe vitamin deficiencies and coagulopathy were present. A computed tomography pulmonary angiogram (CT-PA) revealed bilateral massive pulmonary embolism causing infarction, arising from a left lower limb extensive deep vein thrombosis (DVT). Bone marrow suppression was seen on aspirate. The patient developed severe urosepsis in her immunocompromised state. Prolonged lower limb weakness despite supportive therapy, rehabilitation and strict adherence to a gluten-free diet prompted the magnetic resonance imaging (MRI) confirmed diagnosis of subacute combined degeneration of the spinal cord due to Vitamin-B12 deficiency.

Conclusions: Celiac crisis is a rare and potentially life-threatening presentation of celiac disease, often a diagnosis of exclusion. Subacute combined degeneration of the spinal cord should be considered in patients with chronic Vitamin B12 deficiency presenting with neurological symptoms.

Keywords: Celiac disease, Gluten, Celiac crisis, Subacute degeneration of the spinal cord, Vitamin B12 deficiency, Pulmonary embolism

Background

Celiac disease is a systemic immune-mediated enteropathy characterised by injury to the small intestinal mucosa. It is triggered by dietary intake of gluten in genetically susceptible individuals with class II human leukocyte antigen (HLA) DQ2 and DQ8 [1]. With up to 1% of the population diagnosed, clinical manifestations include diarrhoea, abdominal distension and failure to thrive [2]. It occasionally presents in adults as iron deficiency and osteopenia. The gold standard for diagnosis of celiac disease is duodenal biopsy, revealing lymphocytosis, crypt hyperplasia and villous atrophy in active disease [3]. Celiac disease is treated with a strict gluten-free diet. Celiac crisis, is a rarely documented life-threatening presentation of the disease. Mainly presenting in children, celiac crisis causes profuse intractable diarrhoea with severe metabolic disturbances (such as acidosis and hypokalemia), hypotension, neuromuscular weakness, cardiac arrhythmias and respiratory failure. An adult female presenting with celiac crisis is presented in this report.

Case presentation

A 43-year-old female presented to our facility with profuse diarrhoea, shortness of breath, swollen left leg with ulceration and associated weakness with immobility. This was on a background of 20-kg of unintentional weight loss over a 12-month period. The patient was profoundly emaciated (BMI = 14.7 kg/m^2), hypotensive (87/60 mmHg) with cool peripheries, had a moderately distended abdomen and a discoloured swollen left leg. Her past medical history was significant for biopsy confirmed celiac disease 3-years earlier.

On admission, the patient had a normal anion-gap metabolic acidosis (pH 7.16, (7.35–7.45)) in the setting of chronic malabsorption with ongoing losses. Profound

* Correspondence: Elizabeth.Forrest3@health.qld.gov.au
Diagnostic, Emergency and Medical Services, Gold Coast Hospital and Health Service, Gold Coast University Hospital, 1 Hospital Blvd, Southport, Gold Coast, Queensland 4215, Australia

hypoalbuminemia (< 15 g/L (35–55)) and globalised oedema was noted. Intravenous therapies were used to correct severe electrolyte imbalances including persistent hypokalaemia, hyponatremia, hypomagnesemia and hypophosphatemia. Coagulation profile revealed INR 2.1 (1–2), APTT 45 s (26–39), with thrombocytopenia and anaemia, haemoglobin 78 g/L (120–160). The patient was deficient in iron (Ferritin 19 µg/L (20–200), Transferrin Saturation < 6% (15–45)), Vitamin B12 (164 pmol/L (200–680)), zinc (5 µmol/L (8–18)), copper (5 µmol/L (11–14)) and selenium (0.5 µmol/L (0.7–1.4)). Vitamin B12 and iron deficiencies were treated timely with intramuscular and intravenous replacement, respectively.

Ultrasound of the left leg revealed extensive left lower-limb DVT. CT-PA of the chest revealed bilateral pulmonary embolism, associated pulmonary infarction and two cavitating lung lesions. Provoking factors for her DVT included prolonged pre-hospital immobility and severe hypoalbuminemia. She was subsequently commenced on therapeutic Enoxaparin. Infectious and autoimmune causes including systemic lupus erythematosus, antiphospholipid syndrome, sarcoidosis, tuberculosis, Q-fever, viral hepatitis and human immunodeficiency virus were excluded. Type 1 Diabetes Mellitus was also excluded. A large ulcerative skin lesion developed on the patient's left dorsum foot. Wound healing was impaired by chronic venous stasis, immunosuppression and peripheral oedema.

The patient developed urosepsis requiring treatment with Piperacillin/Tazobactam, Gentamicin and subsequently Ciprofloxacin. Her blood cultures and urine were positive for *Enterobacter cloacae*. Intravenous 5% Albumin infusions were given for hypovolemia and hypoalbuminemia.

Given the patient's profound clinical presentation, the treating clinicians had a strong suspicion for malignancy. A positron emission tomography (PET) scan revealed nil evidence of fludeoxyglucose (FDG) avid malignancy. Subsequent bone marrow and trephine aspirate revealed changes related to copper deficiency and severe iron deficiency (Figs. 1 and 2). Once stable, upper and lower endoscopy was performed to investigate for lymphoma. Histological analysis of gastrointestinal biopsies showed villous atrophy and intraepithelial lymphocytosis consistent with severe active celiac disease in the second part of the duodenum and lymphocytic colitis in the colon (Figs. 3 and 4). Duodenal biopsy Modified Marsh classification was 3c, in keeping with symptomatic celiac disease. Anti-tissue transglutaminase was elevated at 608 units. *Helicobacter pylori* infection was excluded as a cause for the patient's presentation, returning a negative urease (Campylobacter-like organism) test.

The patient was treated with high caloric gluten-free nasogastric and oral feeding regimes, these included elemental and semi-elemental feeds. As the patient was not meeting her target daily oral caloric intake, nasogastric feeds were commenced overnight to assist in weight gain in the context of persistent diarrhoea. A gradual resolution of diarrhoea was noted over a one-month period with a strict gluten-free diet and bridging Loperamide. After comprehensive history taking and investigation, it was concluded that the patient's celiac crisis was likely triggered by poor dietary compliance and consequent severe malnutrition.

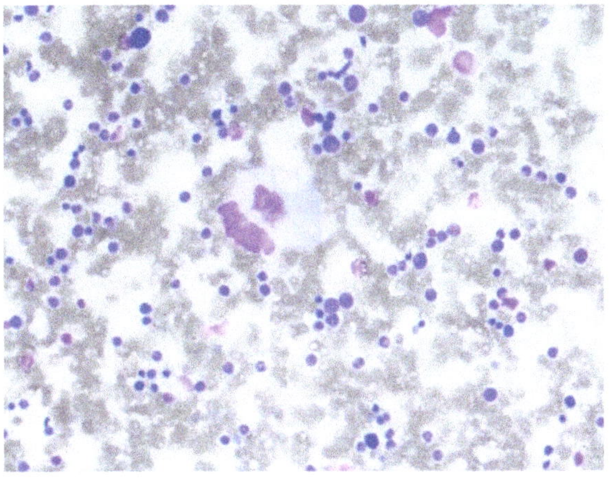

Fig. 1 Bone marrow aspirate showing dysplastic features including bi-nuclear megakaryocyte due to severe copper deficiency

Intensive inpatient rehabilitation was commenced for deconditioning and peripheral neuropathy. Weight gain was recorded over time. Subacute left distal radius and ulnar fractures were discovered, likely from a minor fall one-month prior to admission. Due to the patient's slow progression in rehabilitation and ongoing lower-limb neurological symptoms a magnetic resonance image (MRI) of the spine was performed. Neurologists diagnosed

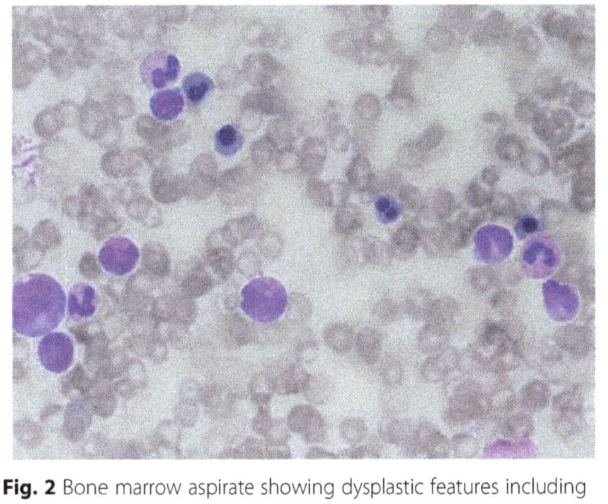

Fig. 2 Bone marrow aspirate showing dysplastic features including bi-nuclearity and nuclear lobulation of red blood cells in bone marrow

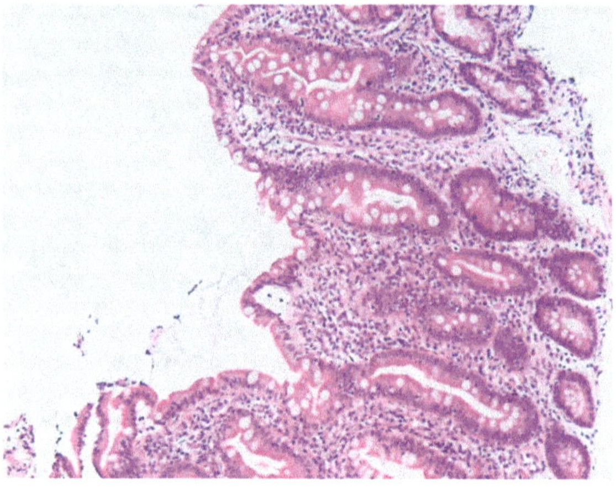

Fig. 3 Duodenal biopsy showing villous atrophy, × 20 magnification, stain hematoxylin and eosin

subacute combined degeneration of the spinal cord, due to chronic Vitamin B12 deficiency. Owing to this diagnosis, the patient continued to be wheelchair-bound and was discharged to a supported care facility. In total, the patient spent 30 days as an acute inpatient and 77 days in inpatient rehabilitation. She is still being followed up by our hospital outpatient haematology, gastroenterology, endocrinology and dietetic service.

Discussion

Celiac disease is a systemic immune-mediated enteropathy characterised by injury to the intestinal mucosa, affecting mostly the small intestine [1]. It is triggered by dietary intake of gluten in genetically susceptible individuals with class II human leukocyte antigen (HLA) DQ2 and DQ8 [2, 3]. Prevalence of celiac disease is most common in Western countries, with up to 1% of the population diagnosed [1]. Celiac disease rarely presents with life-threatening complications, however there have been a handful of documented cases of celiac crisis, mainly in children [4].

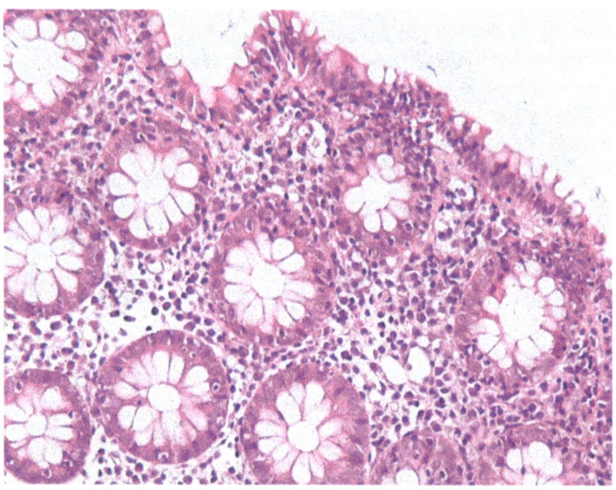

Fig. 4 Colonic biopsy showing microscopic feature of lymphocytic colitis, × 40 magnification, stain hematoxylin and eosin

This is a case of severe presentation of celiac disease which was life-threatening. Such a presentation involving haemodynamic instability, electrolyte imbalance, hypoalbuminemia and acidosis has been described as celiac crisis in the literature. A presentation of celiac disease of such severity is rare and thus can be misdiagnosed, particularly when patients have a variety issues. Due to this, it was paramount in this case to rule out other possible causes of her presentation before it was confidently attributed to celiac crisis.

Corticosteroids have been used in other countries as part of the treatment regime of celiac crisis [4, 5]. Steroids were not given to our patient due to her immunocompromised state and co-current sepsis. The aetiology of celiac crisis is unclear; however, it has been hypothesized that stress stimulus such as surgery, infection or pregnancy can be potential triggers [4].

Celiac crisis is life threatening presentation of celiac disease. With a limited amount of published cases in adults, its pathology is rarely diagnosed and is usually a diagnosis of exclusion. With celiac disease affecting a large proportion of the community, clinicians should be aware of the long-term consequences of celiac crisis, the importance of early diagnosis and its prevention. The most common presentation of celiac crisis is profuse diarrhoea, hypotension and muscle weakness [6]. Hypokalaemia is a key feature on blood work-up. Treatment is with supportive therapies and a strict gluten-free diet. Steroids can be considered, but should be used with caution, having been found to exacerbate hypokalemia [7]. Screening for vitamin and mineral deficiencies should be undertaken in patients presenting with coeliac crisis, as the consequences of prolonged deficiencies can cause significant morbidity. This case demonstrates the results of severe Vitamin B12 deficiency due to malabsorption, with the diagnosis of subacute degeneration of the spinal cord during the patient's rehabilitation journey.

Abbreviations

APTT: Activated partial thromboplastin time; BMI: Body Mass Index; CT-PA: Computed tomography pulmonary angiogram; DVT: Deep vein thrombosis; FDG: Fludeoxyglucose; HLA: Human leukocyte antigen; INR: International Normalised Ratio; MRI: Magnetic resonance imaging; PET: Positron emission tomography

Acknowledgements

The authors would like to acknowledge and thank (anonymously) the patient on whom the case report is based. In addition, the authors would like to thank and acknowledge the Gold Coast Hospital and Health Service for their support in the publication of this case report. We would also like to acknowledge Dr. Melissa Hancock (Haematology), Dr. Sewwandi Francisco (Pathology), Queensland Pathology and all the dedicated allied health and nursing staff involved in the treatment of the patient.

Authors' contributions

EF collected and analysed the patient data and wrote the manuscript. MW, SN, SS all wrote part of the manuscript. All authors read and approved the final manuscript.

Competing interests

The authors declare that they have no competing interests.

References

1. Green PHR, Cellier C. Celiac disease. N Engl J Med. 2007; https://doi.org/10.1056/NEJMra071600.
2. Nijhawan S, Goyal G. Celiac disease review. J Gastrointest Dig Syst. 2015; https://doi.org/10.4172/2161-069X.1000350.
3. Lidums I, Machaber A. First Consult Celiac disease. Clinical Key. Jan 5 2011. https://www-clinicalkey-com-au. Accessed 26 July 2017.
4. Jamma S, Rubio-Tapia A, Kelly CP, Murray J, Najarian R, Sheth S, Schuppan D, Dennis M, Leffler DA. Celiac crisis is rare but a serious complication of celiac disease in adults. Clin Gastroenterol Hepatol. 2010; https://doi.org/10.1016/j.cgh.2010.04.009.
5. Lloyd-Still JD, Grand RJ, Khaw KT, Shwachman H. The use of corticosteroids in celiac crisis. J Pediatr. 1972;81:1074–81.
6. Mones RL, Atienza KV, Youssef NN, Verga B, Mercer GO, Rosh JR. Case Report Celiac crisis in the modern era. J Pediatr Gastoenterol Nutr. 2007; https://doi.org/10.1097/MPG.0b013e318032c8e7.
7. Gupta S, Kapoor K. Steroids in Celiac Crisis: Doubtful Role! Indian Pediatr. 2014;51(9):756–7.

22

Cobalt chloride compromises transepithelial barrier properties of CaCo-2 BBe human gastrointestinal epithelial cell layers

K. M. DiGuilio[1,3], M. C. Valenzano[1], E. Rybakovsky[1] and J. M. Mullin[1,2*]

Abstract

Background: Elevation of the transcription factor HIF-1 is a prominent mediator of not only processes that accompany hypoxia, but also the tumor microenvironment and tissue regeneration. This study uses mediators of "chemical hypoxia" to ask the question whether HIF-1α elevation in a healthy epithelial cell layer leads to leakiness in its tight junctional seals.

Methods: Transepithelial electrical resistance and transepithelial diffusion of ^{14}C–D-mannitol and other radiolabeled probes are used as indicators of transepithelial barrier function of CaCo-2 BBe human gastrointestinal epithelial cell layers cultured on permeable supports. Western immunoblot analyses of integral tight junctional proteins (occludin and claudins) are used as further indicators of barrier function change.

Results: Cobalt, an inhibitor of the prolyl hydroxylase enzymes governing HIF-1α breakdown in the cell, induces transepithelial leakiness in CaCo-2 BBe cell layers in a time and concentration-dependent manner. This increased leakiness is accompanied by significant changes in certain specific integral tight junctional (TJ) proteins such as a decreased level of occludin and increased level of claudin-5. Similar results regarding barrier function compromise also occur with other chemical inhibitors of HIF-1α breakdown, namely ciclopiroxolamine (CPX) and dimethyloxalylglycine (DMOG). The increased leak is manifested by both decreased transepithelial electrical resistance (R_t) and increased paracellular diffusion of D-mannitol (J_m). The induced transepithelial leak shows significant size selectivity, consistent with induced effects on TJ permeability. Less-differentiated cell layers were significantly more affected than well-differentiated cell layers regarding induced transepithelial leak. A genetically modified CaCo-2 variant with reduced levels of HIF-1β, showed reduced transepithelial leak in response to cobalt exposure, further indicating that elevation of HIF-1α levels induced by agents of "chemical hypoxia" is responsible for the compromised barrier function of the CaCo-2 BBe cell layers.

Conclusions: Exposure to inducers of chemical hypoxia elevated HIF-1α levels and increased transepithelial leak. The degree of epithelial differentiation has significant effects on this action, possibly explaining the varying effects of HIF-1 modulation in epithelial and endothelial barrier function in different physiological and pathophysiological conditions.

Keywords: CaCo-2, Tight junction, Claudin, Cobalt, HIF-1, Occludin, Transepithelial, Paracellular, Barrier function

Background

The HIF-1α (hypoxia-inducible factor 1α) monomer in combination with the HIF-1β monomer, constitute in part the HIF-1 heterodimer transcription factor that is responsible for transcriptional regulation of a wide array of genes including those that favor the creation of a (precancerous) tumor microenvironment and survival in hypoxia in general. Increased levels of HIF-1α in the cytosol (e.g., by inhibition of HIF-1α degradation) result in elevated levels of the HIF-1 heterodimer transcriptional factor being formed in the nucleus where its regulation of gene transcription then occurs. Genes whose transcription is increased by HIF-1 include glucose transport proteins, key glycolytic enzymes, Vascular Endothelial Growth Factor (VEGF), Transforming Growth Factor-β1 (TGF-β1), TWIST, c-Met, lysyl oxidase (LOX), and the anti-apoptotic gene, MCL-1. Increased transcription of these genes favors cancer

* Correspondence: mullinj@mlhs.org
[1]Lankenau Institute for Medical Research, 100 Lancaster Avenue, Wynnewood, PA 19096, USA
[2]Division of Gastroenterology, Lankenau Medical Center, Wynnewood, PA 19096, USA
Full list of author information is available at the end of the article

development and metastasis. Regulation of HIF-1 levels has received great attention not only in the field of cancer biology but also in regenerative medicine, autoimmune diseases and hypoxia-related conditions generally [1–5].

Cobalt and other mediators of "chemical hypoxia" such as desferrioxamine (DFO), ciclopirox olamine (CPX), and dimethyloxallylglycine (DMOG) have in common an increase in the cellular content of the protein HIF-1α, achieved in part by these compounds' interference with the prolyl hydroxylase enzyme responsible for initiating the degradation of HIF-1α [6]. Cobalt therefore typically causes increased levels of HIF-1α in cells because degradation of HIF-1α is inhibited while its synthesis is ongoing.

In this current study we sought to ask one question: Does the treatment of intact, functional epithelial cell layer barriers with cobalt weaken, strengthen or have no effect on epithelial barrier function, using a highly investigated in vitro model of human intestinal epithelia, the CaCo-2 BBe cell line [7]. The published literature presents a somewhat bifurcated viewpoint on the issue of HIF-1 and epithelial/endothelial barrier function. There is a great deal of literature using mainly brain capillary endothelial cell culture models that indicates that compounds/conditions that increase HIF-1α levels cause leakiness in tight junctions and consequently cellular barriers [8]. On the other hand, other researchers, using mainly epithelial cell culture and rodent gastrointestinal tissue models have observed that compounds/conditions that increase cellular levels of HIF-1α are supportive of barrier recovery of intestinal cell layers from colitis-like experimental protocols [9]. While it is true that one has quite different cell models here (endothelial vs epithelial), these are two seemingly very opposed sets of findings. However, it needs to be kept in mind that the two disparate findings emerge from different starting conditions — those studies showing HIF-1 to be barrier *compromising* start from a fully functional, intact cell layer barrier. The studies showing HIF-1 to be barrier-enhancing start from an already compromised epithelial barrier that is engaged in repair processes to reinstitute barrier function. We believe this distinction is key to the apparent qualitative difference in outcomes, and we show data examining cobalt's effects on cell layers at different degrees of differentiation that suggest that this is indeed the case.

Methods

Cell culture

The CaCo-2 BBe cell culture, an epithelial cell line derived from human colon adenocarcinoma [7], was obtained from ATCC and was used between passages 52 and 70. Upon confluence, cells were passaged on a weekly basis by trypsinization (0.25% trypsin and 2.2 mM EDTA [Corning Cellgro]) and were seeded at 5×10^5 cells/Falcon 75-cm2 culture flask with 25 ml of Dulbecco-s Modified MEM (25 mM glucose) (Minimum Essential Medium) (Corning Cellgro) supplemented with 2 mM L-Glutamine (Corning Cellgro), 1% Non Essential Amino Acids (Corning Cellgro), 1 mM Sodium Pyruvate (Corning Cellgro) and 10% defined fetal bovine serum (HyClone). Cultures were incubated at 37 °C in 95% air/5% CO2 atmosphere.

Transepithelial permeability measurements

Cells were seeded into sterile Millicell polycarbonate (PCF) permeable supports (30 mm diameter with 0.4 μm pore size) (Millipore, Inc.) on day 0 at a seeding density of 5×10^5 cells/insert. This is approximately 50% of confluent density. Three or 4 sterile Millicell PCF inserts were placed into a 100 mm petri dish. On day 1, all cell layers were refed (2 ml apical/15 ml basal-lateral) with control medium containing 50 U/ml penicillin and 50 μgms/ml streptomycin, followed by refeedings every 2–3 days until treatment, then followed by electrophysiological measurements and radiotracer flux studies.

On the day of transepithelial experiments, the cell layers were refed with fresh control medium and allowed to incubate at 37 °C for 1.5 h prior to electrophysiological readings. All electrophysiological measurements were made in culture medium. Transepithelial potential difference was measured at 37 °C using 1 M NaCl salt bridges in series with calomel electrodes. Transepithelial electrical resistance (R_t) was measured at room temperature using 1 s, 40 μamp direct current pulses (through 1 M NaCl salt bridges in series with Ag/AgCl electrodes) in a custom-made Lexan chamber designed to accept the Millicells, and calculated using Ohm's law. Current-passing and voltage-measuring salt bridges were positioned above and below the center point of the cell layers. As soon as electrical measurements were completed, the basal-lateral medium was aspirated and replaced with 15 ml of medium containing 0.1 mM, 0.1 μCi/ml ^{14}C–D-mannitol (Perkin-Elmer, Boston, MA) or other radiolabeled probe, and incubated at 37 °C. Triplicate basal-lateral medium samples (50 μl) were taken for liquid scintillation counting (LSC) for specific activity determination. Duplicate samples (100 μl) were taken from the apical side at 60 min for LSC to determine flux rates. The flux rate (J_m) (in cpm/min/cm^2 and picomoles/min/cm^2) was calculated for the ^{14}C–D-mannitol diffusing across the cell layer. Flux rate studies involving radiolabeled lactulose and polyethylene glycol also utilized 0.1 mM total concentrations, and flux rates were determined similarly.

Due to our procedure of seeding Millicell PCFs at approximately 50% of confluent density, a 3-day (post seeding) culture is 2-days-post-confluence. A 7-day (post seeding) culture is 6-days-post-confluemnce, and so on. In this publication, cultures are defined by days-post-seeding.

Analyses of tight Junctional proteins

Following transepithelial resistance or transepithelial mannitol diffusion studies, cell layers on Millicell PCF membranes were washed 5X in 4 °C phosphate-buffered saline (PBS) and then harvested by carefully scraping into lysis buffer, followed by sonication and ultra-centrifugation. Samples of these fractions were analyzed by PAGE using a 4–20% gradient Novex Tris-glycine gel at 125 V for 1 h 45 min. 4–12% Novex Tris-glycine gels were used for HIF-1α and HIF-1β determinations. Precision Plus Kaleidoscope Protein Standards (Biorad, Inc.) were also included in each gel. Proteins were transferred at 30 V for 2 h from the gel to a PVDF membrane. The membranes were then stained with MemCode™ reversible protein stain, and densitometry measured. Blots were then washed 3 times with PBS-T (0.3% Tween-20) for 10 min each and blocked with 5% milk/PBS-T for 1 h at RT. Membranes were incubated with the specific primary antibody (anti-claudin-5, anti-claudin-7, anti-occludin [Life Technologies]) at 1.0 μg/ml in 5% milk/PBS-T at 4 °C. For claudin-5 this incubation was for overnight, followed by 2 h at RT. For occludin and claudin-7 there was only a 2 h incubation with the primary antibody at room temperature. The membranes were washed with PBS-T 3X for 10 min each, then incubated with secondary antibody (rabbit anti-mouse or goat anti-rabbit IgG labeled with horseradish peroxidase [Southern Biotechnology]) for 1 h at RT. Membranes were washed with PBS-T (4X for 10 min each), then treated for 1 min with Western Lightning-ECL chemiluminescence reagents (Perkin Elmer). The membranes were then exposed to HyBlot CL autoradiography film (Denville Scientific), which was developed in a Kodak M35A X-OMAT processor. Band densities were quantified by densitometry. Band densities are reported either as absolute values or against normalized averages of corresponding control band densities. All bands are also normalized to a densitometric determination of total protein in that specific immunoblot as visualized by the MemCode reversible staining kit (Thermo Fisher, Inc.). Full length Western immunoblots for all tight junctional proteins (as well as HIF-1a and HIF-1b) are shown in Additional files 1, 2, 3, 4 and 5.

Cell viability

The Cytotox96 cell viability assay was a product of the Promega Corporation. This is a colorimetric-based assay that examines lactate dehydroenase release from non-viable cells.

Statistics

For electrophysiology, radiotracer flux and protein chemistry studies, Co^{++}-treated cell samples (and other experimental treatments) were compared against appropriate matched controls within the same experiment. All data are expressed as the mean ± standard error of the mean (SEM) with the number of replicates provided for each set of studies. Differences between means are evaluated by two-tailed Student's t tests for two groups, or by one-way analysis of variance (ANOVA) followed by Tukey's post-hoc testing for multiple comparisons.

Reagents

Cobalt chloride hexahydrate was a product of Sigma Chemical Co. and was used as a 100 mM stock solution in water. Ciclopirox olamine was also purchased from Sigma and was used as a 250 mM stock in methanol. Dimethyloxalylglycine was used as a 100 mM stock solution in water and was obtained from EMD Millipore. All culture medium and associated reagents were a product of Corning Cellgro (Mediatech, Inc). The fetal bovine serum used in the culture medium was a product of HyClone (Thermo Fisher Corp.).

Results

Exposure of CaCo-2 BBe cell layers to 125 μM $CoCl_2$ on both cell surfaces for 48 h resulted in a small but significant elevation of HIF-1α (Fig. 1a), along with a highly significant (30%) decrease in R_t and a corresponding simultaneous increase in transepithelial paracellular diffusion (leak) of ^{14}C–D-mannitol (J_m) by nearly 100% (Fig. 1b). 250 μM $CoCl_2$ produced a greater elevation of HIF-1α (Fig. 1a). In evaluating the time course of this effect of Co^{++} on CaCo-2 BBe barrier function, cell layers were exposed to 125 μM Co^{++} on both cell surfaces for varying exposure periods out to 72 h, followed by measurement of R_t and J_m. As shown in Fig. 1c, the transepithelial leakiness that ensues from Co^{++} exposure requires 48 h to be detectable by R_t and J_m measurements. Decreased transepithelial leak — evidenced especially by increased R_t — may be occurring at the earliest time points (2 to 6 h) that were measured. R_t decreased to 60% of time-matched controls, and J_m increased to 250% of time-matched controls by 72 h of exposure. The concentration dependence of the Co^{++} effect on R_t and J_m is shown in the graded effects of increasing Co^{++} concentrations seen in Fig. 1d. 125 μM Co^{++} showed statistically significant effects on both R_t and J_m after 48 h of exposure, whereas 50 μM Co^{++} had a significant effect on R_t but not J_m. 250 μM Co^{++} decreased R_t by nearly 50% of control levels, while simultaneously increasing J_m to almost 400% of control levels.

This Co^{++}-induced compromise in barrier function occurred with induced changes in individual tight junctional (TJ) proteins. Occludin was decreased by over 30%, whereas claudin-5 was increased by almost 80%. No significant change occurred in the content of claudin-7 (Fig. 2). Cell layers exhibiting decreased R_t showed no significantly increased cell cytotoxicity as a result of 48 h exposure to 125 or 250 μM Co^{++}, as determined by a lactate dehydrogenase-based viability assay (data not shown). The 125 μM Co^{++} condition showed only a 5% increase in

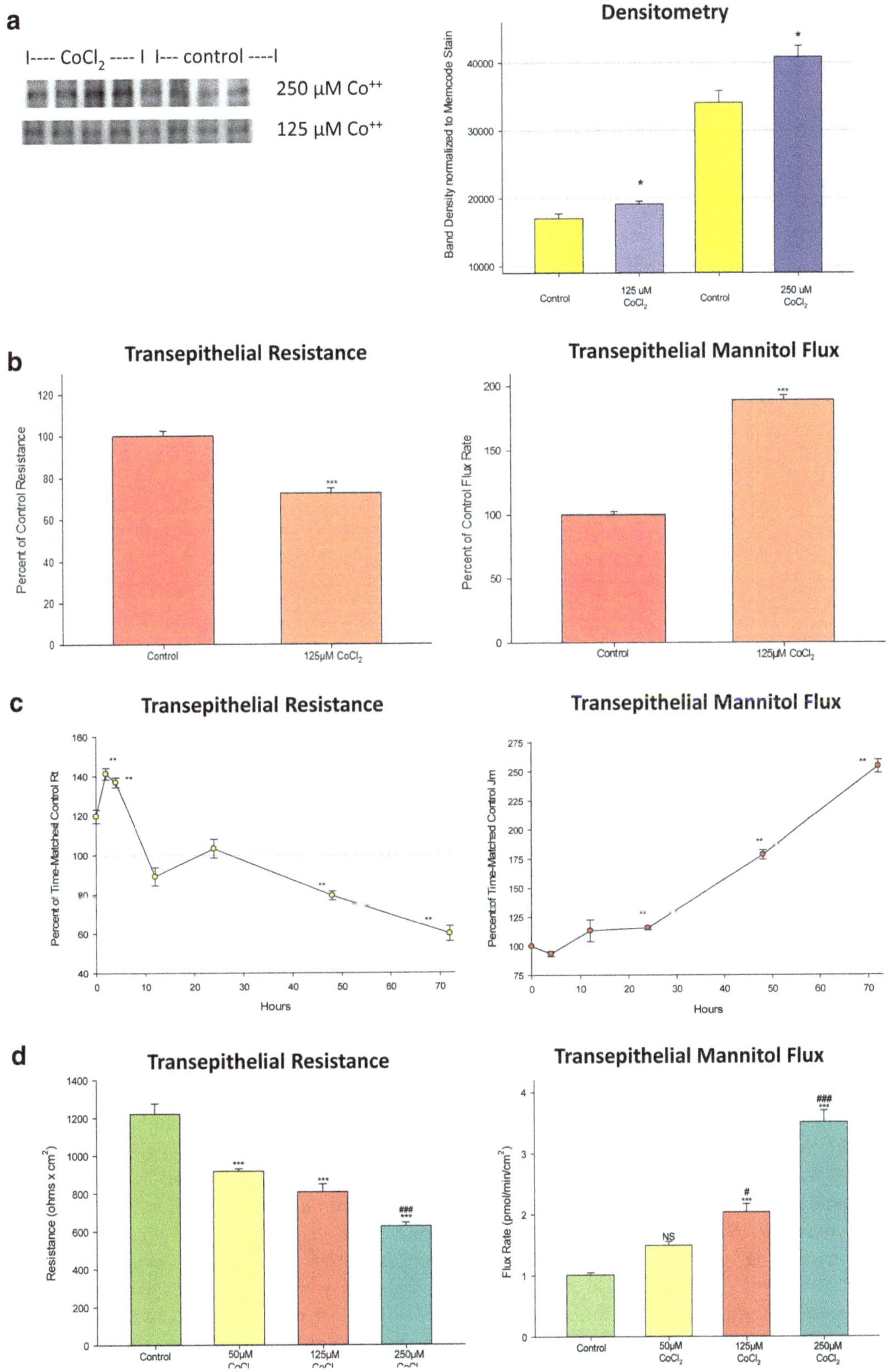

Fig. 1 (See legend on next page.)

(See figure on previous page.)
Fig. 1 The effect of cobalt chloride on CaCo-2 BBe transepithelial electrical resistance and transepithelial flux of ^{14}C–D-mannitol. **a** Western immunoblot data showing the significant increase of HIF-1α levels in whole cell lysates of 4 individual, 7-day post-confluent CaCo-2 BBe cell layers exposed to 125 and 250 μM $CoCl_2$ (or vehicle control) for 48 h. **b** The effect of Co^{++} on barrier function. Seven-day post-confluent CaCo-2 BBe cell layers were refed in control medium or medium containing 125 μM $CoCl_2$ on the apical and basal-lateral sides 48 h prior to electrical measurements. Data shown represent the percent of control resistance expressed as the mean ± SEM of 20 cell layers per condition. After electrical measurements, radiotracer flux studies with 0.1 mmol/L, 0.1 μCi/mL ^{14}C–D mannitol were performed on the same CaCo-2 BBe cell layers, as described in Materials and Methods. Data shown represent the percent of control mannitol flux rate and are expressed as the mean ± SEM of 20 cell layers per condition. ***$P < 0.001$ vs control. (Student's t test, two-tailed). **c** The time course of changes in transepithelial electrical resistance and transepithelial mannitol flux resulting from $CoCl_2$ exposure. Seven-day post-seeding CaCo-2 BBe cell layers on Millicell PCF filters were refed in control medium or medium containing 125 μM $CoCl_2$ (apical and basal-lateral compartments) and transepithelial electrical resistance was recorded at 2, 4, 12, 24, 48, and 72 h (different cell layers were used for each designated time point). Data shown represent the percentage of time-matched resistance (relative to vehicle-treated control cell layers) and are expressed as the mean ± SEM of 4 cell layers per condition. After electrical measurements, radiotracer flux studies with 0.1 mmol/L, 0.1 μCi/mL ^{14}C–D mannitol were performed on the same CaCo-2 BBe cell layers. **$P < 0.01$ (two tailed Student's t test vs time-zero cell layers). **d** The effect of increasing concentrations of $CoCl_2$ on CaCo-2 BBe transepithelial electrical resistance and transepithelial flux of ^{14}C–D-mannitol. Seven-day post-seeding CaCo-2 BBe cell layers on Millicell PCF filters were refed in control medium or medium containing 50 μM, 125 μM, or 250 μM $CoCl_2$ 48 h prior to electrical measurements (apical and basal-lateral compartments). Data shown represent the mean ± SEM of 4 cell layers per condition. After electrical measurements, radiotracer flux studies with 0.1 mmol/L, 0.1 μCi/mL ^{14}C–D mannitol were performed on the same CaCo-2 BBe cell layers used for resistance studies. NS indicates non significance vs control. #$P < 0.05$ vs 50 μM $CoCl_2$; ###$P < 0.001$ vs 50 μM $CoCl_2$; ***$P < 0.001$ vs control. (one-way ANOVA followed by Tukey's post hoc testing)

LDH release (compared to vehicle control), and the 250 μM condition showed only a 4% increase in LDH release. Neither were statistically significant.

Addressing the issue of the epithelial surface from which Co^{++} was able to produce this effect, the experiments of Fig. 1 were repeated, but now adding $CoCl_2$ to culture medium bathing one or the other cell surface or both. As shown in Fig. 3, this effect of Co^{++} was mediated specifically by Co^{++} exposure to the basal-lateral cell surface. Co^{++} exposure to the apical cell surface produced no significant effect on either R_t or J_m. Co^{++} exposure to both cell surfaces simultaneously, produced the same effect as Co^{++} exposure to only the basal-lateral cell surface.

Other "chemical hypoxia" agents known to elevate HIF-1α, namely ciclopirox olamine (CPX) and dimethyloxalylglycine (DMOG), were examined (at concentrations reported to elevate HIF-1α) for their effects on transepithelial barrier function. As shown in Fig. 4, like Co^{++}, CPX (at 15 μM) both significantly decreased R_t and increased J_m in a 48 h exposure. DMOG (1 mM) significantly decreased R_t but the increase it produced in J_m was not statistically significant.

In conditions where Co^{++} produced a 200% increase in J_m (125 μM, 72 h), we examined whether there was a size-selective "sieving" characteristic to the transepithelial leak by observing the transepithelial paracellular diffusion of different-sized molecular probes. Unlike the 200% increase seen for ^{14}C–D-mannitol (182 Da) leak in the presence of Co^{++}, the larger paracellular probe, ^{3}H–lactulose (350 Da) showed only a 45% increase in transepithelial leak (Fig. 5). All flux studies were performed using 0.1 mM concentrations of the radiolabeled probe. The still larger paracellular probe, ^{14}C–polyethyleneglycol (4000 Da) showed only a 20% increase. This suggests that the transepithelial leak produced by Co^{++} possesses sieving characteristics on, at least, a size basis. These comparative flux studies were performed after an extended 72 h incubation with Co^{++}. This longer incubation underscores this point that the effect of Co^{++} on transepithelial leakiness still results in a transepithelial leak that manifests size selectivity. Whether such leak demonstrates charge selectivity has yet to be determined.

CaCo-2 BBe epithelia are known to require significant time after reaching confluence to achieve maximal states of differentiation [10]. In prior work we demonstrated in fact that TJ complexes change as a function of time post confluence [11]. Seven-day cultures have attained near-maximal transepithelial electrical resistance, even though other differentiated features, such as surface membrane hydrolases, SGLT transporters, etc., may require a full 21 days post seeding for maximal expression. We therefore analyzed whether the transepithelial leak in CaCo-2 BBe cell layers produced by Co^{++} is affected by the state of CaCo-2 BBe differentiation. As shown in Fig. 6, less differentiated (3-day) CaCo-2 BBe cell layers were significantly more affected by Co^{++} than more highly differentiated (21 day post seeding) cell layers, in terms of transepithelial leak. A massive 8-fold increase in transepithelial mannitol leak was induced by cobalt in 3-day old cell layers, as opposed to only a 100% increase in 21-day-post-seeding cell layers. An 80% decrease in R_t was induced by Co^{++} in 3-day cell layers, whereas Co^{++} had no significant effect on the R_t of 21-day cell layers. Control 3-day cell layers had an average resistance of approximately 225 $\Omega \times cm^2$, whereas 21-day cell layers manifested average resistances over 1000 $\Omega \times cm^2$.

If the effect of Co^{++} on transepithelial leak was being mediated by the well-described increase in HIF-1α levels caused by Co^{++} inhibition of HIF-1α breakdown, we reasoned that this would in fact be due to downstream effects of the transcriptional regulation exerted by increased levels of the HIF-1α/HIF-1β heterodimer, HIF-1.

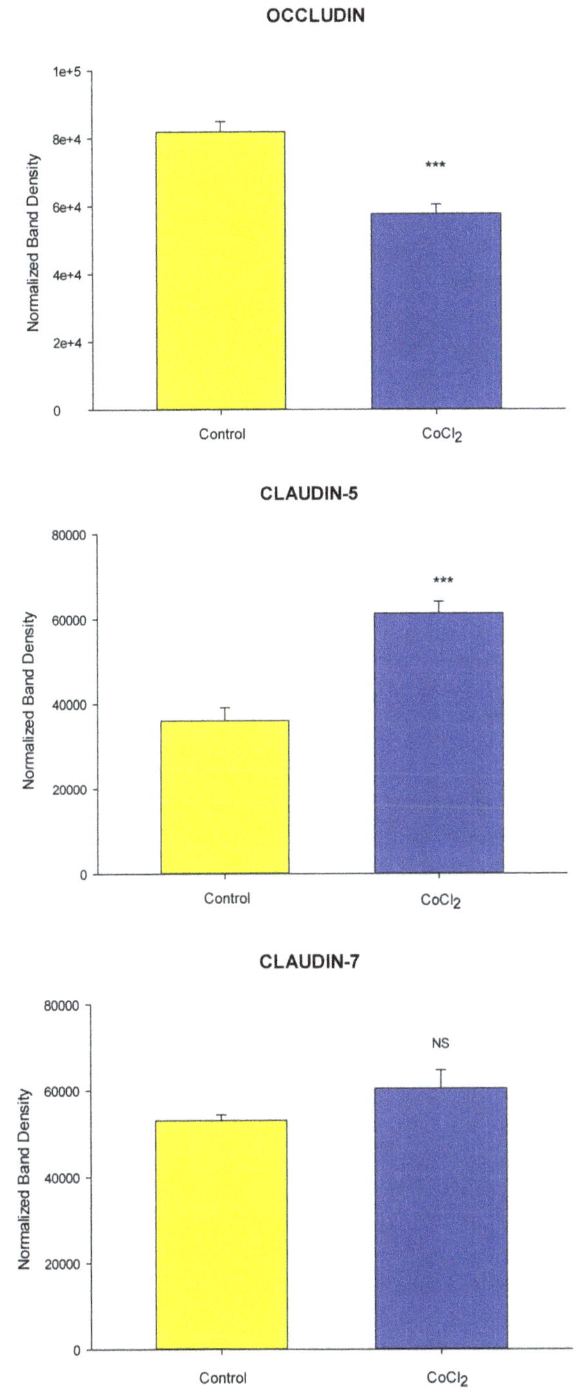

Fig. 2 Effect of 125 μM $CoCl_2$ for 48 h on the abundance of 3 integral tight junction proteins of CaCo-2 BBe cell layers. Seven-day cell layers were harvested from Millicell PCF membranes, and whole cell lysates prepared as described in Methods and Materials. Results shown represent densitometry of western immunoblots expressed as the mean ± SEM of 4 cell layers. *** $P < 0.001$, Student's t test, two-tailed. NS: not significant

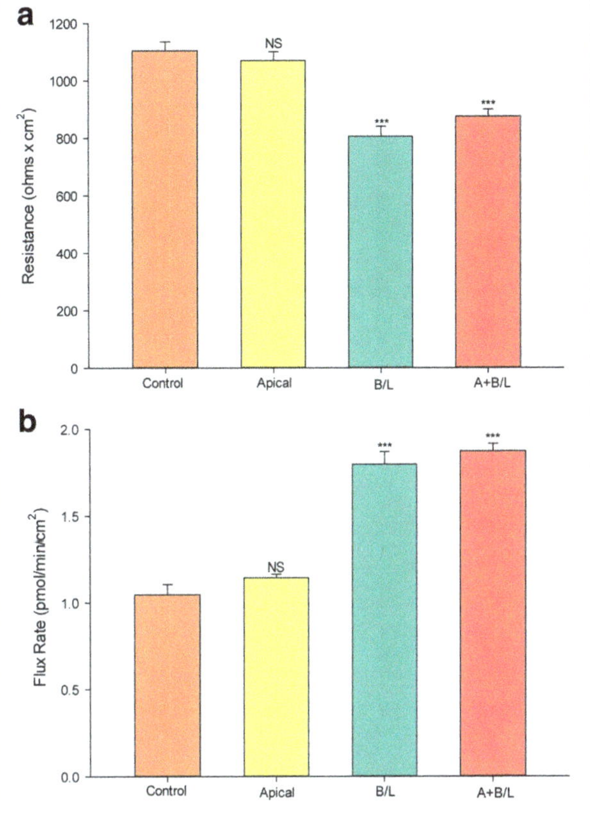

Fig. 3 Sidedness of the $CoCl_2$ effect on CaCo-2 BBe transepithelial electrical resistance and transepithelial flux of ^{14}C-D-mannitol. **a** Seven-day post-confluent CaCo-2 BBe cell layers on Millicell PCF polycarbonate filters were refed in control medium or medium containing 125 μM $CoCl_2$ on the apical-only, basal-lateral-only, or apical and basal-lateral compartments, 48 h prior to electrical measurements. Data shown represent the mean resistance ± SEM of 4 cell layers per condition (3 cell layers used in apical application). **b** After electrical measurements, radiotracer flux studies with 0.1 mmol/L, 0.1 μCi/mL ^{14}C-D mannitol were performed on the same CaCo-2 BBe cell layers represented in A, as described in Materials and Methods. Data represent the mean flux rate ± SEM of 4 cell layers per condition. NS indicates non significance. ***$P < 0.001$ vs control (one-way ANOVA followed by Tukey's post hoc testing)

Therefore a pronounced drawdown of HIF-1β levels in the cell, prior to a stabilization or increase in HIF-1α levels caused by Co^{++}, would result in a diminished effect on transepithelial permeability because of resultant lower levels of the HIF-1 heterodimer. As shown in Fig. 7, exposure of a HIF-1β knockdown variant of CaCo-2 (described in Saeedi et al. [12]) to 125 μM Co^{++} did in fact result in a sharply, significantly diminished response to Co^{++} relative to its transfection-control cell layers, with regard to both R_t and J_m as indicators of increased leak. We observed that this difference between the HIF-1β knockdown and its transfection control, with regard to effect of Co^{++}, was apparent when 3-day-post-seeding cell layers were used, but was not observable when 7-day cell layers were used. In 7-day cell

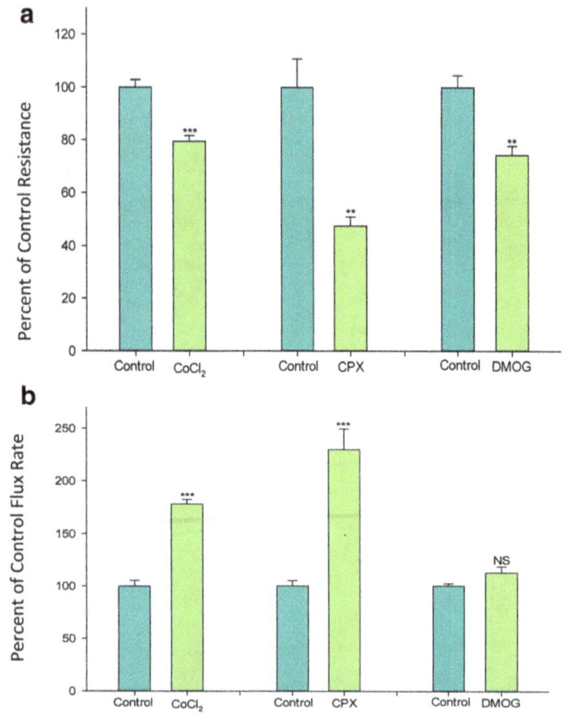

Fig. 4 The effect of the different HIF-1α up-regulators (cobalt chloride, DMOG-Dimethyloxalylglycine, CPX- Ciclopirox olamine) on CaCo-2 BBe transepithelial electrical resistance and transepithelial flux of ^{14}C-D-mannitol. **a** Seven-day post-confluent CaCo-2 BBe cell layers on Millicell PCF filters were refed in control medium or medium containing 125 µM $CoCl_2$ for 48 h, 15 µM CPX for 48 h, or 1.0 mM DMOG for 72 h (apical and basal-lateral compartments) prior to electrical measurements. Data shown represent the percent of control resistance and is expressed as the mean ± SEM of 4 cell layers per condition. **b** After electrical measurements, radiotracer flux studies with 0.1 mmol/L, 0.1 µCi/mL ^{14}C-D mannitol were performed on the same CaCo-2 BBe cell layers represented in A. NS indicates non significance. $^{**}P < 0.01$ and $^{***}P < 0.001$ vs respective controls (Student's t test, two-tailed)

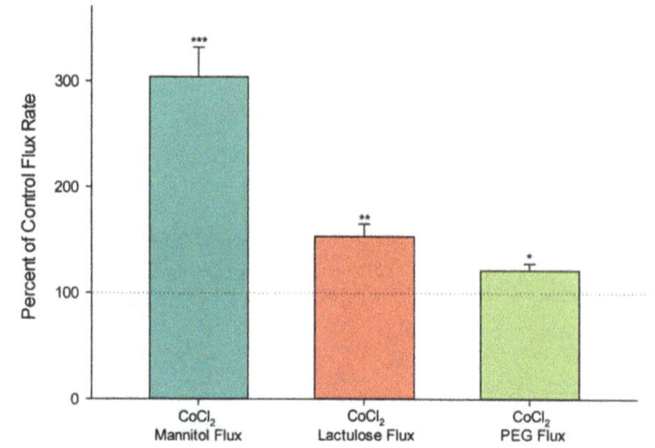

Fig. 5 The effect of $CoCl_2$ on transepithelial flux of ^{14}C-D-mannitol, ^{3}H-lactulose, and ^{14}C-polyethylene glycol across CaCo-2 BBe cell layers. Seven-day post-confluent CaCo-2 BBe cell layers on Millicell PCF filters were refed in control medium or medium containing 125 µM $CoCl_2$ (basal-lateral compartment) 72 h prior to radiotracer flux studies. These studies were performed using 0.1 mmol/L, 0.1 µCi/mL ^{14}C-D-mannitol; 0.1 mmol/L, 0.25 µCi/mL ^{3}H-lactulose; and 0.1 mmol/L, 0.1 µCi/mL ^{14}C-polyethylene glycol as described in Materials and Methods. Data shown represent the percent of control flux rate and is expressed as the mean ± SEM of 4 cell layers per condition. $^{*}P < 0.05$, $^{**}P < 0.01$, $^{***}P < 0.001$ vs respective controls (Student's t test, two-tailed)

layers, Co^{++} caused similar relative increases in J_m and decreases in R_t when comparing the HIF-1β knockdown to its transfection control culture.

Discussion

On a cursory review of the biomedical literature regarding the effect of HIF-1α on tight junctional permeability/barrier function, there seems to be an apparent contradiction. A very large body of mostly endothelial literature suggests that stabilization of (increased) HIF-1α levels induce increased leakiness in cellular barriers, an outcome with an array of pathophysiological implications (reviewed in Engelhardt et al. [8]). An excellent example of this literature is the study by Yan et al. [13] showing that the hyperglycemic induction of transendothelial (TJ) leak is mediated at least in part by HIF-1α. In fact, cobalt chloride stabilization of HIF-1α was shown to be one means of inducing endothelial barrier leak in this model. Yeh et al. [14] observed that pharmacologic inhibition of hypoxia-induced elevation of HIF-1α reduced the tight junctional disruption and barrier leak that ensued. This barrier-compromising action of HIF-1α is in fact not limited to reports using endothelial models. Cao et al. [15] report that the barrier-protective effects of berberine correlated with a suppression of HIF-1α activation in CaCo-2 epithelial cell layers.

On the other hand there is also compelling evidence in the literature that hypoxia and chemical hypoxia-mediated increases in HIF-1α levels can be supportive of barrier function. It is noteworthy here that this evidence of a barrier-friendly role for HIF-1 occurs in the context of barriers that have been already compromised in protocols mimicking the colitis condition. Karhausen et al. [16] noted in hapten-induced murine colitis, that decreased HIF-1 expression associated with more severe clinical symptoms regarding colon length, weight loss, etc. In dextran-sodium sulfate-induced murine colitis, the hydroxylase inhibitor, DMOG, was found to be protective regarding similar parameters [17]. In TNBS-induced murine colitis, another prolyl hydroxylase inhibitor stabilized HIF-1α levels and afforded protection in a similar manner [18]. Intestinal Trefoil Factor, one of many genes whose transcription can be upregulated by HIF-1, was found to reduce the barrier compromise induced by hypoxic conditions for CaCo-2 cell layers [19]. These findings regarding protective actions of HIF-1 in the context of hypoxia and colitis have been recently reviewed [9].

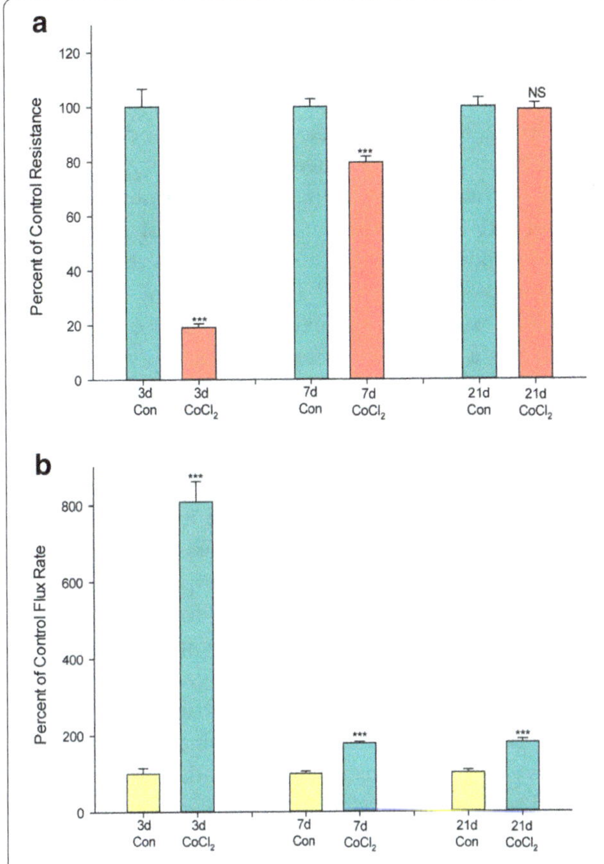

Fig. 6 The effect of $CoCl_2$ on CaCo-2 BBe transepithelial electrical resistance and transepithelial flux of ^{14}C–D-mannitol as a function of the differentiation state of the cell layer. **a** Three-day, 7-day, and 21-day CaCo-2 BBe cell layers were treated on the apical and basal-lateral sides with 125 μM $CoCl_2$ for 48 h before electrical measurements. Data shown represent the percent of control resistance and are expressed as the mean ± SEM of 8 cell layers per condition in the 3-day and 21-day experiments and 4 cell layers per condition in the 7-day experiment. **b** After electrical measurements, radiotracer flux studies with 0.1 mmol/L, 0.1 μCi/mL ^{14}C–D mannitol were performed on the same CaCo-2 BBe cell layers represented in A. NS indicates non significance vs control. ***$P < 0.001$ vs respective controls (Student's t test, two-tailed)

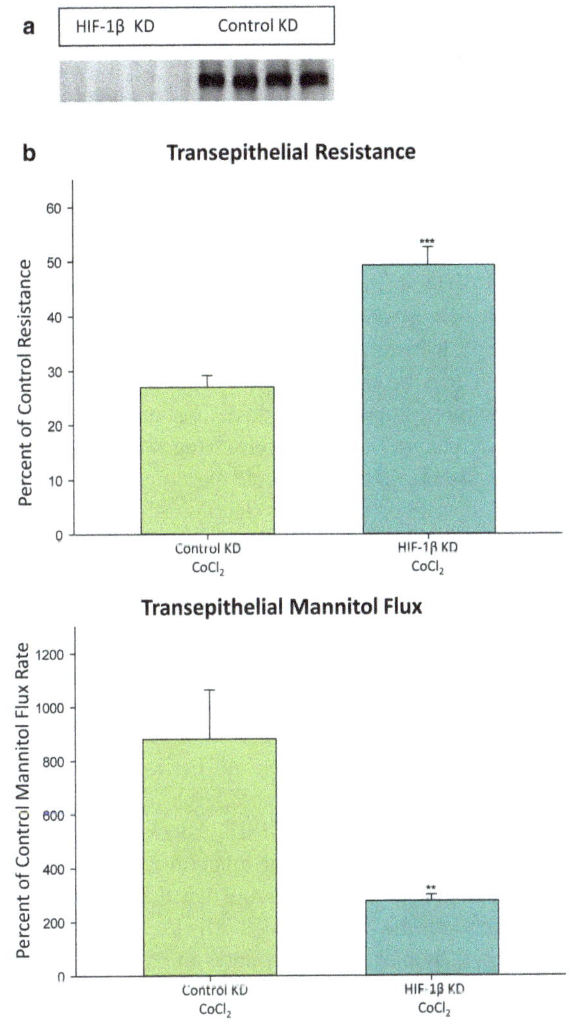

Fig. 7 The effect of $CoCl_2$ on transepithelial electrical resistance and transepithelial flux of ^{14}C–D-mannitol of HIF-1β knockdown CaCo-2 cell layers. **a** Western immunoblot data showing the levels of HIF-1β protein in whole cell lysates of 4 control CaCo-2 cell layers (lanes 5–8) vs 4 HIF-1β knockdown cell layers (lanes 1–4). **b** Three-day-post-seeding control cell layers and 3 HIF-1β knockdown CaCo-2 cell layers (also 3-day-post-seeding) on Millicell PCF polycarbonate filters were refed in control medium or medium containing 125 μM $CoCl_2$ on the apical and basal-lateral sides, 48 h prior to electrical measurements. Data shown represent the percent of respective control resistance and are expressed as the mean ± SEM of 8 cell layers per condition. After electrical measurements, radiotracer flux studies with 0.1 mmol/L, 0.1 μCi/mL ^{14}C–D mannitol were performed on the same CaCo-2 cell layers for which resistance measurements were performed. Data shown represent the percent of respective control mannitol flux rate and are expressed as the mean ± SEM of 8 cell layers per condition. **$P < 0.01$, ***$P < 0.001$ vs cobalt treated control knockdown. (Student's t test, two-tailed)

Our own data, obtained using the procedures we have detailed, support a barrier-compromising role for HIF-1. Three different prolyl hydroxylase inhibitors (Co^{++}, DMOG, CPX) all increased transepithelial leak. The leak correlated with increased HIF-1α levels. Leak was reduced when HIF-1β levels were lowered, reducing the cells' ability to form the needed HIF-1 complex. Increased leak was demonstrated by both significant decreases in R_t and significant increases in J_m, and correlated with modified levels of integral TJ proteins, namely occludin and claudin-5. The leakiness was seemingly not attributable to induced cell death. This interpretation is supported by the size selectivity of the induced leak.

Additional work clearly still needs to be performed to develop a connection between increased HIF-1 levels and increased barrier leak in functional CaCo-2 cell layers. First, immunolocalization of increased HIF-1 specifically in the nucleus needs to be performed. Secondly, it would be very informative to analyze for HIF-1-mediated changes in transcription generally in these cells by performing chip assays focused on HIF-1 binding to various promoters.

We caution against over-interpretation of the TJ protein data presented here, wherein one might conclude e.g. that increased claudin-5 levels are not consistent with decreased barrier function. First, these are whole cell lysates being analyzed, and we therefore don't know the contribution of cytosolic claudin-5. Secondly, it is not simply the level of claudin-5 (or any single claudin) that can predict the robustness of TJ barrier function. The heterotypic interactions of claudin-5 with other claudins — possibly also in play with cobalt treatment — may be even more important. Therefore it may be changes in ratios of claudin pairs that may be far more important in predicting or explaining TJ permeability changes than are the changes in any specific individual claudin. Lastly, it should be noted that CaCo-2 has many other TJ proteins than claudins –5, –7 and occludin. This is an incomplete presentation meant merely to show that HIF-1 modulation is modifying the TJ complex.

The involvement of HIF-1 in this action of Co^{++} that is presented here is supported by 3 pieces of evidence: 1) the increased levels of HIF-1α after Co^{++} exposure, a typical effect of Co^{++} in cultured cells [20, 21]; 2) the barrier compromise brought about by other agents of chemical hypoxia; and 3) the reduced effect of Co^{++} on barrier function in a CaCo-2 cell layer containing reduced levels of HIF-1β.

It is true that whereas HIF-1β knockdown is near complete, Co^{++} effects on barrier function were diminished but still apparent. One could reason that if Co^{++} action on barrier function is mediated through HIF-1 complex, the lack of the HIF-1β subunit should preclude an effect of Co^{++} on barrier function unlike the still significant effect that is shown here in Fig. 7. However Co^{++} has cellular effects other than the elevation of HIF-1α mediated by prolyl hydroxylase inhibition. Cobalt inhibition of the microsomal cytochrome P450 system and protein turnover in the cell is one example of a known effect of cobalt that could still be impacting the TJ complex in the absence of a HIF-1 elevation [22].

The peculiar polarity manifested in the action of Co^{++} on CaCo-2 BBe barrier function (Fig. 3) may simply be a result of polarized distribution of Co^{++} transporters in differentiated CaCo-2 cells, with greater Co^{++} entry into the cell across the basal-lateral membrane. This exact information regarding polar distribution of Co^{++} transporters in intestinal enterocytes or CaCo-2 cells is currently unknown.

Our finding that the state of differentiation of the CaCo-2 BBe cell population weighs significantly on the action of Co^{++} on barrier function (Fig. 6) may shed light on why HIF-1 can be viewed as barrier-unfriendly in some studies by certain research groups, while being barrier-friendly in others. We clearly observe that Co^{++} is unable to affect the barrier function of fully differentiated CaCo-2 BBe cell layers (21-day-post-seeding), yet has pronounced (negative) effects on the barrier function of less-differentiated cell layers (3-day-post-seeding). Therefore, the state of differentiation of a given cell culture or tissue model may matter tremendously in the exact effect observed. One should however note that the greater disruptive effect of Co^{++} on the barrier function of the less-differentiated, 3-day, cell layers — compared to the effect on the more differentiated, 21-day, cell layers (Fig. 6) — runs counter to the apparent barrier-supportive effect of HIF-1α in colitis models. In colitis models, the already wounded and disrupted gastrointestinal barrier should be less differentiated than its healthy counterpart mucosal barrier. However, there is more to the colitis state than simply a less-differentiated epithelial layer, and these other factors (inflammatory mediators, altered vascularization, etc.) could play significant roles in why HIF-1α could be barrier-supportive here.

The molecular mechanism(s) why cobalt action on 3-day cell layers is greater than on the more fully differentiated (21-day) cell layers could have many possible explanations. These could range from a different disposition of cobalt transporters, to different intracellular levels of HIF-1α or -β, to differentiation-dependent changes in junctional proteins or junctional-associated proteins. In addition, future work should also examine whether cobalt affects the cell cycling/division of CaCo-2 BBe cells, since such an effect would be disproportionately on the 3-day cell layers, as opposed to the 21-day cell layers, which are fully differentiated and likely not in the cell cycle.

In addition, it should be considered that there are a host of other factors that can impact not only HIF-1α and HIF-1 levels, but also the levels of downstream "players" such as VEGF that may themselves be directly impacting barrier function. This can be not only the rates of glycolysis and glucose concentrations in the cellular model [13, 23], but also the myriad factors that may impact the level of activation of the various PKC isoforms in the cell [24]. We feel it would be prudent to approach the issue in the biomedical literature from the perspective that both sets of studies are valid — those showing HIF-1 to positively as well as negatively affect barrier function. That being the case, it relies on future research to parse out the differences in methodologies, experimental conditions and cellular models that would result in these qualitative differences. Increased understanding of the mechanisms by which HIF-1 regulates barrier function will result.

Conclusion

Exposure of CaCo-2 BBe cell monolayers to cobalt chloride resulted in elevated HIF-1α as well as increased transepithelial leak manifested by a decrease in transepithelial electrical resistance and an increase in the paracellular diffusion of D-mannitol. Along with the increased leak, we observed changes in TJ protein levels — decreased occludin and increased claudin-5 — that, accompanied by size selectivity of the leak, indicates an effect of cobalt on tight junctional permeability. The fact that this barrier compromise was seen using alternative inhibitors of HIF-1α breakdown, CPX and DMOG, and that a reduced effect of cobalt treatment was seen in a HIF-1β knock-down, both point to a role for HIF-1 in the impaired epithelial barrier function.

Additional files

Additional file 1: Representative western immunoblot probed for Claudin-5, showing effect of cobalt exposure of CACO-2 cell layers.

Additional file 2: Representative western immunoblot probed for Claudin-7, showing effect of cobalt exposure of CACO-2 cell layers.

Additional file 3: Representative western immunoblot probed for HIF-1a, showing effect of cobalt exposure of CACO-2 cell layers.

Additional file 4: Representative western immunoblot probed for HIF-1b, comparing CACO-2 control cell layers vs CACO-2 HIF-1b knockdown cell layers.

Additional file 5: Representative western immunoblot probed for Occludin, showing effect of cobalt exposure of CACO-2 cell layers.

Abbreviations

CPX: Ciclopirox olamine; DMOG: Dimethyloxalylglycine; HIF1: Hypoxia inducible factor-1; J_m: Transepithelial mannitol flux; LSC: Liquid scintillation counting; PAGE: Polyacrylamide gel electrophoresis; PBS: Phosphate-buffered saline; RT: Room temperature; Rt: Transepithelial electrical resistance; SEM: Standard error of the mean; TJ: Tight junction

Acknowledgements

The authors are very grateful to Dr. Sean Colgan, Director of the Mucosal Inflammation Program at the School of Medicine of the University of Colorado, for his gift of the CaCo-2 HIF-1β knockdown model for use in our study. We are appreciative of the insights and comments of Dr. Sunil Thomas, Lankenau Institute for Medical Research, for advice in the preparation of this manuscript, and of the technical support of Ms. Anna Culbertson, Drexel University. Financial support from the Lankenau Hospital Foundation made these studies possible.

Funding

Funding to support these studies came from the Lankenau Foundation.

Authors' contributions

JMM was responsible for overall direction of the study and manuscript preparation. MCV performed all protein chemistry studies. KMD and ER performed all cell culturing and transepithelial permeability studies. KMD made significant input to study interpretation and manuscript preparation. All authors have read and approved the final manuscript.

Authors' information

Not applicable.

Competing interests

The authors declare that they have no competing interests.

Author details

[1]Lankenau Institute for Medical Research, 100 Lancaster Avenue, Wynnewood, PA 19096, USA. [2]Division of Gastroenterology, Lankenau Medical Center, Wynnewood, PA 19096, USA. [3]Present Address: Philadelphia College of Osteopathic Medicine, 4170 City Avenue, Philadelphia, PA 19131, USA.

References

1. Masoud GN, Li W. HIF-1alpha pathway: role, regulation and intervention for cancer therapy. Acta Pharm Sin B. 2015;5(5):378–89.
2. Nagaraju GP, Bramhachari PV, Raghu G, El-Rayes BF. Hypoxia inducible factor-1alpha: its role in colorectal carcinogenesis and metastasis. Cancer Lett. 2015;366(1):11–8.
3. Gilkes DM, Semenza GL. Role of hypoxia-inducible factors in breast cancer metastasis. Future Oncol. 2013;9(11):1623–36.
4. Khong TL, Thairu N, Larsen H, Dawson PM, Kiriakidis S, Paleolog EM. Identification of the angiogenic gene signature induced by EGF and hypoxia in colorectal cancer. BMC Cancer. 2013;13:518.
5. Flamant L, Notte A, Ninane N, Raes M, Michiels C. Anti-apoptotic role of HIF-1 and AP-1 in paclitaxel exposed breast cancer cells under hypoxia. Mol Cancer. 2010;9:191.
6. Milosevic J, Adler I, Manaenko A, Schwarz SC, Walkinshaw G, Arend M, Flippin LA, Storch A, Schwarz J. Non-hypoxic stabilization of hypoxia-inducible factor alpha (HIF-alpha): relevance in neural progenitor/stem cells. Neurotox Res. 2009;15(4):367–80.
7. Peterson MD, Mooseker MS. Characterization of the enterocyte-like brush border cytoskeleton of the C2BBe clones of the human intestinal cell line, Caco-2. J Cell Sci. 1992;102(Pt 3):581–600.
8. Engelhardt S, Al-Ahmad AJ, Gassmann M, Ogunshola OO. Hypoxia selectively disrupts brain microvascular endothelial tight junction complexes through a hypoxia-inducible factor-1 (HIF-1) dependent mechanism. J Cell Physiol. 2014;229(8):1096–105.
9. Colgan SP, Taylor CT. Hypoxia: an alarm signal during intestinal inflammation. Nat Rev Gastroenterol Hepatol. 2010;7(5):281–7.
10. Hidalgo IJ, Raub TJ, Borchardt RT. Characterization of the human colon carcinoma cell line (Caco-2) as a model system for intestinal epithelial permeability. Gastroenterology. 1989;96(3):736–49.
11. Valenzano MC, DiGuilio K, Mercado J, Teter M, To J, Ferraro B, Mixson B, Manley I, Baker V, Moore BA, et al. Remodeling of tight junctions and enhancement of barrier integrity of the CACO-2 intestinal epithelial cell layer by micronutrients. PLoS One. 2015;10(7):e0133926.
12. Saeedi BJ, Kao DJ, Kitzenberg DA, Dobrinskikh E, Schwisow KD, Masterson JC, Kendrick AA, Kelly CJ, Bayless AJ, Kominsky DJ, et al. HIF-dependent regulation of claudin-1 is central to intestinal epithelial tight junction integrity. Mol Biol Cell. 2015;26(12):2252–62.
13. Yan J, Zhang Z, Shi H. HIF-1 is involved in high glucose-induced paracellular permeability of brain endothelial cells. Cell Mol Life Sci. 2012;69(1):115–28.
14. Yeh WL, DY L, Lin CJ, Liou HC, WM F. Inhibition of hypoxia-induced increase of blood-brain barrier permeability by YC-1 through the antagonism of HIF-1alpha accumulation and VEGF expression. Mol Pharmacol. 2007;72(2):440–9.
15. Cao M, Wang P, Sun C, He W, Wang F. Amelioration of IFN-gamma and TNF-alpha induced intestinal epithelial barrier dysfunction by berberine via suppression of MLCK-MLC phosphorylation signaling pathway. PLoS One. 2013;8(5):e61944.
16. Karhausen J, Furuta GT, Tomaszewski JE, Johnson RS, Colgan SP, Haase VH. Epithelial hypoxia-inducible factor-1 is protective in murine experimental colitis. J Clin Invest. 2004;114(8):1098–106.
17. Cummins EP, Seeballuck F, Keely SJ, Mangan NE, Callanan JJ, Fallon PG, Taylor CT. The hydroxylase inhibitor dimethyloxalylglycine is protective in a murine model of colitis. Gastroenterology. 2008;134(1):156–65.
18. Robinson A, Keely S, Karhausen J, Gerich ME, Furuta GT, Colgan SP. Mucosal protection by hypoxia-inducible factor prolyl hydroxylase inhibition. Gastroenterology. 2008;134(1):145–55.
19. Furuta GT, Turner JR, Taylor CT, Hershberg RM, Comerford K, Narravula S, Podolsky DK, Colgan SP. Hypoxia-inducible factor 1-dependent induction of intestinal trefoil factor protects barrier function during hypoxia. J Exp Med. 2001;193(9):1027–34.
20. Chen C, Pore N, Behrooz A, Ismail-Beigi F, Maity A. Regulation of glut1 mRNA by hypoxia-inducible factor-1. Interaction between H-ras and hypoxia. J Biol Chem. 2001;276(12):9519–25.

23

Pneumatosis cystoides intestinalis

Yong juan Wang[1†], Yu ming Wang[2†], Yan min Zheng[2], Hui qing Jiang[1] and Jie Zhang[2*]

Abstract

Background: Pneumatosis cystoides intestinalis (PCI) is characterized by gas-filled cysts in the intestinal submucosa and subserosa. There are few reports of PCI occurring in duodenum and rectum. Here we demonstrated four different endoscopic manifestations of PCI and three cases with intestinal stricture all were successfully managed by medical conservative treatment.

Case presentation: There are 6 cases of PCI with varied causes encountered, in which the etiology, endoscopic features, treatment methods and prognosis of patients were studied. One case was idiopathic, while the other one case was caused by exposing to trichloroethylene (TCE), and the remaining four cases were secondary to diabetes, emphysema, therioma and diseases of immune system. Of the six patients, all complained of abdominal distention or diarrhea, three (50%) reported muco-bloody stools, two (33.3%) complained of abdominal pain. In four other patients, PCI occurred in the colon, especially the sigmoid colon, while in the other two patients, it occurred in duodenum and rectum. Endoscopic findings were divided into bubble-like pattern, grape or beaded circular forms, linear or cobblestone gas formation and irregular forms. After combination of medicine and endoscopic treatment, the symptoms of five patients were relieved, while one patient died of malignant tumors.

Conclusion: PCI endoscopic manifestations were varied, and radiology combined with endoscopy can avoid misdiagnosis. The primary bubble-like pattern can be cured by endoscopic resection, while removal of etiology combined with drug therapy can resolve majority of secondary cases, thereby avoiding the adverse risks of surgery.

Keywords: Pneumatosis Cystoides intestinalis, Diagnosis, Endoscopy, Therapy

Background

Pneumatosis cystoides intestinalis (PCI) is characterized by gas-filled cysts in the intestinal submucosa and subserosa. It is a rare disease with reported incidence of 0.03% and can occur in any age group [1]. PCI was first described by DuVernoi in 1783 and later subcategorized by Koss in 1952 [2]. It can be divided into primary or idiopathic (15%) type, which refers to air pockets that are cystic in appearance and imply to a chronic, benign idiopathic etiology [3], and secondary type (85%), which refers to radiological findings of linear, microvesicular, or more circumferential appearing intramural gas caused by various predisposing factors [3, 4]. The pathogenesis of PCI remains unclear; however, six pathophysiologic mechanisms have been proposed including inflammation, physical damage of intestinal mucosa, nutritional imbalance and dysbacteriosis, gastrointestinal dysmotility, and immune dysfunction [5, 6]. PCI can occur anywhere within the gastrointestinal tract from the esophagus to the rectum. It was previously reported that mainly involve the terminal ileum, but Morris later reported that PCI localized to large intestine in 46% of the cases, the small intestine in 27% of the cases, the stomach in 5% of the cases and the large combined with small intestine in 7% of the cases [7]. PCI can be found incidentally in asymptomatic patients, while some cases presented as abdominal pain, diarrhea, abdominal distention, constipation, bloody stool, flatus, loss of appetite, weight loss, and even life-threatening illnesses including bowel necrosis and perforation [8].

Several reports of endoscopic ultrasonography (EUS) in the evaluation of bumps in the colon have clarified the diagnosis of PCI [9, 10], while computed tomography scan

* Correspondence: Zhangjiezhj1024@yahoo.com
†Yong juan Wang and Yu ming Wang contributed equally to this work.
[2]Department of Gastroenterology and Hepatology, The General Hospital of Tianjin Medical University, Tianjin, China
Full list of author information is available at the end of the article

is regarded as the most sensitive imaging modality for detection. However, some patients who frequently presented with non-specific gastrointestinal symptoms were often prone to be misdiagnosed or maltreated and even underwent surgical resection, which resulted in several adverse events. Herein, we reported the etiological characteristics, endoscopic features, treatment and prognosis of 6 PCI cases to recognize the endoscopic characteristics and investigate the proper treatment methods for PCI.

Case presentation

Case 1

A 56-year-old man was admitted to the hospital with abdominal distension and diarrhea for several days. Physical examination revealed no abnormality. Routine laboratory examinations, bacterial and parasitic stool examinations and viral serology were negative. Chest and abdomen X-ray showed no obvious abnormality. However, endoscopic examination disclosed scattered bubble-like or cystoid nodules, which distributed in transverse colon (Fig. 1b). Meantime, narrow band imaging (NBI) showed clear texture of intestinal wall vessels (Fig. 1c). Considered PCI was idiopathic, we used high frequency electrosurgical resection of the gas cysts, and the cysts were collapsed after the gas was discharged (Fig. 1a). The patient was treated with Bifidobacterium (420 mg/bid) to improve his intestinal function (Table 1). We also advised him to eat less gas-producing foods without using any antibiotic. The patient was symptom-free after one week and the lesions disappeared completely after three months of follow-up (Fig. 3a, b).

Case 2

A 48-year-old woman complained of constipation for 5 days, and then turned into diarrhea with discontinuous abdominal distension. She was hospitalized because of

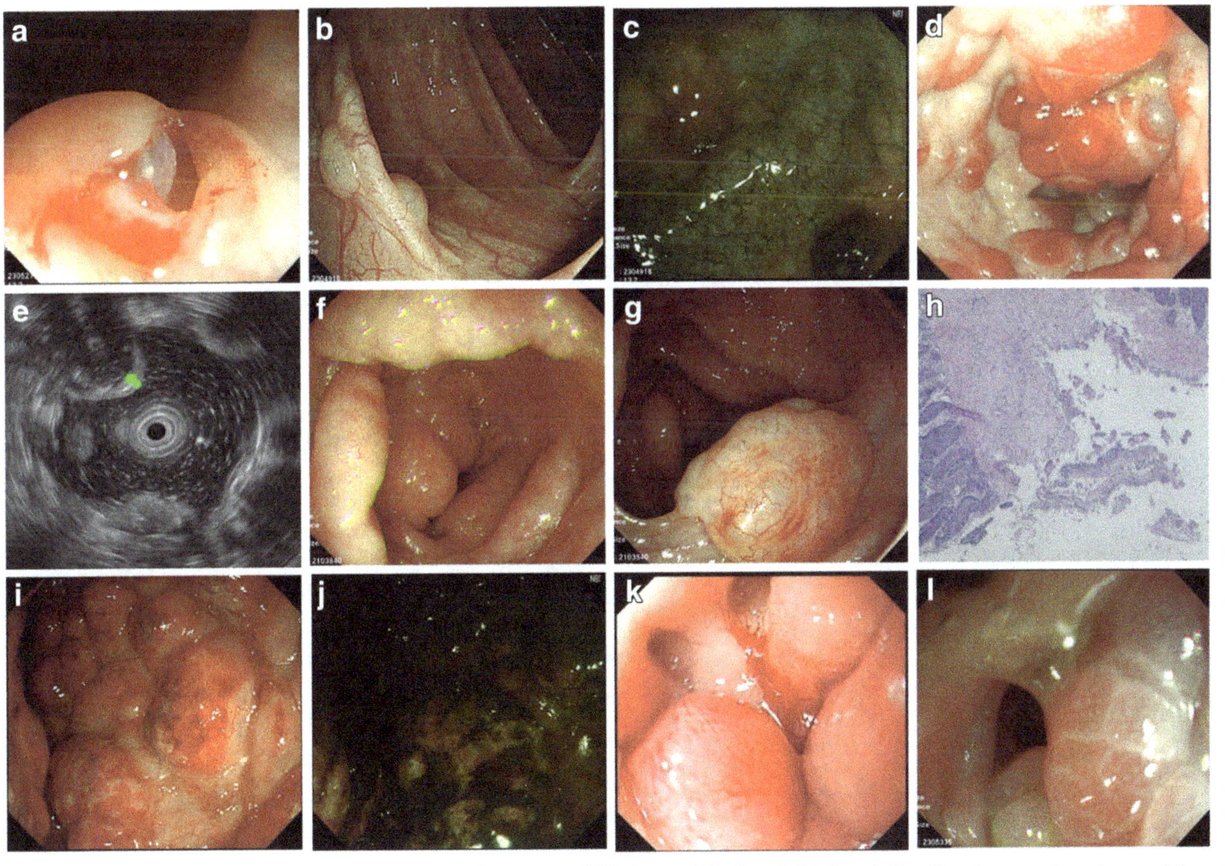

Fig. 1 Endoscopic features of PCI. Case 1: (**a-c**); Case 2: (**d**, **e**); Case 3: (**f-h**); Case 4: (**i**, **j**); Case 5: (**k**); Case 6: (**l**). **a** Biopsies were done to reveal the nature of the cystic lesions underneath the mucosa; **b** Scattered bubble-like or cystoid nodules were seen, which needed to be distinguished from polyps; **c** NBI showed clear texture of intestinal wall vessels; **d** Grape-like or beaded subepithelial lesions were identified in the colon, some with erythematous mucosa; **e** The endoscopic ultrasonography showed low echo of cystic below the mucosal layer; **f** Line or pebble like sessile cysts were distributed around the colon, with normal overlying mucosa; **g** Irregular forms were disclosed, which needed to be distinguished from malignant tumor; **h** The pathologic findings revealed submucosal cystic structure; **i** Irregular forms needed to be distinguished from Crohn's disease; **j** NBI showed unclear vascular texture on mucosal surface; **k** Gastroscope demonstrated duodenal gas cyst, leading to lumen stenosis; **l** Appearance of air cysts in the rectum, honeycomb-like

Table 1 General conditions, clinical manifestations, endoscopic features, treatment and prognosis of patients with PCI

No.	Age	Gender	symptoms	Etiology	Loc.	Endoscopic findings	PCI treatment	Outcome	Follow-up (mo)
1	56	M	abdominal distension diarrhea	–	Transverse ascending	bubble-like	Bifidobacterium endoscopic treatment	remission	3
2	48	F	Constipation, diarrhea, muco-bloody stools, abdominal distension farting more	exposure to TCE (1 year)	Sigmoid descending	grape or beaded	tinidazole, Bifidobacterium endoscopic treatment	remission	4
3	66	F	constipation, diarrhea muco-bloody stools abdominal pain	AA (20 years) UCTD (2 years)	Sigmoid	linear or bullous	Bifidobacterium aluminum phosphate	remission	10
4	72	F	constipation, diarrhea muco-bloody stools abdominal distension farting more	diabetes (10 years)	Sigmoid ascending	irregular forms	rifaximin metronidazole Bifidobacterium	remission	6
5	64	M	abdominal distension abdominal pain	emphysema (1 year)	Duodenal- bulb	bubble-like	Bifidobacterium	remission	8
6	27	F	abdominal distension diarrhea abdominal pain	peritoneal carcinoma	Rectum	grape or beaded	Bifidobacterium	died	

TCE trichloroethylene, *AA* aplastic anemia, *UCTD* Undifferentiated connective tissue disease

severe diarrhea (7 times/ d) with muco-bloody stools for one week. The stool frequency was five times a day. Her previous medical history revealed exposure to trichloroethylene (TCE) for one year. (Table 1) Physical examination at admission revealed extensive abdominal tenderness. Fecal occult blood tests were positive. Other serological markers for autoimmunity and viral serology were normal, as was stool examination for bacteria and parasites. However, abdominal X-ray showed multiple intraluminal gas pockets in the left colon (Fig. 2a). Coronal reconstruction confirmed the widespread serosal intestinal air cysts involving long segment of colon (Fig. 2b). Colonoscopy revealed grape-like or beaded subepithelial lesions, and some with erythematous mucosa distributed in the sigmoid. Given the narrowing of the lumen secondary to these lesions the colonoscopy was incomplete (Fig. 1d). The endoscopic ultrasonography showed low echo of cystic below the mucosal layer (Fig. 1e). We used high frequency electrosurgical resection of the gas cysts; But considering that extensive endoscopic therapy might lead to infection, we used only partial treatment. Since the narrow lumen of the patient, we restricted her food intake and used parenteral nutrition. One week later, the patient started to have a half-fluid diet. Ornidazole (500 mg/bid) and vitamin B2 (10 mg/bid) were given to regulate intestinal anaerobes, while bifidobacterium (420 mg/bid) was given at intervals of half an hour. We also advised him to eat less gas-producing foods. The patients' condition improved after 2 weeks (Table 1). One month later the lesions disappeared completely (Fig. 3c) and NBI demonstrated visible patchy erythema and yellow nodules (Fig. 3d). After four months of follow up, the patient was still no symptoms, and findings at colonoscopy were normal.

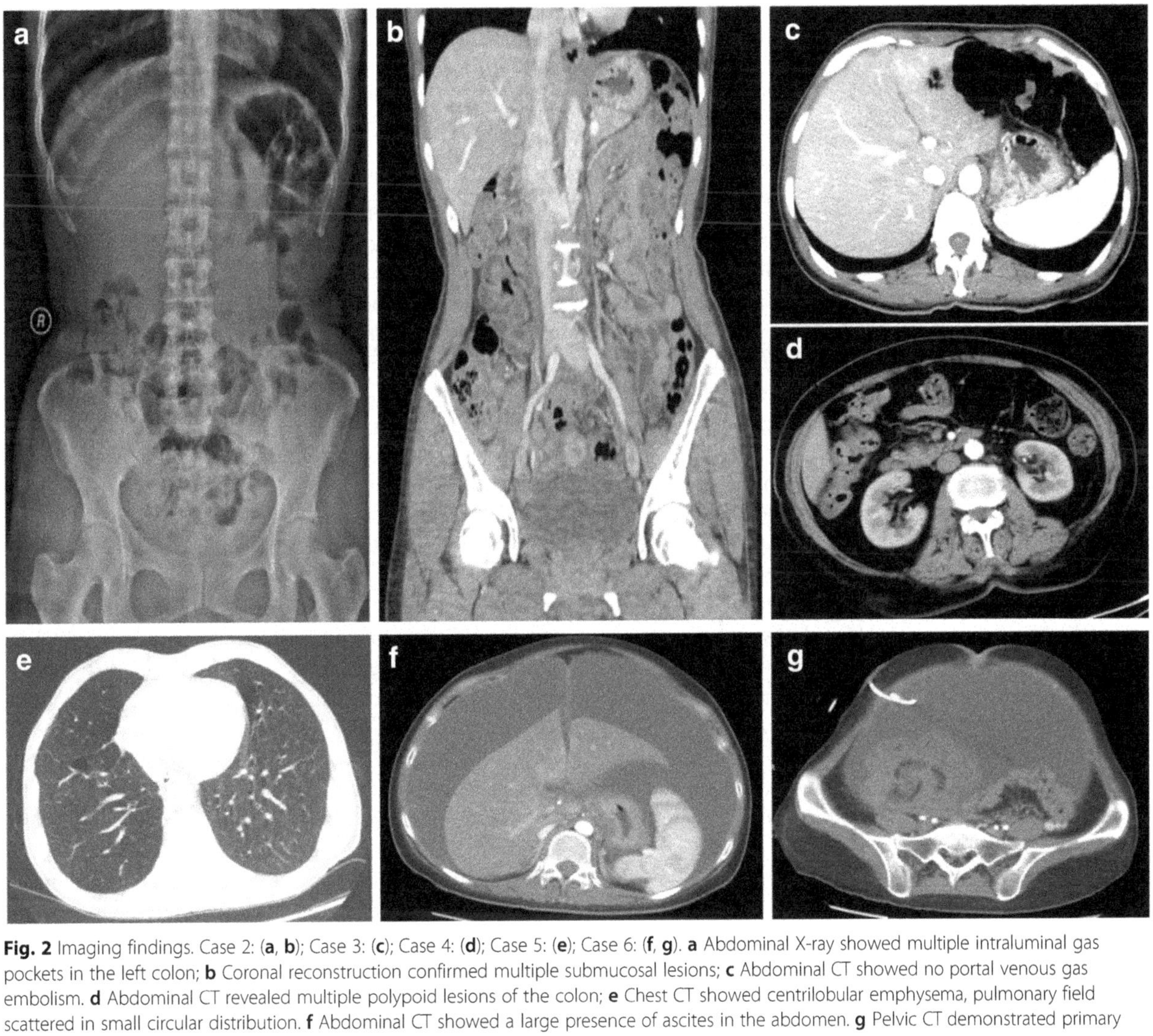

Fig. 2 Imaging findings. Case 2: (**a**, **b**); Case 3: (**c**); Case 4: (**d**); Case 5: (**e**); Case 6: (**f**, **g**). **a** Abdominal X-ray showed multiple intraluminal gas pockets in the left colon; **b** Coronal reconstruction confirmed multiple submucosal lesions; **c** Abdominal CT showed no portal venous gas embolism. **d** Abdominal CT revealed multiple polypoid lesions of the colon; **e** Chest CT showed centrilobular emphysema, pulmonary field scattered in small circular distribution. **f** Abdominal CT showed a large presence of ascites in the abdomen. **g** Pelvic CT demonstrated primary peritoneal carcinomatosis with balloon like structures in the rectum

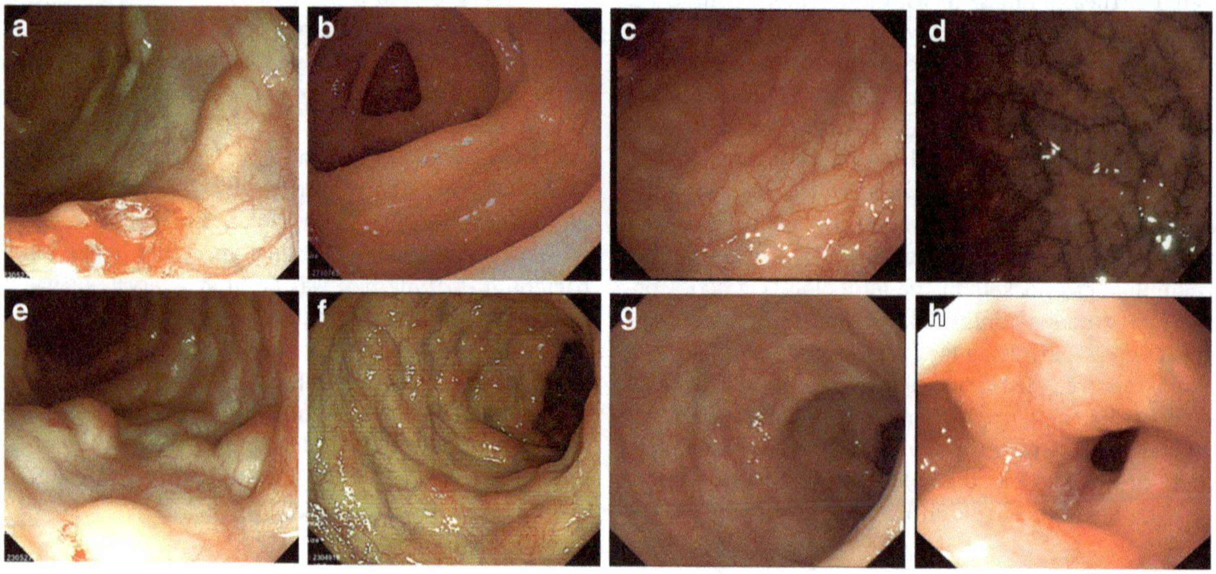

Fig. 3 Endoscopic manifestations after treatment. Case 1: (**a**, **b**); Case 2: (**c**, **d**); Case 3: (**e**); Case 4: (**f**, **g**); Case 5: (**h**). **a** Biopsies were performed, with the release of "air" and cyst collapse; **b** Gas cyst completely disappeared after treatment; **c** The cyst of the colon disappeared; **d** NBI demonstrated visible patchy erythema and yellow nodules; **e** Gas-filled cysts flattened; **f** The cyst of the colon improved, but mucosal surface redness still existed; **g** Colonic gas cyst was full recovery; **h** Duodenal descending presented as stenosis due to gas cyst

Case 3

A 66-year-old woman was admitted to the gastroenterology ward because of alternate constipation and diarrhea with muco-bloody stools. She had a history of undifferentiated connective tissue disease (UCTD) for 20 years and aplastic anemia (AA) for 1 year. In the past, she was mainly treated with glucocorticoid, and subsequently developed AA. Recently she presented with a diffuse pain in the abdomen with muco-bloody stools. Physical examination at admission revealed extensive abdominal tenderness. The biochemical tests revealed cytopenia due to AA and no obvious abnormality in stool culture for pathogens. Blood cultures were also negative. Computer tomography (CT) examination showed no portal venous gas embolism (Fig. 2c). Colonoscopic examination disclosed line or pebble like sessile cysts and irregular forms, which mainly distributed in sigmoid (Fig. 1f, g). Irregular forms of PCI with large bulge should be distinguished from malignant tumor (Fig. 1g). Given the narrowing of the lumen secondary to these lesions, the colonoscopy was incomplete. The pathologic findings revealed submucosal cystic structure (Fig. 1h). We used high frequency electrosurgical resection of the gas cysts. Because of the history of AA, she was treated with aluminum phosphate (20 g/bid) and bifidobacterium (420 mg/bid) without any antibiotics. We also advised him to eat less gas-producing foods. Symptoms of diarrhea improved significantly after one month, and gas-filled cysts became flattened (Fig. 3e). After ten months of follow-up the clinical symptoms were still resolved.

Case 4

A 72-year-old woman complained of constipation for several days, and then turned to diarrhea for one month. She was hospitalized for muco-bloody stools and severe abdominal distension. She had a history of diabetes for 10 years and was mainly treated with acarbose and insulin. Physical examination at admission revealed extensive abdominal tenderness. Routine laboratory examinations, bacterial and parasitic stool examinations and viral serology were negative. Abdominal X-ray showed multiple intraluminal gas pockets in sigmoid and ascending colon. Computer tomography (CT) examination showed multiple polypoid lesions of the colon (Fig. 2d). Colonoscopy showed irregular forms of lesions that were covered with mucosa of normal appearance in sigmoid and ascending colon (Fig. 1i). Irregular forms of PCI and mucosal lesions with erosion should be distinguished from Crohn's disease. Given the narrowing of the lumen secondary to these lesions, the colonoscopy was incomplete. NBI showed mucosal redness, which appeared as punctate labelling, and the blood vessels of intestine were clear (Fig. 1j). We used high frequency electrosurgical resection of the gas cysts. She was banned from using acarbose, continued to use insulin treatment for diabetes. The patient was initially treated with ornidazole (500 mg/bid) and bifidobacterium (420 mg/bid). In view of the older age of the patient and a history of diabetes, the antibiotic was changed to rifaximin (200 mg/qid) to avoid antibiotic resistance. We also advised him to eat less gas-producing foods. The patients' condition was improved after one month and the findings at endoscopy were improved (Fig. 3f). After 6 months of follow up, the cysts gas disappeared (Fig. 3g).

Case 5

A 64-year-old man was admitted to the hospital with wheezes and exertional dyspnea, which he had suffered from for several months, but without abdominal symptoms. He was diagnosed with emphysema pulmonum 1 years ago. Physical examination revealed double diffuse rales. Serological markers for autoimmunity and viral serology were normal, so as was the stool examination. Chest CT showed centrilobular emphysema, pulmonary field scattered in small circular distribution (Fig. 2e). A chest X-ray and CT examination showed the improvement of emphysema pulmonum. Endoscope showed stenosis due to gas cyst in duodenal descending (Fig. 1k). Emphysema as the primary disease, it is mainly used seretide for treatment. The PCI was treated successfully with intensive (but not hyperbaric) oxygen therapy and bifidobacterium (420 mg/bid). The findings at endoscopy were improved after eight months of follow-up (Fig. 3h).

Case 6

A 27-year-old woman was hospitalized because of ascites and abdominal pain for 3 months. She was diagnosed as Budd-Chiari syndrome (BCS) before admission. Physical examination at admission revealed pronounced abdominal tenderness and abdominal mass. Routine laboratory examinations, bacterial and parasitic stool examinations and viral serology were negative, while the level of serum C125 increased significantly up to 1560 U/ml. Abdominal X-ray and Abdominal CT showed a large presence of ascites in the abdomen (Fig. 2f). CT showed massive hydrops of abdominal cavity, multiple intraluminal gas pockets in the rectum and ovarian mass (Fig. 2g), which was limited to the ovarian surface without invasion. Abdominal ultrasonography revealed massive hydrops in the abdominal cavity, and abdominal paracentesis indicated bloody ascites. Colonoscopy showed grape or beaded lesions (Fig. 1l). Finally, primary peritoneal carcinoma (PPC) was diagnosed by peritoneal biopsy. After this the patient was given nutritional support. Finally, she was transferred to a hospital near her home and unfortunately died.

Discussion and conclusion

PCI is a rare condition characterized by gas-filled cysts in the intestinal submucosa and subserosa. Various predisposing factors have been associated with PCI: postsurgery [11], chemotherapy [12], Acarbose [13], Trichloroethylene (TCE) [14], scleroderma [15], and pulmonary illness [16]. In this report, there were total 6 patients studied, which included one case of idiopathic, one case induced by TCE, one case with UCTD, one case induced by emphysema, one case caused by diabetes and one case with PPC. Exposure to TCE results in primary PCI that previously reported in Japan, and the pathogenesis may be related to intestinal mucosal toxicity [14]. Patients with UCTD can be combined with PCI, including systemic sclerosis (SS), systemic lupus erythematosus (SLE), etc., which may be related to abnormal immune function regulation [17] and long-term use of glucocorticoids resulted in intestinal mucosal atrophy and defects, which promoted the formation of cysts in the intestinal submucosa. PCI has been associated with pulmonary disease in the absence of gastrointestinal disorder [16]. Recently, several reports have mentioned that the α-GI, voglibose or Acarbose, might be a causative factor for PCI [13, 18, 19]. It is generally understood that α-GI causes flatulence, because it suppresses absorption of carbohydrates in the colon, and intestinal bacteria then generates a large volume of gas by carbohydrate fermentation [20]. Recently, application of rituximab in patients with squamous cell carcinoma [21], sunitinib in patients with renal cell carcinoma, gefitinib in patients with lung adenocarcinoma and chemotherapy drugs, such as fluorouracil in patients with colorectal cancer were suggested to be associated with the development of PCI [22]. In this study, one of patient was suffering from peritoneal cancer, but did not use chemotherapy drugs, so the relationship between the tumor and the intestinal gas cyst requires further study. Recently, molecular-targeted agents such as anti-vascular endothelial growth factor (VEGF) agents and epidermal growth factor receptor (EGFR) tyrosine kinase inhibitors have been suspected to increase intestinal toxicity as well, which is interrelated to PCI [23].

Patients with PCI can be asymptomatic or present with non-specific gastrointestinal symptoms such as abdominal distention, diarrhea, constipation, abdominal pain and weight loss [5]. Although PCI was previously reported to occur more frequently in the terminal ileum of the gastrointestinal tract, Horiuchi A's studies showed that PCI occurred 61.8% in colon,15.4% in the small intestine, which was more common in the sigmoid colon [24]. In this study, in 4 (66.7%) patients, PCI occurred in the colon, especially the sigmoid colon, while in other two (33.3%) patients, it occurred in duodenum and rectum, which was relatively rare. We looked up a lot of literature and found that there were fewer reports of PCI occurred in duodenum and rectum, so more clinical evidence needed further study. Since the lack of specificity in clinical manifestations, it should be differentiated from the duodenal diverticulum when PCI occurred in that duodenum. It has been reported that PCI can be found in mesentery, omentum, ligamentum hepatogastricum, but rarely found in esophagus and stomach. Endoscopic findings were divided into bubble-like pattern, grape or beaded circular forms, linear or cobblestone gas formation and irregular forms. The bubble-like lesion was often idiopathic, which needed to be distinguished from polyps. The grape-like or beaded subepithelial lesions should be differentiated from intestinal tuberculosis. Irregular shapes need attention to distinguish from tumors and Crohn's disease. In previously described cases, linear gas formations were an ominous sign [25]. The radiological findings of diffuse and extensive intraluminal cysts within the walls of the colon are classic for PCI. Contrast-enhanced CT has an advantage in revealing gas within the portal venous system [26]. Endoscopic ultrasonography findings of the mucosal layer low echo below the cystic in the diagnosis of PCI is superior [27], which can avoid the risk of CT examination and distinguish from other diseases, such as polyps, carcinoma, lymphoma, liquid cysts, Gardner syndrome, Cronkhite-Canada syndrome, Peutz-Jehers syndrome, Crohn's disease, etc. [28]. Overall, the diagnosis of PCI and its adverse events including bowel perforation, portal venous gas (PVG) [29], intestinal hemorrhage, sepsis or peritonitis is very important.

PCI is a benign lesion and very few patients face cancer risk. There is no unified standard for treatment of PCI. The most of PCI cases are usually managed conservatively, while exploratory laparotomy is considered if peritoneal irritation or persistent bowel obstruction occurs in PCI. Joseph D. Feuerstein proposed that PCI could be effectively alleviated with hyperbaric oxygen therapy at 2.5 atmospheres for 2.5 h for at least three sessions [30, 31]. In our cases, we gave oxygen therapy to PCI patients with emphysema, but without hyperbaric oxygen, which can alleviate the patient's COPD, meanwhile regarded as the treatment methods of PCI associated with emphysema. Electronic colonoscopy forceps can facilitate the treatment of bubble-like pattern PCI, however blindly using argon knife excision may cause an explosion considering the possible existence of methane and other combustible gases. In addition, ornidazole and Bifidobacterium can be used to regulate intestinal flora, which can obviously improve the symptoms. The mechanism of antibiotic therapy is to inhibit the growth of harmful intestinal bacteria and thus to inhibit the production of hydrogen. The application of Bifidobacterium is to regulate the dysbacteriosis and improve the function of gastrointestinal tract. Knechtle reported that low pH (< 7.3), low serum bicarbonate (< 20 mmol/L) and elevated serum lactic acid (LA) (> 2 mmol/L) are associated with poor prognosis [32]. Alexander J found that surgical treatment of PCI patients with PVG could decrease the risk of death as compared to other PCI patients, so he recommended that surgical treatment was needed if the patient was not responsive to conservative treatment or had developed serious adverse events. Through the study of 123 cases of PCI, Ho-Su Lee et al. concluded that patients with both peritoneal irritation and decreased or absent enhancement of bowel wall on CT should be observed, and we should establish a simple and novel risk score that predicted mortality in patients with PCI [33]. The treatment of primary diseases is imperative for secondary PCI. Long-term follow-up of patients with PCI will facilitate understanding of the disease prognosis.

In this article, we demonstrated 6 cases of PCI with varied causes and 3 of 6 cases with intestinal stricture all were successfully managed by medical conservative treatment. PCI endoscopic manifestations were varied, and radiology combined with endoscopy could avoid misdiagnosis. The primary bubble-like pattern can be cured with endoscopic resection, while removal of etiology combined with drug therapy can resolve majority of secondary cases, thereby avoiding the adverse risks of surgery.

Abbreviations

AA: Aplastic anemia; BCS: Budd-Chiari syndrome; CT: Computer tomography; EGFR: Epidermal growth factor receptor; EUS: Endoscopic ultrasonography; LA: Lactic acid; PCI: Pneumatosis cystoides intestinalis; PPC: Primary peritoneal carcinoma; PVG: Portal venous gas; SLE: Systemic Lupus erythematosus; SS: Systemic sclerosis; TCE: Trichloroethylene; UCTD: Undifferentiated connective tissue disease; VEGF: Anti-vascular endothelial growth factor

Acknowledgements

We thank the patients for their cooperation. We gratefully acknowledge the financial supports by the National Science Foundation of China under Grant numbers 81570489. Thanks are due to Yi xiang Chang for assistance with the ultrasonography and to Hao ran Song for guidance in iconography.

Funding

This report received grant from the National Science Foundation of China under Grant numbers 81570489.

Authors' contributions

YJW, YMW and JZ contributed to the concept and design of the study. YJW drafted the manuscript, YMW and YMZ contributed to treatment of the patient. HQJ and JZ revised it critically. YJW, YMW, YMZ, HQJ and JZ reviewed and revised the manuscript, and approved the final manuscript as submitted. All authors approved the final manuscript as submitted.

Competing interests

The authors declare that they have no competing interests.

Author details
[1]Department of Gastroenterology and Hepatology, The Second Affiliated Hospital of Hebei Medical University, Hebei, China. [2]Department of Gastroenterology and Hepatology, The General Hospital of Tianjin Medical University, Tianjin, China.

References

1. Heng Y, Schuffler MD, Haggitt RC, Rohrmann CA. Pneumatosis intestinalis: a review. Am J Gastroenterol. 1995;90:1747–58.
2. KOSS LG. Abdominal gas cysts (pneumatosis cystoides intestinorum hominis); an analysis with a report of a case and a critical review of the literature. AMA Arch Pathol. 1952;53(6):523–49.
3. Greenstein AJ, et al. Pneumatosis intestinalis in adults: management, surgical indications, and risk factors for mortality. J Gastrointest Surg. 2007; 11(10):1268–74.
4. Gelman SF, Brandt LJ. Pneumatosis intestinalis and AIDS: a case report and review of the literature. Am J Gastroenterol. 1998;93(4):646–50.
5. Pear BL. Pneumatosis intestinalis: a review. Radiology. 1998;207:13–9.
6. St PS, Abbas MA, Kelly KA. The spectrum of pneumatosis intestinalis. Arch Surg. 2003;138:68–75.
7. Morris MS, Gee AC, Cho SD. Management and outcome of pneumatosis intestinalis. Am J Surg. 2008;195(5):679–82.
8. Kreiss C, et al. Pneumatosis intestinalis complicating C. Difficile pseudomembranous colitis. Am J Gastroenterol. 1999;94(9):2560–1.
9. Castro-Pocas F, Araujo T, Pedroto I. Endoscopic ultrasound of pneumatosis cystoides intestinalis. Endoscopy. 2015;(47 Suppl 1 UCTN):E274.
10. Rodríguez MGC. Colon polyps. Little bumps, big significance. Mayo Clin Health Lett. 2003;21(11):1–3.
11. Neesse A, Nimphius W, Schoppet M, Gress TM. Abdominal pain following percutaneous mitral valve repair (MitraClip). Pneumatosis intestinalis (PI) of the ascending colon. Gut. 2015;64:458. 494
12. Petrides C, Kyriakos N, Andreas I, Konstantinos P, Chrysanthos G, Athanasios P, et al. Pneumatosis cystoides intestinalis after cetuximab chemotherapy for squamous cell carcinoma of parotid gland. Case Rep Surg. 2015;2015:530680.
13. Rottenstreich A, Agmon Y, Elazary R. A rare case of benign Pneumatosis intestinalis with portal venous gas and pneumoperitoneum induced by Acarbose. Intern Med. 2015;54:1733–6.
14. Yamaguchi K, Shirai T, Ueno K, Shimakura K, Akamatsu T. 12 cases of pneumatosis cystoides intestinalis with the etiological implication of trichloroethylene. Nihon Shokakibyo Gakkai Zasshi. 1983;80:1659.
15. Devgun P, Hassan H. Pneumatosis cystoides intestinalis: a rare benign cause of pneumoperitoneum. Case Rep Radiol. 2013;2013:353245.
16. Natarajan D. Primary PCI for acute anterior wall MI with pulmonary edema and left anterior descending artery ostial stenosis. Indian Heart J. 2010;62:90–1.
17. Sagara A, Kitagawa K, Furuichi K, Kitajima S, Toyama T, Okumura T, et al. Three cases of pneumatosis intestinalis presenting in autoimmune diseases. Mod Rheumatol. 2012;22:610–5.
18. Yanaru R, Hizawa K, Nakamura S, et al. Regression of pneumatosis cystoides intestinalis after discontinuing of alpha-glucosidase inhibitor administration. J Clin Gastroenterol. 2002;35:204–5.
19. Tsujimoto T, Shioyama E, Moriya K. Pneumatosis cystoides intestinalis following alpha-glucosidase inhibitor treatment: a case report and review of the literature. World J Gastroenterol. 2008;14(39):6087–92.
20. Miyagawa M, Kanemasa H, Nakagawa S. A case of pneumatosis cystoides intestinalis after treatment with an α-glucosidase inhibitor. Gastroenterol Endosc. 2006;48:329–33.
21. Petrides C, Kyriakos N, Andreas I. Pneumatosis cystoides intestinalis after cetuximab chemotherapy for squamous cell carci- Noma of parotid gland. Case Rep Surg. 2015;2015:530680.
22. Ohtake S, Namura K, Fujikawa A. A case of pneumatosis cystoides intestinalis secondary to sunitinib treatment for renal cell carcinoma. Hinyokika Kiyo. 2014;60(2):75–8.
23. Coriat R, Ropert S, Mir O, Billemont B, Chaussade S, Massault PP, et al. Pneumatosis intestinalis associated with treatment of cancer patients with the vascular growth factor receptor tyrosine kinase inhibitors sorafenib and sunitinib. Investig New Drugs. 2011;29:1090–3.
24. Horiuchi A, Akamatsu T, Mukawa K, Ochi Y, Arakura N, Kiyosawa K. Review case report: pneumatosis cystoides intestinalis associated with post-surgical bowel anastomosis: a report of three cases and review of the Japanese literature. J Gastroenterol Hepatol. 1998;13:534–7.
25. Pohl J. Pneumatosis Cystoides intestinalis. Video Journal and Encyclopedia of GI Endoscopy. 2013;1:393–4.
26. Fujikawa T, Murai S. Portal venous gas after a caudal block. BMJ Case Rep. 2014;2014
27. Castro-Pocas F, Araujo T, Pedroto I. Endoscopic ultrasound of pneumatosis cystoides intestinalis. Endoscopy. 2015;47(Suppl 1 UCTN):E274.
28. Santos-Antunes J, Ramalho R, Lopes S, Guimaraes S, Carneiro F, Macedo G. Asymptomatic pneumatosis cystoides intestinalis diagnosed in the follow-up of a dysplastic polyp. Endoscopy. 2014;46(Suppl 1 UCTN):E425–6.
29. Fukumori D, Sasaki T, Matsumoto H, et al. Necrotizing enteritis with hepatic portal venous gas and pneumatosis intestinalis: report of a case[J]. Eur J Gastroenterol Hepatol. 2003;15(2):201–3.
30. Feuerstein JD, White N, Berzin TM. Pneumatosis intestinalis with a focus on hyperbaric oxygen therapy. Mayo Clin Proc. 2014;89:697–703.
31. Masterson JS, Fratkin LB, Osler TR, Trapp WG. Treatment of pneumatosis cystoides intestinalis with hyperbaric oxygen. Ann Surg. 1978;187:245–7.
32. Knechtle SJ, Davidoff AM, Rice RP. Pneumatosis intestinalis. Surgical management and clinical outcome. Ann Surg. 1990;212:160–5.
33. Lee HS, Cho YW, Kim KJ, Lee JS, Lee SS, Yang SK. A simple score for predicting mortality in patients with pneumatosis intestinalis. Eur J Radiol. 2014;83:639–45.

24

Combined activity of COX-1 and COX-2 is increased in non-neoplastic colonic mucosa from colorectal neoplasia patients

Thorbjørn Søren Rønn Jensen[1,2*], Badar Mahmood[1,2], Morten Bach Damm[1,2], Marie Balslev Backe[2], Mattias Salling Dahllöf[2], Steen Seier Poulsen[2], Mark Berner Hansen[1] and Niels Bindslev[2]

Abstract

Background: Cyclooxygenase (COX) activity is increased in endoscopic normal colonic mucosa from patients with colorectal neoplasia (CRN). COX-2 is thought to be the predominant COX isozyme involved in neoplasia. Meanwhile, relative contributions of COX-1 and COX-2 isoforms are unknown. Knowledge about their mutual activity in colonic mucosa is important for diagnostics and targeted therapy for CRN. The aim of this study was to assess the relative function, expression and localization of COX-1 and COX-2 enzymes in colonic non-neoplastic human mucosa and thereby to potentially reveal a mucosal disease predisposition for better treatment.

Methods: Biopsies were pinched from normal appearing colonic mucosa in patients undergoing endoscopy. Ussing chamber technique was applied for an indirect assessment of epithelial activity, RT-qPCR for expression and immunohistochemistry for localization of COX-1 and COX-2 enzymes in patients without (ctrls) and with a history of CRN (CRN-pts).

Results: Combined COX-1 and COX-2 activity was higher in CRN-pts, $p = 0.036$. COX-2 was primarily localized in absorptive cells, while COX-1 appeared to be restricted to nonenteroendocrine tuft cells of the colonic epithelium.

Conclusions: In biopsies from endoscopic normal appearing colonic mucosa, combined activity of COX-1 and COX-2 enzymes is increased in CRN-pts compared with ctrls. This indicates that COX-1 and COX-2 together contribute to an increased proliferation process. Of note, in colonic epithelial cell lining, the COX-1 enzyme seems localized in tuft cells.

Keywords: Short circuit current (SCC), Cyclooxygenase, Endoscopic, Biopsy, Carcinogenesis, Tuft cells

Background

In the Western world, colorectal cancer (CRC) caused some 694,000 deaths in 2012, making it the third most common type of cancer and the second leading cause of cancer-related death [1]. Observation and documentation of possible altered signaling in pre-neoplastic colorectal mucosa from humans are essentials for future development of targeted pharmacotherapy against CRC and colorectal neoplasia (CRN).

Epidemiological studies show that daily intake of non-steroidal anti-inflammatory drugs (NSAIDs) reduces long-term incidence of developing CRC [2, 3]. Based primarily on these data, the United States Preventive Services Task Force (USPSTF) recently recommended routine use of low-dose aspirin for chronic disease prophylaxis, including CRC prevention, among adults between ages 50 and 59 with a > 10% risk of cardiovascular events [4, 5].

The mechanism behind NSAIDs's chemoprevention is most likely due to inhibition of cyclooxygenase (COX) enzymes, although other mechanisms of aspirins CRN-prevention are possible [6]. COX enzymes convert arachidonic acid into various metabolites including prostaglandin E2 (PGE_2). PGE_2 appears to be involved in neoplastic changes owing to its proinflammatory properties. Further, PGE_2 has been demonstrated to promote proliferation, cell migration, angiogenesis and reduce

* Correspondence: tjens07@gmail.com
[1]Digestive Disease Center K, Bispebjerg Hospital, DK-2400 Copenhagen, NV, Denmark
[2]Department of Biomedical Sciences, Faculty of Health Sciences, University of Copenhagen, DK-2200 Copenhagen N, Denmark

apoptosis in colonic mucosal lining [7, 8]. The COX enzyme exists in two major and clinically relevant isoforms: COX-1 and COX-2. COX-1 is known to have constitutive activity, while COX-2 is an infectious and injury-inducible enzyme.

Our research group has previously identified up-regulated indomethacin-sensitive COX activity in biopsies taken from endoscopically normal appearing colonic mucosa when compared between patients with a history of or present CRN to controls [9]. Another study by us showed a significantly augmented expression of two potential PGE_2 inward transporters, OATP2B1 and OATP4A1, in colonic biopsies from patients with CRN compared to patients without CRN. This up-regulated expression points to a compensatory increased basolateral PGE_2 uptake into colonic columnar epithelial cells associated with neoplasia [10]. This study also suggested the ABCC5 transporter as the epithelial cell PGE_2 exporter rather than the ABCC4 transporter.

The importance of COX enzyme subtypes for development of CRC is generally assumed to be due to an increased activity of the COX-2 isozyme [11]. However, this view is mostly based on studies on transformed cells or malignant tissue samples. It is well-known that the expression and activity of effector molecules, such as enzymes, transporters and receptors, often are dramatically altered in cell lines and in cancerous tissues as a byproduct of the cancer process itself. So far, to our knowledge, the relative contribution of COX-1 and COX-2 subtypes to an up-regulated COX activity, causing CRN, has not yet been fully elucidated. Accordingly, we decided to determine possible altered activity of both COX-1 and COX-2 in endoscopically normal appearing colonic mucosa from individuals with CRN when compared to controls. Choosing a comparison between normal appearing mucosa from both patient groups, further give a potential opportunity to evaluate if the colonic mucosa in patients with CRN is predisposed for development of the disease.

We hypothesized that activity of both COX isozymes might be up-regulated even in normal appearing mucosa and thereby together contribute to development of CRN, Fig. 1.

Accordingly, the aim of this study was to assess the relative functional importance, expression and localization of COX-1 and COX-2 enzymes in endoscopically normal appearing colonic mucosa from patients without (ctrls) and with colorectal neoplasia (CRN-pts), and furthermore to potentially reveal a mucosal predisposition for the disease.

Methods

Study population

Adult patients (≥ 18 years), referred for colonoscopy, were invited to participate. Patients were pooled into the neoplasia group if they presented a history of CRN. Patients with no present endoscopic signs or history of CRN served as ctrls. Patients with hemorrhagic diathesis or inflammatory bowel disease were excluded from the study. For each patient, we noted medication, body mass index (BMI), previous illnesses, all signs of earlier colorectal disease and the findings during the colonoscopy.

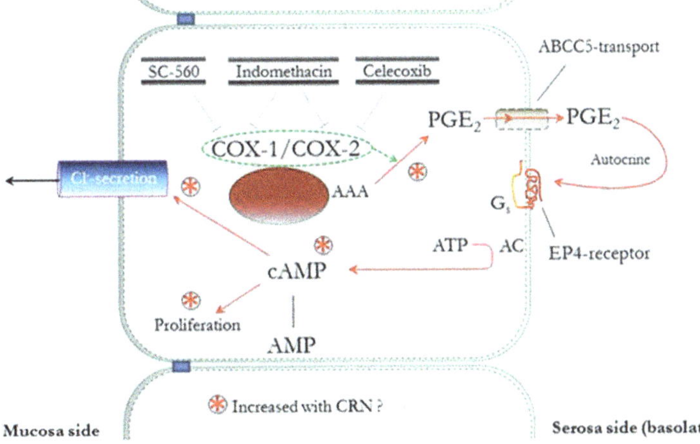

Fig. 1 A simplified scheme for involvement of COX enzymes in development of CRN. COX-1 and COX-2 convert active arachidonic acid (AAA) into PGE_2, which at the basolateral side is transported out off the cell via an ABCC5-transporter. Through a Gs-protein-coupled EP-4-receptor, PGE_2 mediates conversion of ATP to cAMP, thus inducing mucosal Cl^- secretion and cell proliferation. COX isozymes may be inhibited selectively by SC-560 and celecoxib or non-selectively by indomethacin. Pathways with ⊛ markers are hypothetically increased in CRN, thereby increasing cell proliferation and carcinogenesis. PGE_2: prostaglandin E2, cAMP: cyclic adenosine monophosphate, AMP: adenosine monophosphate, ATP: adenosine triphosphate, COX: cyclooxygenase, CRN: colorectal neoplasia, G_s: stimulatory heterotrimeric G protein, ABCC5: ATP-binding cassette transporter C5, EP4: prostaglandin receptor subtype 4, SC-560: selective COX-1 inhibitor, celecoxib: selective COX-2 inhibitor

Forty three patients were enrolled in the study (19 women). For Ussing chamber studies, biopsies from randomly selected 22 CRN-pts (10 women) and 21 ctrls (9 women) were examined. In the real time polymerase chain reaction study (RT-qPCR), biopsies from randomly selected 11 CRN-pts (6 women) and 7 ctrls (4 women) were included. For immunohistochemistry, biopsies from randomly selected 8 CRN-pts (3 women) and 7 ctrls (3 women) were assessed. Eleven patients, both CRN-pts (2 women, 3 men) and ctrls (3 women, 3 men), had co-morbidity such as diabetes, hypertension, atrial fibrillation, prostatic cancer, chronic obstructive pulmonary disease and dyslipidemia.

The study protocol was approved by the scientific Ethical Committee of Copenhagen (H-3-2013-107) and the Danish Data Protection Agency approved the study protocol (BBH-2013-024, I-suite no: 02342). The study was conducted in accordance with the Helsinki declaration. Patient information and data were collected and stored in locked containers.

Statistical analysis

Mann-Whitney Rank Sum test or unpaired t-test was used for the calculation of p-values depending on the results of normality and equal variance tests. P-values less than 0.05 were considered significant. All statistics were done with SigmaPlot 12.3 for Windows (Systat Software Inc., USA/Canada). Data are presented as mean (±SEM).

Chemicals

Theophylline, indomethacin, prostaglandin E2 (PGE_2), SC-560 and celecoxib were purchased from Sigma-Aldrich (Seelze, Germany). Amiloride, bumetanide and ouabain were purchased from Sigma (Vallensbaek Strand, Denmark).

The antibody for COX-2 (cat. no.: SB-M3210) was obtained from Nordic BioSite ApS (Täby, Sweden) and antibodies for COX-1 from Santa Cruz Biotechnology (cat. no.: sc-1752, sc-7950, and sc-19998; Santa Cruz, CA, USA) and Abcam Cambridge (cat. no.: ab109025; Cambridge, UK). Fluorescence double labeling was conducted with antibodies for the following entities: serotonin (cat. no.: M075801-2) and chromogranin A (cat. no.: M086929-2) were purchased from Dako (Glostrup, Denmark); proprotein convertase-1 and -2 (PC1 and PC2; cat. no.: alx-210-518-R100 and alx-210-519-R100) from Enzo Life Sciences (Varazdin, Croatia); somatostatin (cat. no.: sc-13099) from Santa Cruz Biotechnology (Santa Cruz, CA, USA); gastric inhibitory polypeptide (GIP, cat. no.: ABS021-04-02) from Thermo Scientific (Rockford, USA) and glucagon-like peptide-1 (GLP-1; cat. no.: 87805-34) from Tocris Bioscience (Bristol, UK).

Primer sequences were synthesized by TAG Copenhagen (Copenhagen, Denmark). All other chemicals were of analytical grade.

Biopsy procedure

Six biopsies were obtained from each patient. Of the six biopsies, one was used for RT-qPCR, one for immunohistochemistry and four biopsies were mounted in modified air-suction Ussing chambers [9]. During endoscopy, biopsies were pinched from normal appearing mucosa approximately 30 cm orally from the anal verge and at least 10 cm from abnormal tissue on retraction of the endoscope. Standard biopsy forceps (Boston Scientific, Radial Jaw 4, outside diameter of 2.2 mm) were used. Biopsies were placed in iced Ringer-solution and immediately transferred to the laboratory for mounting in Ussing chambers.

Three experimental techniques were employed:

Ussing chamber (A), RT-qPCR (B) and immunohistochemistry (C)

A. *Functional studies*

Biopsies were mounted within 30 min in Ussing chambers [9]. Mounting was carried out at 10 times magnification by means of a stereomicroscope to secure correct mucosa-serosa orientation and proper fixation. Both sides of the tissue were bathed in bicarbonate-Ringer solution containing (in mM) 140 Na^+, 4 K^+, 121 Cl^-, 1 Ca^{2+}, 0.5 Mg^{2+}, 0.5 SO_4^{2-}, 25 HCO_3^-, and 5.5 D-glucose. Solutions were oxygenated with 95% O_2/5% CO_2, i.e., buffered to pH 7.4, and circulated by gas-lifts. Temperature was maintained at 37 °C by water jackets. Short circuit current (SCC, $\mu A \cdot cm^{-2}$) and slope conductance (G, $mS \cdot cm^{-2}$) were recorded continuously using an automated voltage-clamp device. Correction for solution resistance was performed immediately before specimens were mounted. The slope conductance was only used as a control for acceptable slit fixation ranging between 60 and 120 mS per sq. cm.

Experiments were initiated following a minimum equilibration period of 10 min. Amiloride (20 μM, apical side) was added to inhibit sodium channels (ENaCs). Theophylline (400 μM, both sides) was then added to raise the level of cAMP due to inhibition of phosphodiesterase activity and thus optimizing the effect of COX subtype inhibitors. When the SCC was stable, a selective inhibitor of either COX-1 (SC-560, 500 nM, both sides) or COX-2 (celecoxib, 500 nM, both sides) was added. After 30 min or when the SCC reached a plateau, indomethacin was added (13 μM, both sides). Again, after 30 min or when SCC had stabilized, PGE_2 (100 nM, serosal side) was added. Finally, at the end of the experiment, bumetanide (25 μM, serosal side) was added as a measure for induced chloride secretion and followed by ouabain (200 μM, serosal side) as a control of biopsy viability. Selection of half-chamber concentrations for the various drugs was based on pharmacodynamic experience from previous studies.

B. *Expression studies*

From each patient included here, one biopsy was obtained and immediately transferred to RNAlater (Life Technologies, Naerum, Denmark). Biopsies were homogenized using a TissueLyser II (Qiagen, Copenhagen, Denmark), and subsequently RNA was extracted using NucleoSpin RNA® (Macherey-Nagel, Düren, Germany). Concentration and purity of RNA were determined using a NanoDrop® ND-1000 (NanoDrop Technologies, Wilmington, DE, USA), the latter by the A_{260}/A_{280} and A_{260}/A_{230} absorbance ratios. RNA was converted to cDNA using the iScript™ cDNA Synthesis Kit (BioRad, Copenhagen, Denmark) according to the manufacturer's protocol. Primers against genes of interest and ß-actin were designed using Primer3 (http://frodo.wi.mit.edu/primer3/input.htm) based on sequences obtained from Ensembl (www.ensembl.org). The primer sequences were synthesized by TAG Copenhagen (Copenhagen, Denmark): COX-1 forward (5'-GAGCAGCTTTTCCAG ACGA -3'); COX-1 reverse (5'- TCCTCGATGACAATC TTGATG -3'); COX-2 forward (5'- ACTAGAGCCCTT CCTCCTGTG -3'); COX-2 reverse (5'- GGGATCAGG GATGAACTTTCT -3'); ß-Actin forward (5'-ACCCAG CACAATGAAGATCA-3'); ß-Actin reverse (5'-CGTCA TACTCCTGCTTGCTG-3'). Dilution series of cDNA from HEK293 cells were run to verify acceptable amplification efficiencies and specificities by standard and dissociation curves for all primer sets. cDNA was amplified on a 7900HT Fast Real-Time PCR System (Applied Biosystems, Foster City, CA, USA) using Fast SYBR® Green Master Mix (Applied Biosystems) in accordance with the manufacturer's manual. Samples were run in triplicates with ß-actin primers as reference gene on all plates. Results were analyzed using SDS 2.3 (Applied Biosystems), and expression was calculated by the $2^{-\Delta CT}$ method.

C. *Localization and abundance studies*

Immunohistochemical staining was performed to localize and quantify the two COX isoforms. One colonic biopsy from each patient, included for this part, was put aside in 4% neutral buffered formaldehyde right after the endoscopy procedure. Biopsies were subsequently embedded in paraffin and cut in 4 μm thin slices. The sections were deparaffinated and rehydrated, followed by heat treatment in a microwave oven in order to unmask epitopes. The sections were blocked with a 2% bovine serum albumin solution for 10 min to rule out unspecific antibody adhesion, followed by incubation with a primary antibody at 4 °C overnight. Images were recorded using a Zeiss Axioplan 2 plus microscope (Jena, Germany) fitted with a Photometrics CoolSNAP camera (Tucson, AZ, USA) and analysis was performed using Image-Pro Plus 7.0 software.

Immunohistochemical staining of COX-1 turned out insufficient for three of the antibodies and a fourth (sc-1752) stained single, open enteroendocrine-like cells in the epithelium, Fig. 3. To verify that the coloring was of non-enteroendocrine cells, double labeling immunofluorescence with sc-1752 and various markers for endocrine cells was performed. The following antibody concentrations were used: COX-1 (sc-1752) 1:800, COX-2 1:400, GLP-1 1:375, serotonin 1:100, somatostatin 1:2500, PC1 1:1250, PC2 1:1600, chromogranin A 1:10000 and GIP 1:1750.

For COX-2, all biopsies were quantified by a blinded investigator. Quantification images were recorded at 20× magnification and the area measured represented 186,000 μm^2 of the tissue. The area of stained structures was quantified by selecting a colored region of interest. Automatically, areas with same color were measured. One image from each biopsy was measured. Blinded quantification of COX-2 was repeated 3 times. Data were calculated as mean area $\mu m^2 \pm$ SEM for each group. Images for localization were recorded using a Zeiss Axio10 Imager A1 microscope (Jena, Germany) fitted with a Zeiss AxioCam ICc 3 camera (Jena, Germany) and analysis was performed using Image-Pro 9.1 software. Only mucosal layers were analyzed.

Results

Study population

We found no differences in comorbidity or in medication between the two patient groups. BMI and age was higher in CRN-pts compared to ctrls with BMI displaying statistically significance (BMI: CRN-pts 27.2 (±1.2) vs ctrls 23.2 (±1.2), $p = 0.048$. Age: CRN-pts 69.5 (±4.1) years vs ctrls 58.4 (±5.4) years, $p = 0.062$).

A. *Function*

Baseline SCC and differential effects of amiloride, theophylline, indomethacin, PGE_2, bumetanide and ouabain on SCC are listed in Table 1. Inhibition of SCC by amiloride was more pronounced in CRN-pts compared to ctrls, $p = 0.006$. Stimulation of SCC by theophylline was significantly more efficacious in CRN-pts compared to ctrls, $p = 0.025$.

Total SCC response to COX inhibition was calculated by adding the response of either selective inhibitor to

Table 1 Drug-induced changes in short circuit current (SCC)

	CRN-pts Mean ΔSCC, SEM (µA·cm^{-2})	CRN-pts N/n	Ctrls Mean ΔSCC, SEM (µA·cm^{-2})	Ctrls N/n	*p*-value
Baseline SCC	91 ± 10.1	22/42	95 ± 26.6	21/30	0.518
Amiloride	−77 ± 13.4	17/38	−30 ± 15.1	13/22	0.006 *
Theophylline	73.5 ± 7.1	17/38	50.5 ± 6.9	13/22	0.025 *
SC-560 + Celecoxib	−66.7 ± 3.5	17/38	−54.7 ± 4.3	13/22	0.036 *
PGE_2	87.5 ± 32.3	15/26	73.0 ± 17.3	10/19	0.275
Bumetanide	−41.5 ± 5.3	15/32	−55.0 ± 9.4	7/18	0.261
Ouabain	−70.5 ± 14.4	13/24	−93.0 ± 14.7	7/18	0.431

Baseline SCCs are absolute values, while amiloride (20 µM, apical), theophylline (400 µM, both sides), SC-560 + Celecoxib (500 µM, both sides), prostaglandin (PGE_2) (100 nM, serosal), bumetanide (13 µM, serosal) and ouabain (200 µM, serosal) effects are changes from prestimulatory SCC (ΔSCC). SC-560 and Celecoxib are selective COX-1 and COX-2 inhibitors. SC-560 + Celecoxib represent the combined SCC inhibition data of both COX-1/indomethacin and COX-2/indomethacin application. CRN-pts values represent SCC or ΔSCC in biopsies from colorectal neoplasia patients and ctrls values are for patients without colorectal neoplasia. *N* = number of patients, *n* = number of biopsies, in parenthesis (N/n). * *p*-value < 0.05

the ensuing response of indomethacin. The decrease in SCC to either of the selective COX-inhibitors was normalized based on total COX inhibition for the individual biopsy. Examples of Ussing chamber experiments of inhibition of either COX subtype can be seen in Fig. 2. No difference in SCC inhibition between patients group was observed for either of the two selective COX inhibitors. By contrast, the SCC response of combined COX-1 and COX-2 inhibition, after indomethacin application, was significantly larger in CRN-pts compared to ctrls, $p = 0.036$, Table 1. This significant data difference corroborates a significantly larger drop in

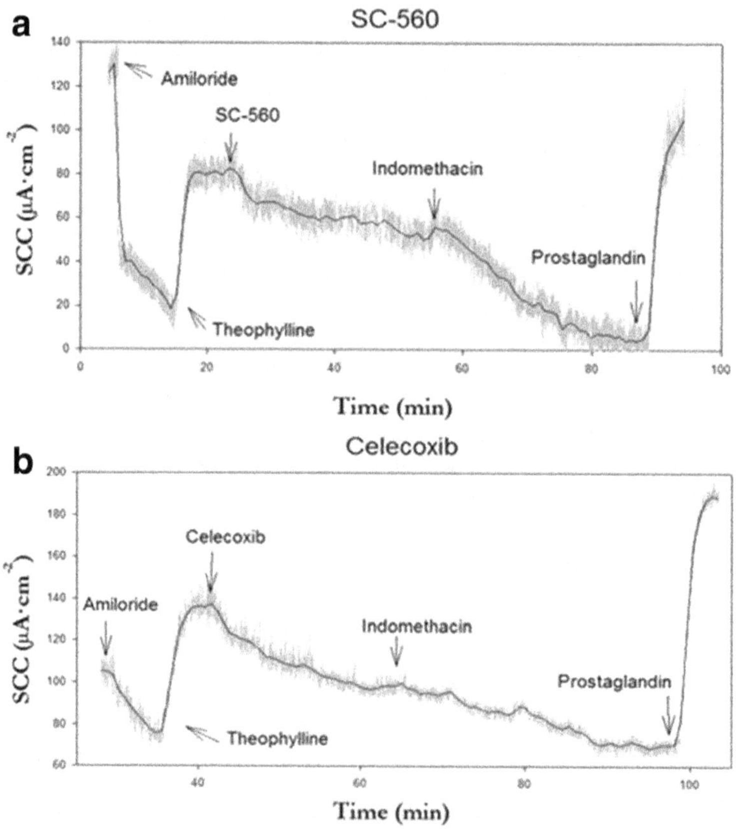

Fig. 2 Examples of typical recording in Ussing Chamber experiments on short circuit current (SCC) following exposure to COX-1 (cyclooxygenase) inhibitor SC-560 (**a**) and COX-2 inhibitor celecoxib (**b**). Compounds were added to biopsies in the following concentrations: amiloride (20 µM, mucosal side), theophylline (400 µM, both sides), either COX-1 inhibitor (SC-560, 500 nM, both sides) or COX-2 inhibitor (celecoxib, 500 nM, both sides), indomethacin (13 µM, both sides) and prostaglandin (PGE_2, 100 nM, serosal side)

SCC to indomethacin found in a previous study for CRN-pts compared to ctrls [9].

When comparing the fractional contribution of COX-1 and COX-2, both normalized with total COX activity, COX-1 contribution was significantly higher compared to COX-2 both for ctrls ($p = 0.028$) and CRN-pts ($p = 0.035$), Table 2.

B. *Expression*

Using RT-qPCR, we examined the expression of COX-1 and COX-2 in colonic mucosa from CRN-pts and ctrls. We further wanted to compare the combined expression of COX-1 and COX-2 between the two patient groups.

The expression of COX-1 was significantly higher compared to COX-2 both in CRN-pts (COX-1 = 0.024 (±0.003) vs COX-2 = 0.007 (±0.002), $p = 0.012$) and in ctrls (COX-1 = 0.020 (±0.003) vs COX-2 = 0.005 (±0.002), $p < 0.001$). Comparing CRN-pts with ctrls, mRNA-expression of both COX-1 and COX-2 was numerically higher in CRN-pts, although upregulation of both genes failed to reach statistical significance (COX-1: $p = 0.249$, COX-2: $p = 0.431$), Table 3. Combined expression of the COX isozymes was defined as the summed expression of COX-1 and COX-2. Comparing combined COX expression for CRN-pts and ctrls showed no statistical significant difference (CRN-pts = 0.015 (±0.003) vs ctrls = 0.012 (±0.003), $p = 0.353$).

C. *Localization and abundance*

Localization of COX-2 was immunohistochemically delimited to cytoplasm of absorptive cells, Fig. 3a. Quantification of COX-2 showed no significant difference between CRN-pts and ctrls, CRN-pts: 1472 ± 168 μm^2 and ctrls: 1398 ± 132 μm^2, $p = 0.362$.

Since neither of the classical makers for endocrine cells co-stained with sc-1752 for the COX-1 enzyme, we conclude that the sc-1752 antibody marks tufts cells in the

Table 2 Percentage drop in total COX-induced short circuit current by selective inhibitors, COX-1 (SC-560) and COX-2 (Celecoxib)

	SC-560 Inhibition, SEM (%)	Celecoxib Inhibition, SEM (%)	*p*-value
CRN-pts (N/*n* = 15/26)	68.8 ± 4.5	53.7 ± 5.1	0.035*
Ctrls (N/*n* = 10/19)	80.6 ± 4.8	52.6 ± 10.3	0.028*
p-value	0.10	0.91	

Horizontal *p*-values to the right show inhibition by SC-560 compared to inhibition by Celecoxib for CRN-pts and ctrls. Vertical *p*-values at the bottom show CRN-pts compared to ctrls for SC-560 inhibition and Celecoxib inhibition. Inhibition calculated as percentage selective COX-inhibition of total COX-inhibition. Total COX-inhibition defined as selective COX-inhibition + indomethacin inhibition. Percentage drop reflects the overall decreased activity. CRN-pts represent values for biopsies from colorectal neoplasia patients and ctrls values are for biopsies from patients without colorectal neoplasia. *N* = number of patients, *n* = number of biopsies, in parenthesis (N/n). * *p*-value < 0.05

Table 3 COX-1 and COX-2 expression based on real time polymerase chain reaction in colonic biopsies from CRN-pts and ctrls

	COX-1 expression, SEM	COX-2 expression, SEM	*p*-value
CRN-pts (N/*n* = 11/11)	0.024 ± 0.003	0.007 ± 0.002	0.012 *
Ctrls (N/*n* = 7/7)	0.020 ± 0.003	0.005 ± 0.002	< 0.001 *
p-value	0.24	0.43	

Horizontal *p*-values to the right compare COX-1 expression with COX-2 expression for CRN-pts and ctrls. Vertical *p*-values at the bottom compare CRN-pts with ctrls for COX-1 and COX-2 expression. Total or combined expression of COX enzyme is defined as expression of COX-1 + COX-2. The combined COX expression was 0.015 ± 0.003 for CRN-pts and 0.012 ± 0.003 for ctrls; $p = 0.35$. CRN-pts represent values for biopsies from colorectal neoplasia patients and ctrls values are for biopsies from patients without colorectal neoplasia. *N* = number of patients, *n* = number of biopsies, in parenthesis (N/n). * *p*-value < 0.05

epithelial lining as also reported by Gerbe et al. ([12], and their supplemental material Fig. S1A). Use of two other antibodies gave either smeared stains or no staining.

Double fluorescence staining was made with COX-1 antibody sc-1752 and antibodies for the following endocrine cell-markers: chromogranin A, GIP, serotonin, GLP-1, somatostatin, PC1 and PC2. None of the markers for endocrine cells were found to co-localize with COX-1, see Fig. 3c, thus confirming the coloring of non-enteroendocrine epithelial cell, identified as tuft cells, and also of unspecified solitary stromal cells. In a preliminary enhanced fluorescence immuno-histochemical study of COX-1 in human colonic biopsies in our laboratory, there is a clear subepithelial localization of the protein in solitary cells with a morphology resembling myofibroblasts (Dr. Hanne Borger Rasmussen and Christian Hunnicke Petersen, unpublished results).

Discussion

Our study seeks to evaluate parameters related to the content and impact of PGE_2 in normal human colonic mucosa. We chose to study normal appearing colonic mucosa from ctrls and CRN-pts in order to try to evaluate a possible predisposition for the disease in normal tissue from CRN-pts when compared with ctrls. Thus, in biopsies from this mucosa, we looked at a functional parameter, indomethacin-sensitive short circuit current (IS-SCC) in the presence of amiloride, including COX enzyme subtype-specific SCC inhibition. Although IS-SCC is indirectly related to the effects of PGE_2, it is well-established as a measure of PGE_2 activity working through a COX enzyme-adenylate-cyclase-Gs-cAMP pathway, Fig. 1. There are several advantages of IS-SCC, as a measure of functionality. Thus, IS-SCC is solely related to the epithelial cell layer and with superior sensitivity as compared for instance with enzymatic assays for the content of PGE_2 and/or signaling pathway entities, most often determined

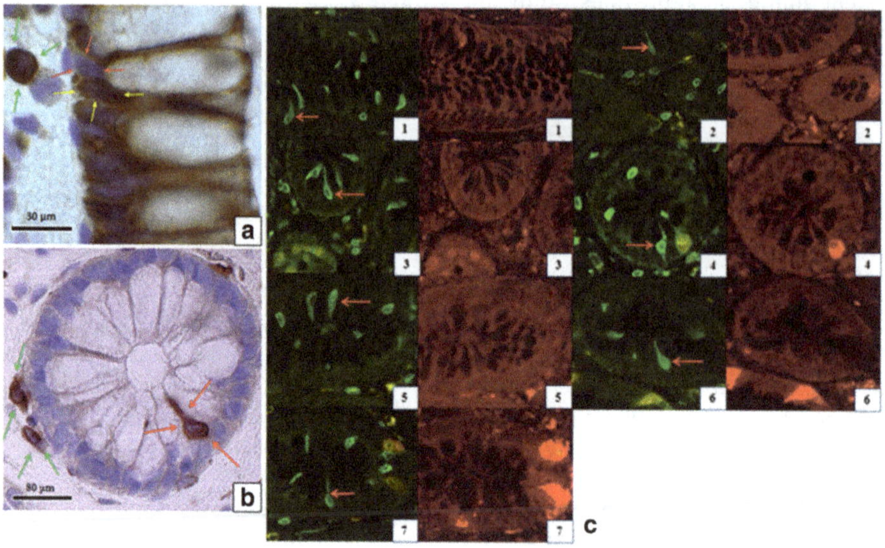

Fig. 3 Immunohistochemical staining of colonic mucosa with cyclooxygenase (COX) subtype specific antibodies in patients with colorectal neoplasia. **a** COX-2 immunohistochemical staining appears localized to the cytoplasm of absorptive cells (yellow arrows). No staining is seen in goblet cells (red arrows). A pericryptal stromal cell is marked (green arrow). **b** COX-1 immunohistochemical staining, here with antibody sc-1752, appears to stain morphological appearing tuft cells (red arrows) and in the lamina propria proposedly myofibroblasts (green arrow). **c** Fluorescence double labeling shows no co-localization between COX-1 (green) and specific markers for endocrine cells (red). Arrows point at COX-1 positive tuft cells. Subfigures 1, 2, 3, 5 and 7 have proportions of 100 µm per centimeter, subfigures 4 and 6 have proportions of 50 µm per centimeter. 1: Glucagon-like peptide-1, 2: Somatostatin, 3: Gastric Inhibitory Polypeptide, 4: Proprotein Convertase-1, 5: Proprotein Convertase-2, 6: Serotonin, 7: Chromogranin A

for the entire mucosa, with low accuracy and thus limited by indirect congruency with epithelial functionality.

COX-1 and COX-2 isozymes

A previous functional study from our laboratory reported an increased total COX activity in endoscopic normal appearing mucosa from patients with diagnosis of CRN [9]. The present study supports this observation, since the combined activity of COX-1 and COX-2 in colonic mucosa is significantly increased with CRN and cancer, though neither COX-1 nor COX-2 alone showed a significantly augmented activity.

Up-regulation of COX-2 is associated with increased cell adhesion, phenotypic changes, resistance to apoptosis and tumor angiogenesis [13–17]. These changes are possibly due to a raised prostaglandin E2 production, a notion supported by two laboratories, where Eberhart et al. found levels of prostaglandin E2 to be 3-4 fold increased in CRC tissue [18, 19]. PGE_2 is known to inhibit apoptosis, to stimulate both tumor growth and angiogenesis and to act as an immunosuppressant in patients with CRC [13, 20, 21]. Even though COX-2 is a well-known enhancer of carcinogenesis in CRC, it has been proposed that both COX-1 and COX-2 pathways are involved in intestinal tumorigenesis [17]. This statement is strongly supported by experimental animal studies as the loss of either COX-1 or COX-2 genes blocks intestinal polyposis in mouse models of familial adenomatous polyposis by approximately 90% [22, 23].

Knowledge about overexpression of various enzymes in neoplastic tissue is well established, but our study additionally indicates that NSAID-sensitive mechanisms are over-activate not only in neoplastic tissue, but also in endoscopic normal appearing mucosa in CRN-pts, thereby representing tissue with an predisposed potential condition for neoplastic development.

In the present study, expressional levels of constitutive COX-1 were statistically higher compared to COX-2 in both CRN-pts and ctrls, Table 3 horizontal p-values. This finding may be contrasted by considerations about the characteristics of the two isozymes. COX-1 gene is considered the "housekeeping enzyme" and is highly and constitutively expressed in platelets and in gastric epithelial cells. In the latter, it helps in cytoprotection through the generation of prostanoids [24, 25]. In contrast, the COX-2 enzyme is inducible by many factors: e.g., bacterial endotoxins, cytokines and growth factors. Accordingly, the COX-2 activity is typically transient [26]. Of note, this differentiation between the cyclooxygenase isozymes, more than often turns out to be too simplistic [27, 28].

COX-1 detection and tuft cells

One of three employed COX-1 antibodies stained the biopsy mucosa specifically in sporadic epithelial cells. By double-staining for COX-1 and enteroendocrine cells (EECs), we could exclude a labeling of EECs, Fig. 3c. Therefore, we rationalized that the COX-1 staining detected tuft cells as also concluded in several mouse colon studies with COX-1 immunostaining [12, 29–31]. These cells (also known as brush cells) have previously been found in endoderm-derived epithelia [12]. Tuft cells have long and blunt microvilli with a protruding root system along a well-built tubulovesicular system in the cytoplasm near the nucleus [32]. Fairly recently, tuft cells have been acknowledged as an important part of the intestinal lining with an immunological role to play in helminthic infections [33], while a more strict combination of specific tuft cell markers is still debated [12, 29, 33, 34]. Functional studies of tuft cells related to human colon cancer are still scarce [35], while colonic tuft cells appear related to the defense against worm infections [12]. To conclude, the COX-1-dependent PGE_2 production in human colonic mucosa seems likely derived solely from epithelial tuft cells and probably as well supplied from subepithelial immune cells, which also stained with COX-1 antibody, data not shown. This proposal and a quantification of tuft cells in CRN-pts compared with ctrls, requires a separate study.

PGE_2-producing stromal cells, colored by COX-1 and COX-2 antibodies in Fig. 3a, b, and c, are possibly myofibroblast, as suggested by Powell et al. [36], immune cells, mesenchymal stem cells and other non-identified stromal cells. As mentioned in the Result section, there is also an expression of the COX-1 protein in solitary subepithelial myofibroblast-like cells of human colonic mucosa, although with a much fainter coloring than for other stromal cells and epithelial tuft cells shown in Fig. 3b and c. This finding of COX-1 in subepithelial myofibroblasts is in line with earlier findings in the mouse small intestine and of myofibroblasts cultured from a mucosal biopsy of human neonatal colon [36, 37]. Of note, some of the produced PGE_2 in human colonic mucosa is most likely also produced by stromal myofibroblasts as demonstrated for cultured colonic myofibroblasts from mice [38].

Study population

Due to differences in the basic characteristics of our two patient groups, our study presents certain potential limitations. BMI and age were apparently slightly higher in the CRN study population. These observations are in line with obesity and increasing age being known risk factors for developing CRN and CRC [39]. Furthermore, SCC inhibition with amiloride and stimulation with theophylline differed between the study groups, Table 1. The colonic SCC response to amiloride is known for its variability and dependence on food ingredients, e.g., salt intake [40, 41]. The observed difference in SCC induced by amiloride can therefore be an unrelated variation in salt intake in our human study cohort and needs to be clarified in future studies. The characteristic of a significantly larger stimulatory effect of theophylline in CRN-pts is currently under study in our laboratory with results indicating lower SCC response to phosphodiesterase 4, PDE4, inhibition in colonic mucosa from CRN-pts. The increased theophylline response found in CRN-pts in this study, Table 1, could therefore also be a result of compensatory elevated phosphodiesterase activity in patients with CRN [42].

Perspective on the use of aspirin and other NSAIDs

In the last decade, the mechanism of daily low-dose aspirin as a CRN-preventive measure has been questioned. Originally, the benefits of low-dose aspirin intake were thought primarily due to its COX enzyme inhibitor effects [2, 43]. Also, the recently published USPSTF's recommendation for aspirin use in the prevention of CRN and CRC has not yet reached a general endorsement, as additional groupings, conditions and more evidence are still needed for a broad acceptance [5]. Our study here adds experimental human data, which support medication with non-selective COX-inhibitors for the prevention and/or treatment of CRN and CRC.

The subject of aspirin supplementation is now further complicated by recent realizations about the mechanisms behind beneficial effects of aspirin treatment involving integrated and intracellular multi-signaling pathways, such as pathological Wnt-beta-catenin and MAPKinase signaling as well as dysregulated non-coding long-RNA epigenetics and platelet functions [3, 6, 44].

Notwithstanding, a supposed major CRC prevention mechanism is still the inhibition of COX enzymes elicited by aspirin and other NSAID drugs. The level of mucosal PGE_2 is lifted with CRN due to increased COX activity and possibly also reduced catabolism by not of a 15-hydroxy-prostaglandin-dehydrogenase PGE_2 breakdown [31]. NSAID-inhibition in effect reduces a lifted PGE_2 level presumed to drive an immunosuppression or immune evasion, that establishes an oncogenic milieu [45].

Therefore, it is still important to study the PGE_2 metabolism, including steps of its synthesis and catabolism, as well as its pertinent signaling pathways. And also, bring these studies from the culture dish and animal cage to human individuals for a comparison between these PGE_2 parameters obtained from normal colonic mucosa of affected patients and controls. The research presented here is such a study and has revealed an equal importance of the two COX enzyme subtypes, COX-1 and COX-2, for the development of CRN, as the combined COX-1 and COX-2 displayed higher activity in CRN-pts. As the study is a pilot study with few participants, it certainly warrants confirmation by similar studies with much larger cohort numbers.

Full consensus for the use of daily low-dose aspirin to prevent CRC development, in the USPSTF recommendation, is still limited by uncertainties about the balance between advantageous and adverse effects for prophylactic use of NSAID chemo-preventive medicine against colorectal neoplasia [5]. This is due to variable setups and outcomes of several large clinical trials together involving more than 70,000 test persons. Furthermore, in this context it is still a hope to obtain better individualized medication, precision medicine, and molecular bio-markers for a more accurate assessment of risk stratification [46].

There is an ongoing dramatic development in studies on the COX-2 downstream-enzyme mPGES-1 (microsomal prostaglandin E2 synthase 1) with associated research for its selective and clinically relevant inhibitors. Discovery of such mPGES-1 inhibitors are intensely chased for the prevention of COX-2 dependent PGE 2 production and their installment as therapeutics [47]. While we wait for clinically approved mPGES-1 inhibitors for CRN, our study rather point to a possible use of low-dose non-specific COX inhibitors. Other alternative approach for treating CRN and CRC involving PGE_2 may come from the bourgeoning studies on the gut microbiota, where the microorganism *Fusobacterium nucleatum* is linked with development of CRC and suspected of inducing microRNA-21 to increase the levels of IL-10 and prostaglandin E2 [48, 49].

Conclusions

We find that COX-1 and COX-2 jointly contribute to COX-overactivity in colonic mucosa from patients with colorectal neoplasia. The clinical implications of the study are important for possible medical treatment of colorectal neoplasia with COX inhibitors, as it points to the use of non-selective COX inhibitors rather than specific COX-2 inhibitors. Immunohistochemically, COX-2 localizes to the cytoplasm of absorptive cells, while cells morphologically appearing like endocrine cells, non-identifiable with ordinary endocrine cell markers, seem to be COX-1 positive. However, for the normal epithelium of human colon, confirmation of COX-1 enzyme localization needs additional studies.

Abbreviations

BMI: Body mass index; COX: Cyclooxygenase; CRC: Colorectal cancer; CRN: Colorectal neoplasia; CRN-pts: Colorectal neoplasia patients; Ctrls: Patients without colorectal neoplasia; EECs: Enteroendocrine cells; ENaCs: Epithelial sodium channel; GIP: Gastric inhibitory polypeptide; GLP-1: Glucagon-like peptide-1; IS-SCC: Indomethacin-sensitive short circuit current; mPGES-1: mincrosomal prostaglandin E2 synthase 1; NSAID: Non-steroid anti-inflammatory drug; PC: Proprotein convertase; PGE_2: Prostaglandin E_2; RT-qPCR: Real time polymerase chain reaction; SCC: Short circuit current; USPSTF: United States Preventive Services Task Force

Acknowledgements

Laboratory technicians Katrine Qvist and Heidi Marie Paulsen are acknowledged for assistance with the immunohistochemical study. We thank all the participating patients for tissue donations as well as consultant and endoscopist Svend Knuhtsen and the staff at endoscopy unit of Digestive Disease Center at Bispebjerg Hospital for general support. Dr. Hanne Borger Rasmussen is thanked for helpful discussions.

Funding

This work was kindly supported by Højmosegård Foundation (jr no. F-12310-01-32-01), Beckett Foundation (jr. no. 37569/37570), Krista Krista and Viggo Petersens Foundation (jr. no. 5793/97), Else and Mogens Wedell-Wedellsborgs Foundation (jr. no. 25-15-1), Ingeborg Roikjers Foundation (jr. no. 51289-1) and Bispebjerg and Frederiksberg Hospital's intern start-up scholarship.

Authors' contributions

TSRJ was the principal investigator and took part in every aspect of this study and was a major contributor in writing the manuscript. MMBD and BM were major contributors in analyzing the functional, expressional and immunohistochemical data. MBB and MSD contributed as experts in performing and analyzing the expressional data. SSP contributed as an expert in performing and analyzing the immunohistochemical data. MBH contributed as an expert in the functional part of the study and study design and contributed in writing the manuscript. NB contributed as an expert in the functional part of the study and served as the supervisor of the project while contributed in writing the manuscript. All authors read and approved the final manuscript.

Competing interests

The authors declare that they have no competing interests.

References

1. Siegel RL, Miller KD, Jemal A. Cancer statistics, 2016. CA Cancer J Clin. 2016; 66:7–30.
2. Thun MJ, Namboodiri MM, Heath CW. Aspirin use and reduced risk of fatal colon cancer. N Engl J Med. 1991;325:1593–6.
3. Drew DA, Cao Y, Chan AT. Aspirin and colorectal cancer: the promise of precision chemoprevention. Nat Rev Cancer. 2016;16:173–86.
4. Chan AT, Ogino S, Fuchs CS. Aspirin and the risk of colorectal cancer in relation to the expression of COX-2. N Engl J Med. 2007;356:2131–42.
5. Chan AT, Ladabaum U. Where do we stand with aspirin for the prevention of colorectal cancer? The USPSTF recommendations. Gastroenterology. 2016;150:14–8.
6. Guo H, Liu J, Ben Q, Qu Y, Li M, Wang Y, et al. The aspirin-induced long non-coding RNA OLA1P2 blocks phosphorylated STAT3 homodimer formation. Genome Biol. 2016;17:24.
7. Stack E, DuBois RN. Role of cyclooxygenase inhibitors for the prevention of colorectal cancer. Gastroenterol Clin N Am. 2001;30:1001–10.
8. Chell S, Kaidi A, Kadi A, Williams AC, Paraskeva C. Mediators of PGE2 synthesis and signalling downstream of COX-2 represent potential targets for the prevention/treatment of colorectal cancer. Biochim Biophys Acta. 2006;1766:104–19.
9. Kaltoft N, Tilotta MC, Witte A-B, Osbak PS, Poulsen SS, Bindslev N, et al. Prostaglandin E2-induced colonic secretion in patients with and without colorectal neoplasia. BMC Gastroenterol. 2010;10:9.
10. Kleberg K, Jensen GM, Christensen DP, Lundh M, Grunnet LG, Knuhtsen S, et al. Transporter function and cyclic AMP turnover in normal colonic mucosa from patients with and without colorectal neoplasia. BMC Gastroenterol. 2012;12:78.
11. Ahmed M, Hussain AR, Siraj AK, Uddin S, Al-Sanea N, Al-Dayel F, et al. Co-targeting of Cyclooxygenase-2 and FoxM1 is a viable strategy in inducing anticancer effects in colorectal cancer cells. Mol Cancer. 2015;14:131.
12. Gerbe F, van Es JH, Makrini L, Brulin B, Mellitzer G, Robine S, et al. Distinct ATOH1 and Neurog3 requirements define tuft cells as a new secretory cell type in the intestinal epithelium. J Cell Biol. 2011;192:767–80.
13. Wang D, Dubois RN. The role of COX-2 in intestinal inflammation and colorectal cancer. Oncogene. 2010;29:781–8.
14. Nie D, Honn KV. Cyclooxygenase, lipoxygenase and tumor angiogenesis. Cell Mol Life Sci. 2002;59:799–807.

15. Tsujii M, Kawano S, DuBois RN. Cyclooxygenase-2 expression in human colon cancer cells increases metastatic potential. Proc Natl Acad Sci. 1997;94:3336–40.
16. Fujita T, Matsui M, Takaku K, Uetake H, Ichikawa W, Taketo MM, et al. Size- and invasion-dependent increase in cyclooxygenase 2 levels in human colorectal carcinomas. Cancer Res. 1998;58:4823–6.
17. Marnett LJ. Aspirin and the potential role of prostaglandins in colon cancer. Cancer Res. 1992;52:5575–89.
18. Eberhart CE, Coffey RJ, Radhika A, Giardiello FM, Ferrenbach S, Dubois RN. Up-regulation of cyclooxygenase 2 gene expression in human colorectal adenomas and adenocarcinomas. Gastroenterology. 1994;107:1183–8.
19. Pugh S, Thomas GA. Patients with adenomatous polyps and carcinomas have increased colonic mucosal prostaglandin E2. Gut. 1994;35:675–8.
20. Shao J, Jung C, Liu C, Sheng H. Prostaglandin E2 stimulates the beta-catenin/T cell factor-dependent transcription in colon cancer. J Biol Chem. 2005;280:26565–72.
21. Balch CM, Dougherty PA, Cloud GA, Tilden AB. Prostaglandin E2-mediated suppression of cellular immunity in colon cancer patients. Surgery. 1984;95:71–7.
22. Oshima M, Dinchuk JE, Kargman SL, Oshima H, Hancock B, Kwong E, et al. Suppression of intestinal polyposis in Apc delta716 knockout mice by inhibition of cyclooxygenase 2 (COX-2). Cell. 1996;87:803–9.
23. Chulada PC, Thompson MB, Mahler JF, Doyle CM, Gaul BW, Lee C, et al. Genetic disruption of Ptgs-1, as well as of Ptgs-2, reduces intestinal tumorigenesis in min mice. Cancer Res. 2000;60:4705–8.
24. Smyth EM, Grosser T, Wang M, Yu Y, FitzGerald GA. Prostanoids in health and disease. J Lipid Res. 2009;50:423–8.
25. Patrono C, Patrignani P, García Rodríguez LA. Cyclooxygenase-selective inhibition of prostanoid formation: transducing biochemical selectivity into clinical read-outs. J Clin Invest. 2001;108:7–13.
26. Kang Y-J, Mbonye UR, DeLong CJ, Wada M, Smith WL. Regulation of intracellular cyclooxygenase levels by gene transcription and protein degradation. Prog Lipid Res. 2007;46:108–25.
27. Kirkby NS, Chan MV, Zaiss AK, Garcia-Vaz E, Jiao J, Berglund LM, et al. Systematic study of constitutive cyclooxygenase-2 expression: role of NF-κB and NFAT transcriptional pathways. Proc Natl Acad Sci U S A. 2016;113:434–9.
28. Takeuchi K, Kita K, Hayashi S, Aihara E. Regulatory mechanism of duodenal bicarbonate secretion: roles of endogenous prostaglandins and nitric oxide. Pharmacol Ther. 2011;130:59–70.
29. Bjerknes M, Khandanpour C, Möröy T, Fujiyama T, Hoshino M, Klisch TJ, et al. Origin of the brush cell lineage in the mouse intestinal epithelium. Dev Biol. 2012;362:194–218.
30. Schütz B, Jurastow I, Bader S, Ringer C, von Engelhardt J, Chubanov V, et al. Chemical coding and chemosensory properties of cholinergic brush cells in the mouse gastrointestinal and biliary tract. Front Physiol. 2015;6:87.
31. von Moltke J, Ji M, Liang H E, Locksley RM. Tuft-cell-derived IL-25 regulates an intestinal ILC2-epithelial response circuit. Nature. 2016;529:221–5.
32. Höfer D, Drenckhahn D. Identification of brush cells in the alimentary and respiratory system by antibodies to villin and fimbrin. Histochemistry. 1992; 98:237–42.
33. Gerbe F, Sidot E, Smyth DJ, Ohmoto M, Matsumoto I, Dardalhon V, et al. Intestinal epithelial tuft cells initiate type 2 mucosal immunity to helminth parasites. Nature. 2016;529:226–30.
34. Gerbe F, Legraverend C, Jay P. The intestinal epithelium tuft cells: specification and function. Cell Mol Life Sci. 2012;69:2907–17.
35. Westphalen CB, Asfaha S, Hayakawa Y, Takemoto Y, Lukin DJ, Nuber AH, et al. Long-lived intestinal tuft cells serve as colon cancer-initiating cells. J Clin Invest. 2014;124:1283–95.
36. Powell DW, Mifflin RC, Valentich JD, Crowe SE, Saada JI, West AB. Myofibroblasts. II. Intestinal subepithelial myofibroblasts. Am J Phys. 1999; 277:183–201.
37. Cohn SM, Schloemann S, Tessner T, Seibert K, Stenson WF. Crypt stem cell survival in the mouse intestinal epithelium is regulated by prostaglandins synthesized through cyclooxygenase-1. J Clin Invest. 1997;99:1367–79.
38. Berschneider HM, Powell DW. Fibroblasts modulate intestinal secretory responses to inflammatory mediators. J Clin Invest. 1992;89:484–9.
39. Maskarinec G, Harmon BE, Little MA, Ollberding NJ, Kolonel LN, Henderson BE, et al. Excess body weight and colorectal cancer survival: the multiethnic cohort. Cancer Causes Control. 2015;26:1709–18.
40. Clauss W, Arnason SS, Munck BG, Skadhauge E. Aldosterone-induced sodium transport in lower intestine. Effects of varying NaCl intake. Pflügers Arch Eur J Physiol. 1984;401:354–60.
41. Geraedts MCP, Troost FJ, De Ridder RJ, Bodelier AGL, Masclee AAM, Saris WHM. Validation of Ussing chamber technology to study satiety hormone release from human duodenal specimens. Obesity. 2012;20:678–82.
42. Mahmood B, Matthiesen M, Damm B, Søren T, Jensen R, Balslev Backe M, et al. Phosphodiesterases in non-neoplastic appearing colonic mucosa from patients with colorectal neoplasia. BMC Cancer. 2016;16:938.
43. Rothwell PM, Wilson M, Price JF, Belch JF, Meade TW, Mehta Z. Effect of daily aspirin on risk of cancer metastasis: a study of incident cancers during randomised controlled trials. Lancet. 2012;379:1591–601.
44. Thun MJ, Jacobs EJ, Patrono C. The role of aspirin in cancer prevention. Nat Rev Clin Oncol. 2012;9:259–67.
45. Wang D, DuBois RN. The role of prostaglandin E2 in tumor-associated immunosuppression. Trends Mol Med. 2016;22:1–3.
46. Cuzick J, Thorat MA, Bosetti C, Brown PH, Burn J, Cook NR, et al. Estimates of benefits and harms of prophylactic use of aspirin in the general population. Ann Oncol. 2015;26:47–57.
47. Koeberle A, Laufer SA, Werz O. Design and development of microsomal prostaglandin E2 Synthase-1 inhibitors: challenges and future directions. J Med Chem. 2016;59:5970–86.
48. Nosho K, Sukawa Y, Adachi Y, Ito M, Mitsuhashi K, Kurihara H, et al. Association of Fusobacterium nucleatum with immunity and molecular alterations in colorectal cancer. World J Gastroenterol. 2016;22:557–66.
49. Mima K, Ogino S, Nakagawa S, Sawayama H, Kinoshita K, Krashima R, et al. The role of intestinal bacteria in the development and progression of gastrointestinal tract neoplasms. Surg Oncol. 2017;26:368–76.

25

Synchronous polypectomy during endoscopic diagnosis of colorectal cancer – is the risk of tumour implantation at the polypectomy site significant?

W. J. Tan[1,2*†], N. ZP. Ng[1†], Y. D. Chen[1], Y. H. M. Chee[1], F. J. Foo[1,2], C. L. Tang[1] and M. H. Chew[1,2]

Abstract

Background: Synchronous polypectomy in colonic malignancies is contentious due to the perceived risks of tumour implantation at polypectomy sites (PS). We assess the risks of tumour implantation after synchronous polypectomy.

Methods: An analysis of all endoscopies for cancer that were accompanied by synchronous polypectomies from 2005 to 2009 was performed. The incidence of metachronous colorectal cancers located at the same segment of a previous PS was the surrogate for tumour implantation. Data on patient demographics, tumour and polyp location(s) and follow-up outcomes were extracted. The rate of metachronous lesions at the same segment of a previous PS between patients who had all synchronous PS resected (Group A) and patients with PS left in-situ (Group B) were compared.

Results: Two hundred and eighty-four patients had synchronous polypectomy performed during their initial endoscopy for cancer. Three patients were lost to follow-up and, in the remaining 281 patients, 87 (31.0%) were in Group A while 194 (69%) were in Group B. Median age, gender, tumour location, tumour stage, and pathological characteristics were similar between both groups. 2 (0.7%) patients developed local recurrences. Six (2.1%) patients developed metachronous lesions, four of which were located at the same segment where synchronous polypectomy was previously performed. The rates of metachronous lesions at the PS in groups A and B were similar at 1.1% (1/87) and 1.5% (3/194), respectively ($p = 0.795$).

Conclusion: Malignant implantation after synchronous polypectomy in the setting of a newly diagnosed cancer remains unproven. Even if tumor implantation did occur, the incidence is likely low.

Keywords: Colorectal cancer, Synchronous polypectomy, Tumour seeding, Local recurrence, Metachronous tumour

Background

Colonoscopy is an essential component of colorectal cancer diagnosis. Synchronous polyps are detected in up to 15–50% of malignancies during colonoscopy [1–4].

As viable cancer cells exfoliated into the lumen have a recognized role in anastomotic suture line implantation and tumour recurrence with the normal physiological passage of faeces [5–8], many endoscopists prefer not to perform immediate polypectomy of synchronous polyps due to a perceived risk of tumour cell implantation into the raw colonic mucosa left at the polypectomy site. It is uncertain whether doing so protects patients from a theoretical and unquantified risk of tumour implantation. In turn, such an approach subjects patients to a further endoscopic procedure that could have been avoided had a polypectomy been performed during the initial diagnostic colonoscopy. This formed the premise of an earlier systemic review by Sheel et al. [9]. In this review, articles were included if they described human or

* Correspondence: winson.tan.j.h@singhealth.com.sg
†W. J. Tan and N. ZP. Ng contributed equally to this work.
[1]Department of Colorectal Surgery, Singapore General Hospital, 20 College Road, Academia Level 5, Singapore 169856, Singapore
[2]Department of General Surgery, Sengkang General Hospital, 110 Sengkang East Way, Singapore 544886, Singapore

mammalian models related to colorectal cancer cell implantation on normal and damaged colonic mucosa, such as polypectomy sites. The systematic review failed to identify any randomized trials, cohort studies, or retrospective evidence that addressed this clinical question. Available evidence was restricted to that of isolated case reports, the majority of which described implantation on haemorrhoidectomy or fistulectomy wounds. There was only a single case that described a possible cancer cell implantation into an endoscopic biopsy site proximal to a tumour [10].

The scarcity of evidence on this important clinical question prompted a review of our institutional data to decipher if any trends could be derived to guide future management. We decided to use the incidence of metachronous colorectal cancers located at the same colonic segment of previous polypectomy sites (PS) as a surrogate measure for possible tumour implantation. This study aims to compare the incidence of metachronous colorectal cancers in patients with resected PS to those whose PS were left in-situ following their primary colonic resection.

Methods

An analysis of a prospectively maintained database of all patients who underwent curative resection for colorectal cancers from 2005 to 2009 in the Department of Colorectal Surgery at Singapore General Hospital was performed. All patients whose initial diagnostic endoscopy was accompanied by a synchronous polypectomy were included in our study. The study duration was chosen as it ensured that all patients included in the study had at least a 5-year duration of follow-up.

Patients who presented with recurrent cancer, inflammatory bowel disease, familial adenomatous polyposis, or other polyposis syndromes were excluded. We also excluded cases that were diagnosed on presentation with a stage 4 disease and those who underwent an endoscopic removal of malignant colorectal polyps or a local/transanal excision of low rectal cancers. The study protocol was approved by the Institutional Review Board of Singapore General Hospital.

Data on patient demographics, tumour and polyp location(s), biopsy method, size, morphology, histology, and follow-up outcomes were extracted. Patients who developed metachronous lesions during their follow-up were identified and details were sought to determine if these lesions were located at the same colonic region where their previous synchronous polypectomy was performed.

Patients were followed-up to the end of 2016 or to the day of their demise.

The cohort was divided into two groups for statistical analysis. Group A comprised patients who had all synchronous PS resected during their colorectal resection while Group B comprised patients with PS left in-situ.

Follow-up details

The follow-up regime in our department is in accordance with the National Comprehensive Cancer Network guidelines [11]. At each consultation, carcinoembryonic antigen (CEA) levels were measured, and full history and physical examinations (including digital rectal examination) were performed. Patients are followed-up at thrice-monthly intervals for the first 2 years, bi-yearly for the next 3 years, then yearly thereafter. Colonoscopy was performed within 6 months of surgery for patients who did not have a complete colonic evaluation prior to their resection. Those who had an initial complete colonic evaluation would undergo colonoscopy at the first year of follow-up and again at 3-yearly intervals post-operatively if there were no indications for more frequent surveillance. Patients with suspicious symptoms and signs of rising CEA trend on follow-up would be evaluated earlier with colonoscopy and/or radiological imaging (including computerized tomography of the chest, abdomen, and pelvis, bone scan, and positron emission tomography scans if applicable).

Adjuvant therapy regime

Adjuvant therapy was offered for all stage 3 patients who were deemed fit enough to undergo adjuvant chemotherapy. Adjuvant chemotherapy was also offered to stage 2 patients with high risk factors such as perineural invasion, lympho-vascular invasion, and obstructed or perforated tumours. Adjuvant therapy comprised 6 months of fluoropyrimidine (5-fluorouracil or capecitabine) with or without oxaliplatin.

We used metachronous lesions developing at the same colonic segment of the previous polypectomy as a surrogate measure for the possible risk of tumour seeding on PS.

Metachronous colorectal cancer was defined as a secondary colorectal cancer that occurred for more than 6 months after a curative resection of the index cancer [12]. Metachronous lesions developing near the anastomosis were differentiated from local recurrences by using 3 cm as a cut-off. Lesions at or within 3 cm of the anastomosis were considered local recurrences rather than metachronous lesions.

The location of the metachronous tumours detected on surveillance was determined based on their described location in the endoscopy report and computed tomography scan report. In all these lesions, details of the initial endoscopy with synchronous polypectomy were retrieved to determine if the lesion was located at the same colonic region where the synchronous polypectomy was performed.

Statistical analysis

Differences between groups A and B were analysed using Fisher's exact test for categorical variables while Mann-Whitney U test was utilized for continuous variables. Metachronous cancer rates at the colonic segments of previous synchronous polypectomy sites were compared between the two groups.

All statistical analyses were performed using SPSS version 20.

Results

Three thousand, three hundred, and ninety-seven patients underwent surgical resection for colorectal cancer from 2005 to 2009. Two hundred and eighty-four (8.3%) patients had polypectomy(s) performed for synchronous benign polyps at their initial diagnostic colonoscopy. Three patients were subsequently lost to follow-up and, among the remaining 281 patients, 87 (31.0%) had all their PS resected (Group A) while 194 (69%) patients had some or all PS left in-situ (Group B). The patient distribution of the study cohort is illustrated in Fig. 1.

A total of 469 polyps were removed in these 284 patients. The histological distribution of these polyps is illustrated in Table 1.

The demographic characteristics of the patients in groups A and B are illustrated in Table 2. Median age (67 years versus 70 years, $p = 0.25$) and gender distribution (70.1% males versus 63.9% males, $p = 0.348$) were comparable between groups A and B. Both groups did not differ significantly in terms of age, gender, tumour sites, T and N staging, or lympho-vascular and peri-neural invasion.

Metachronous tumours

Two (0.7%) patients developed local recurrences while six (2.1%) patients developed metachronous colorectal tumours. The details of the six patients who developed metachronous lesions are illustrated in Table 3.

Four of the six patients (Patients 1 to 4) with metachronous tumours developed lesions at the same segment of the residual colon where their previous synchronous polypectomy was performed. In the remaining 2 patients (Patients 5 & 6), one had a metachronous tumour at the hepatic flexure (initial polypectomy site in the transverse colon) while the other had a metachronous tumour in the transverse colon (initial polypectomy site in the sigmoid colon).

The rates of metachronous tumours occurring at the same colonic segments of the previous synchronous PS in groups A and B were 1.1% (1 out of 87) and 1.5% (3 out of 194), respectively ($p = 0.795$). Among these four patients, two had initial PS located proximal to the primary cancer (Patient 2 and 4) while the other two had PS located distal to the primary cancer (Patient 1 and 3).

Discussion

This study is one of the first to analyse potential tumour implantation risks after a polypectomy in the setting of a newly diagnosed colorectal malignancy. The decision of concurrent endoscopic polypectomy in a malignant lesion is often variable. Often, endoscopists may remove small polyps during intubation, prior to reaching the cancer, to avoid missing these lesions during withdrawal.

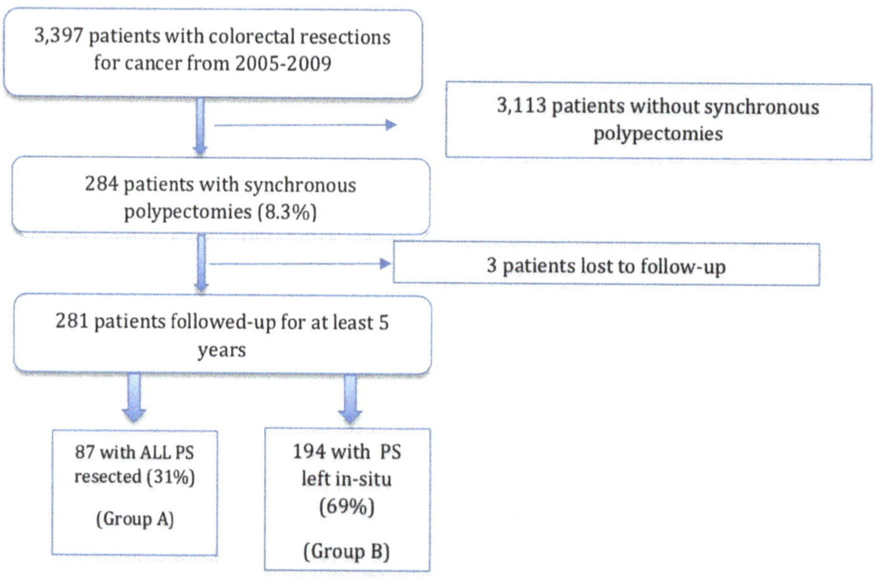

Fig. 1 Flow diagram illustrating patient distribution of study cohort

Table 1 Histology distribution of resected polyps

Polyp histology	Group A*	Group B^	Total Number (%) $n = 469$
Hyperplastic	31	88	119 (25.4)
Serrated adenoma	13	9	22 (4.7)
Tubular adenoma	77	207	284 (60.6)
Tubullovillous adenoma	11	24	35 (7.5)
Villous adenoma	0	1	1 (0.2)
Data missing	3	5	8 (1.7)

Group A - Patients who had all synchronous polypectomy sites resected*
Group B^ - Patients who had synchronous polypectomy sites left in situ

In other circumstances, when a significant polyp is diagnosed synchronously, but at a considerable distance from the cancer, the polyp may be removed to obtain a histology. This will aid the decision for surgery as a malignant histology of a large polyp will require a concurrent bowel resection of the site, or the surgeon may choose to leave a portion of the bowel alone if the histology is benign. This has an important bearing on various technical considerations as performing an anastomosis may be more difficult when bowel lengths are reduced. Furthermore, this decision has important implications for patients as the functional outcomes of patients can be affected adversely in an extensive bowel resection, which can result in copious diarrhoea after surgery.

Table 2 Comparison of demographic characteristics between Groups A* and B^

	Group A * ($n = 87$)	Group B^ ($n = 194$)	*p*-value
Median age (range)	67 (34–92)	70 (32–94)	0.25
Gender			0.348
Male (%)	61 (70.1%)	124 (63.9%)	
Female (%)	26 (29.9%)	70 (36.1%)	
Tumor site, n (%)			0.838
Caecum	4 (4.6%)	13 (6.7%)	
Ascending	5 (5.7%)	21 (10.8)	
Hepatic Flexure	6 (6.9%)	6 (3.1%)	
Transverse	2 (2.3%)	5 (2.6%)	
Splenic Flexure	1 (1.2%)	3 (1.5%)	
Descending	4 (4.6%)	9 (4.6%)	
Sigmoid	27 (31.0%)	47 (24.2%)	
Rectum	38 (43.7%)	90 (46.9%)	
T Stage, n (%)			0.434
T1	17 (19.5%)	21 (10.8%)	
T2	15 (17.2%)	37 (19.1%)	
T3	43 (49.4%)	115 (59.3%)	
T4	12 (13.8%)	21 (10.8%)	
N Stage, n (%)			0.361
N0	50 (57.5%)	102 (52.6%)	
N1	21 (24.1%)	44 (22.7%)	
N2	16 (18.4%)	48 (24.7%)	
Lympho-vascular Invasion, n (%)	25 (28.7%)	60 (30.9%)	0.688
Peri-neural invasion, n(%)	17 (19.5%)	33 (17.0%)	0.625

Group A - Patients who had all synchronous polypectomy sites resected*
Group B^ - Patients who had synchronous polypectomy sites left in situ

Our study has demonstrated that the incidence of tumour seeding at the PS after synchronous polypectomy, if any, is very low. This is evident as the rates of metachronous tumour that developed at the same colonic region of previous synchronous polypectomies were similar in patients from groups A and B (1.1% vs 1.5%, $p = 0.795$). If the incidence of tumour implantation in PS was significant, one would expect those in group B to have a far higher incidence of metachronous tumour when compared to those in group A. This was not the case in our study and alludes that the risk of tumour implantation on PS is likely insignificant. The cited rates of a 5-year local recurrence after curative treatment for colorectal cancer range from 2 to 5% while that of metachronous lesions range from 3 to 10% [13–16]. The metachronous lesion rate of 2.1% in our study cohort, all of whom had synchronous polypectomy performed, lies within the lower limit of these figures. This further reiterates that risks of tumour implantation after synchronous polypectomy is likely to be negligible.

These findings are also consistent with the systematic review by Sheel et al. [9]. In this systematic review, the only identified literature that studied human subjects was an isolated case report [10]. In this case report, a patient was diagnosed with a long segment primary rectal tumour of 1.5 cm to 12 cm from the anal verge and had proximal colonic biopsies during the index colonoscopy. This was performed before the rectal cancer was biopsied. After neoadjuvant radiation treatment, the patient underwent abdominal-perineal resection and was noted to have an area of mucosal irregularity, 12 cm proximal to the tumour. This area was subjected to histopathology analysis, which revealed granulation tissue near the mucosal surface; however, malignant tumoural glandular structures were detected in the submucosa. This led the authors to allude that the findings may be related to tumour seeding. However, another possible explanation could also be a sub-mucosal extension or lymphatic or vascular invasion of the primary lesion, an alternative made even more plausible in view of the poorly differentiated histology of the primary malignant lesion.

The low risk of mucosal implantation of tumour cells has also been demonstrated in mammalian studies. Yu et al. performed a study assessing tumour implantation

Table 3 Characteristics of patients who developed metachronous lesions

Patient	1	2	3	4	5	6
Initial tumour site	HF	Rectum	Caecum & AC	Rectum	DC & SC	AC
Histology/stage	AdenoCa T3N0M0	AdenoCa T3N2M0	AdenoCa T3N2M0	AdenoCa T3N0M0	AdenoCa T2N0M0	AdenoCa T3N2M1
Margins of initial resection	Clear Proximal - 17 cm Distal - 3 cm	Clear Proximal - 13 cm Distal - 2 cm	Clear Proximal - 5.5 cm Distal - 8.5 cm	Clear Proximal - 11.5 cm Distal - 2.5 cm	Clear Proximal - 2 cm Distal - 3.5 cm	Clear Proximal - 20 cm Distal - 6 cm
Surgery	Right Hemicolectomy	Low Anterior Resection	Right Hemicolectomy	Low Anterior Resection	Left Hemicolectomy	Right Hemicolectomy
Synchronous polypectomy numbers	1	4	2	2	1	1
Polypectomy site(s)	DC	a) SC b) SC c) DC d) DC	a) AC b) TC	a) Rectum b) DC	TC	SC
PS Proximal/Distal to tumour	Distal	Proximal	Distal	Proximal	Proximal	Distal
Polyp(s) morphology	Pedunculated	a) Pedunculated b) Pedunculated c) Sessile d) Sessile	a) Sessile b) Sessile	a)Pedunculated b) Sessile	Sessile	Pedunculated
Polyp histology	TA LGD	a) TA LGD b) TA HGD c) HP d) HP	a) HP b) HP	a) TA LGD b) TA LGD	TA LGD	TVA HGD
Size (mm)	15	a) 15 b) 12 c) 6 d) 7	a) 3 b) 3	a) Missing b) Missing	3	10
All PS included in resection	No (Group B)	No (Group B)	No (Group B)	Yes (Group A)	No (Group B)	No (Group B)
Site of metachronous tumour	DC	DC	TC	DC	HF	TC
Interval to development of metachronous lesion (months)	32	11	11	36	83	9
Metachronous lesion at colonic segment of previous synchronous PS?	Yes	Yes	Yes	Yes	No	No

HF **Hepatic flexure,** ***AC*** **Ascending colon,** ***DC*** **Descending colon,** ***SC*** **Sigmoid colon,** ***AdenoCa*** **Adenocarcinoma,** ***TC*** **Transverse colon,** ***TA LGD*** **Tubulo-adenoma with low grade dysplasia,** ***TA HGD*** **Tubulo-adenoma with high grade dysplasia,** ***HP*** **Hyperplastic,** ***TVA HGD*** **Tubulo-villous adenoma with high grade dysplasia,** ***TVA LGD*** **Tubulo-villous adenoma with low grade dysplasi**

in rabbits and failed to demonstrate any cases of mucosal implantation in the study [17]. Tumour implantation appeared to predominantly occur in areas where the serosa of the bowel was breached, with the tumour in-growth from the serosa inwards. In another study, Broyn et al. assessed the risks of tumour implantation in the damaged colonic mucosa of rats and similarly concluded that damaged colonic mucosa is extremely resistant to tumour seeding [18].

Two factors ought to be considered in the mechanism of tumour implantation in the colonic mucosa: 1) the presentation of viable malignant cells and 2) the susceptibility of the mucosa to allow the proliferation of malignant cells. In addition to the intrinsic ability of the colonic mucosa to resist tumour implantation, the distribution pattern of exfoliated cancer cells may also explain the low incidence of mucosal implantation in clinical settings. Maeda et al. assessed the distribution of exfoliated colonic tumour cells and concluded that malignant cells were predominantly found within 5 cm from the primary tumour [19]. Within 5 cm proximal and distal to the primary tumour, exfoliated malignant cells were found in 25 to 90% of the specimens compared to in 5 to 15% at distances beyond 5 cm. The findings suggest that PS at the greatest risk of exposure to exfoliated malignant cells lie within 5 cm from the primary tumour [20]. 5 cm is the current recommended resection margin for colon cancer and thus the at-risk mucosa in these regions would usually have been resected in an oncological resection.

There are several limitations to our study.

Data on the location (colonic segment) of the polyps removed were based mainly on endoscopists' descriptions, which are prone to an error rate of close to 20% [21]. In mitigation, this error rate is likely to be evenly balanced during the comparisons between groups A and B. There is also evidently treatment bias in this study as significant polyps or polyps with high risks of implantation due to the proximity of the tumours may have been removed surgically, thus not completely excluding this hypothesis. The use of metachronous tumors as a surrogate for PS implantation is also contentious and ideally, the metachronous cancers that were detected should be subjected to genomic analysis and compared to the initial malignant lesion to determine true malignant implantation. However, this would be costly and we did not have the necessary funding to pursue this verification.

It would also be interesting if the metachronous cancer rate of our study cohort could be compared with the other 3113 patients with colorectal cancer without synchronous polypectomy (Fig. 1). Unfortunately, we do not have the complete follow up data for these 3113 patients for comparison. In addition, with our study cohort demonstrating such a low metachronous cancer rate of 2.1%, it is highly unlikely that the patients without synchronous polypectomy would have a metachronous cancer rate that is significantly lower. Nonetheless, this study represents an invaluable addition to literature on the possible risks of tumour implantation after synchronous polypectomy in the setting of a newly diagnosed colorectal cancer. The incidence of mucosal implantation after synchronous polypectomy is so infrequent that it would be impractical to expect evidence in the form of randomized controlled trials to guide our clinical practice. A meta-analysis of published clinical studies represents the most practical alternative once a critical mass of studies is available.

Conclusion

Malignant implantation after synchronous polypectomy in the setting of a newly diagnosed cancer remains unproven. Even if tumour implantation did occur, the incidence is likely low.

Abbreviations

CEA: Carcinoembryonic antigen; PS: Polypectomy sites

Authors' contributions

WJT and NZPN collected and analysed and date and contributed equally in the preparation of the manuscript. YDC and YHMC performed data collection, assisted in statistical analysis and participated in drafting of the manuscript. FJF, CLT and MHC participated in the study conceptualization and design as well as the drafting and editing of the manuscript. All authors read and approved the final manuscript.

Competing interests

The authors declare that they have no competing interests.

References

1. Brullet E, Montane JM, Bombardo J, Bonfill X, Nogue M, Bordas JM. Intraoperative colonoscopy in patients with colorectal cancer. Br J Surg. 1992;79(12):1376–8.
2. Burns FJ. Synchronous and metachronous malignancies of the colon and rectum. Dis Colon Rectum. 1980;23(8):578–9.
3. Kim MS, Park YJ. Detection and treatment of synchronous lesions in colorectal cancer: the clinical implication of perioperative colonoscopy. World J Gastroenterol. 2007;13(30):4108–11.
4. Langevin JM, Nivatvongs S. The true incidence of synchronous cancer of the large bowel. A prospective study. Am J Surg. 1984;147(3):330–3.
5. Hasegawa J, Nishimura J, Yamamoto S, Yoshida Y, Iwase K, Kawano K, Nezu R. Exfoliated malignant cells at the anastomosis site in colon cancer surgery: the impact of surgical bowel occlusion and intraluminal cleaning. Int J Color Dis. 2011;26(7):875–80.
6. Loktionov A. Cell exfoliation in the human colon: myth, reality and implications for colorectal cancer screening. Int J Cancer. 2007;120(11): 2281–9.
7. Rosenberg IL. The aetiology of colonic suture-line recurrence. Ann R Coll Surg Engl. 1979;61(4):251–7.
8. Tsunoda A, Shibusawa M, Tsunoda Y, Choh H, Takata M, Kusano M. Implantation on the suture material and efficacy of povidone-iodine solution. Eur Surg Res. 1997;29(6):473–80.
9. Sheel AR, Artioukh DY. Endoscopic excision of synchronous large bowel polyps in the presence of colorectal carcinoma: is the fear of malignant cell implantation justified? A systematic review of the literature. Color Dis. 2015; 17(7):559–65.

10. Basha G, Ectors N, Penninckx F, Filez L, Geboes K. Tumor cell implantation after colonoscopy with biopsies in a patient with rectal cancer: report of a case. Dis Colon Rectum. 1997;40(12):1508–10.
11. National Comprehensive Cancer Network (NCCN) Guidelines in Clin Oncol 2016.
12. Park IJ, Yu CS, Kim HC, Jung YH, Han KR, Kim JC. Metachronous colorectal cancer. Color Dis. 2006;8(4):323–7.
13. Bouvier AM, Launoy G, Bouvier V, Rollot F, Manfredi S, Faivre J, Cottet V, Jooste V. Incidence and patterns of late recurrences in colon cancer patients. Int J Cancer. 2015;137(9):2133–8.
14. Laubert T, Habermann JK, Hemmelmann C, Kleemann M, Oevermann E, Bouchard R, Hildebrand P, Jungbluth T, Burk C, Esnaashari H, et al. Metachronous metastasis- and survival-analysis show prognostic importance of lymphadenectomy for colon carcinomas. BMC Gastroenterol. 2012;12:24.
15. Scholefield JH, Steele RJ, British Society for G, Association of Coloproctology for Great B, Ireland. Guidelines for follow up after resection of colorectal cancer. Gut. 2002;51(Suppl 5):V3–5.
16. Tziris N, Dokmetzioglou J, Giannoulis K, Kesisoglou I, Sapalidis K, Kotidis E, Gambros O. Synchronous and metachronous adenocarcinomas of the large intestine. Hippokratia. 2008;12(3):150–2.
17. Yu SK, Cohn I Jr. Tumor implantation on colonmucosa. Arch Surg. 1968; 96(6):956–8.
18. Broyn T. Tumour implantation in ischemic, thermic and mechanical lesions of the colonic mucosa. An experimental study in rats. Acta Chir Scand. 1972; 138(2):202–6.
19. Maeda K, Hanai T, Sato H, Masumori K, Koide Y, Matsuoka H, Katsuno H, Kuroda M. Intraluminal exfoliated cancer cells and effectiveness of bowel ligatures during sigmoidectomy for sigmoid colon cancer. Surg Today. 2014; 44(2):297–301.
20. Nelson H, Petrelli N, Carlin A, Couture J, Fleshman J, Guillem J, Miedema B, Ota D, Sargent D, National Cancer Institute expert P. Guidelines 2000 for colon and rectal cancer surgery. J Natl Cancer Inst. 2001;93(8):583–96.
21. Neri E, Turini F, Cerri F, Faggioni L, Vagli P, Naldini G, Bartolozzi C. Comparison of CT colonography vs. conventional colonoscopy in mapping the segmental location of colon cancer before surgery. Abdom Imaging. 2010;35(5):589–95.

26

Therapeutic preferences and outcomes in newly diagnosed patients with Crohn's diseases in the biological era in Hungary: a nationwide study based on the National Health Insurance Fund database

Zsuzsanna Kurti[1†], Akos Ilias[1†], Lorant Gonczi[1], Zsuzsanna Vegh[1], Petra Fadgyas-Freyler[2], Gyula Korponay[2], Petra A. Golovics[1], Barbara D. Lovasz[1,4] and Peter L. Lakatos[1,3,5*]

Abstract

Background: Accelerated treatment strategy, including tight disease control and early aggressive therapy with immunosuppressives (IS) and biological agents have become increasingly common in inflammatory bowel disease (IBD). The aim of the present study was to estimate the early treatment strategy and outcomes in newly diagnosed patients with Crohn's disease (CD) between 2004 and 2008 and 2009–2015 in the whole IBD population in Hungary based on the administrative database of the National Health Insurance Fund (OEP).

Methods: We used the administrative database of the OEP, the only nationwide state-owned health insurance provider in Hungary. Patients were identified through previously reported algorithms using the ICD-10 codes for CD in the out-, inpatient (medical, surgical) non-primary care records and drug prescription databases between 2004 and 2015. Patients were stratified according to the year of diagnosis and maximum treatment steps during the first 3 years after diagnosis.

Results: A total of 6173 (male/female: 46.12%/53.87%) newly diagnosed CD patients with physician-diagnosed IBD were found in the period of 2004–2015. The use of 5-ASA and steroids remained common in the biological era, while immunosuppressives and biologicals were started earlier and became more frequent among patients diagnosed after 2009. The probability of biological therapy was 2.9%/6.4% and 8.4%/13.7% after 1 and 3 years in patients diagnosed in 2004–2008/2009–2015. The probability of hospitalization in the first 3 years after diagnosis was different before and after 2009, according to the maximal treatment step (overall 55.7%vs. 47.4% ($p = 0.001$), anti-TNF: 73%vs. 66.7% ($p = 0.103$), IS: 64.6% vs. 56.1% ($p = 0.001$), steroid: 44.2%vs. 36.8% ($p < 0.007$), 5-ASA: 32.6% vs. 26.7% $p = 0.157$)). In contrast, surgery rates were not significantly different in patients diagnosed before and after 2009 according to the maximum treatment step (overall 16.0%vs.15.3%($p = 0.672$) anti-TNF 26.7%vs.27.2% ($p = 0.993$), IS: 24.1%vs22.2% ($p = 0.565$), steroid 8.1%vs.7.9% ($p = 0.896$), 5-ASA 10%vs. 11% ($p = 0.816$)).

(Continued on next page)

* Correspondence: kislakpet99@gmail.com; peter.lakatos@mcgill.ca
†Equal contributors
[1]1st Department of Medicine, Semmelweis University, Budapest H-1083, Hungary
[3]Division of Gastroenterology, McGill University Health Centre, 1650 Ave. Cedar, D16.173.1, Montreal, QC H3G 1A4, Canada
Full list of author information is available at the end of the article

(Continued from previous page)

Conclusions: IS and biological exposure became more frequent, while hospitalization decreased and surgery remained low but constant during the observation period.
Use of steroids and 5-ASA remained high after 2009. The association between the maximal treatment step and hospitalization/surgery rates suggests that maximal treatment step can be regarded as proxy severity marker in patients with IBD.

Keywords: Treatment strategy, Crohn's disease, Inflammatory bowel disease, Biological therapy, Surgery, Administrative database, Nationwide

Background

Inflammatory bowel diseases (IBD) are chronic conditions affecting the patient's quality of life, leading to disability; moreover, a significant proportion of patients require surgery. In the past decades, the prevalence of IBD increased worldwide [1–3]. However, development of medical therapy improved patients' perspectives significantly. In recent years, treatment strategies and therapeutic targets have evolved: "treat-to-target" has become an important in-patient management and therapeutic goals have been determined [4]. Additionally, accelerated treatment strategy, including tight disease control and early aggressive therapy with immunosuppressives (IS) and biological agents (mostly anti-TNFs) have become increasingly common in IBD. Emerging data suggest that earlier introduction of IS and biologicals may be associated with improved outcomes including lower risk for surgery and hospitalization [5–9]. These improvements in the management of IBD are reflected by clinical guidelines as well [10]. Nevertheless, it is important to investigate how these changing paradigms affect every day clinical practice and clinical outcomes.

The recent ECCO-EpiCom studies based on the 2010 and 2011 inception cohorts provided data about up-to-date IBD incidences, treatment steps and initial disease course of IBD in the biological era in Europe. Differences were reported between Western and Eastern Europe, not only in the prevalence of IBD, but also regarding treatment strategy and disease outcomes [11–13]. Data on the natural history and therapeutic strategies of Crohn's disease was also reported in population-based studies from North-America, including data from the Mayo clinic, Olmsted Country, Minnesota and the Manitoba Cohort, Canada [8, 14, 15]. It is essential to note, that direct comparison of the above studies may be difficult due to differences in health care insurance systems and data acquisition.

In Hungary, previous population-based studies on the epidemiology and treatment strategy in IBD were reported in the Veszprem population-based IBD database. Nevertheless, data on medical strategy were reported from the pre-biological era [16, 17]. Recently, our group reported nationwide estimate of IBD prevalence from the administrative database of the National Health Insurance Fund [18]. However, the effect of medical therapy on disease outcomes has not been studied yet.

Therefore, the aim of the present study was to investigate the early treatment strategy and outcomes in newly diagnosed patients with Crohn's disease (CD) between 2004 and 2015 in Hungary. Since the prescription regulations changed significantly at the end of 2008 with easier access to biologicals, it has been aimed to evaluate surgical outcomes and hospitalization rates before and after the change of prescription-regulations in the administrative database of the National Health Insurance Fund (OEP) which is the only (state-owned) health insurance provider in Hungary.

Methods

We used the administrative database of the National Health Insurance Fund (OEP). Patients were identified through previously reported algorithms using the ICD-10 codes for Crohn's disease (K50..) in the out- and in-patient (medical, surgical) non-primary care records and drug prescription databases between 1st of January 2004 and 1st of January 2015 [18]. Hospitalizations, surgical episodes and drug prescriptions were identified through the database of the OEP, which contains data on in- and outpatient stays, outpatient procedures and filled drug prescriptions. Any event with a CD-related ICD-10 code was regarded as related.

New patients with Crohn's disease was defined as no CD-related outpatient visits and/or IBD-related drug prescriptions in the last 3 years before the start of the observational period and at least 2 CD-related outpatient visits and/or IBD-related drug prescription during the observational period. Patients with less than 3 years follow up were excluded from the study. Patients were stratified according to the year of diagnosis and the maximum treatment step during the first 3 years after diagnosis.

We determined time to prescription of different drug classes, (5-ASA, steroid, IS and biologicals) and stratified patient groups according to the maximal therapeutic step (1. group – maximum therapeutic step: 5-ASA therapy (oral and/or topical 5-ASA treatment), 2. group – maximum therapeutic step: steroid therapy (systemic or topical steroids), 3. group – maximum therapeutic step:

IS therapy (azathioprine, 6-mercaptopurine, cyclosporine or methotrexate), 4. group – maximum biological therapy (infliximab or adalimumab)). Finally, we calculated hospitalization and surgery rates according to the maximal treatment step and the diagnostic period (diagnosis in 2004–2008 vs. 2009–2015).

Statistical methods

SPSS® 20 (SPSS Inc., Chicago, IL) was used for statistical analysis. Khi-square test and Fischer-exact tests were used to compare categorical variables. Kaplan-Meier analysis and Cox-Mantel LogRank test was used for time dependent change of the categorical variables. Time from diagnosis were weighted to 30-days periods in the Kaplan-Meier analysis. A p value of < 0.05 was regarded as statistically significant.

Results

Patient characteristics

A total of 6173 (male/female: 46.12%/53.87%) newly diagnosed CD patients with physician-diagnosed Crohn's disease were found between 2004 and 2015. 4458 and 1715 newly diagnosed CD patients with an available 3-year follow up period were identified between 01.01.2004 and 31.21.2008 and between 01.01.2009 and 01.01.2015. Distribution of age at diagnosis was similar in the two diagnostic eras, the most prevalent age group at the diagnosis of Crohn's disease was the 20–29 years old group in both gender and in both diagnostic eras (Fig. 1).

Therapeutic strategy

Drug exposures were calculated in a time dependent analysis. The cumulative probability of 5-ASA, steroid, IS and biological therapy were 95.7, 74.8, 37.1 and 4% after 12 months and 97.7, 81.3, 49.4 and 9.9% after 3 years from diagnosis (Fig. 2).

The use of 5-ASA was 93%/90.8% after 3 months and 97.9%/97.1% after 3 years from the diagnosis in the whole patient groups diagnosed before and after 2009, and it did not differ according to the different maximal treatment steps. Use of 5-ASA was similar in the two diagnostic eras in each patient group.

Cumulative steroid exposure was also comparable in both groups (64.4%/66% after 3 months, 72.6%/74.2% after 12 months, 79.8%/79.9% after 3 years in patients diagnosed before and after 2009). Probability of early steroid exposure was different according to the maximum treatment step but not according to the year of

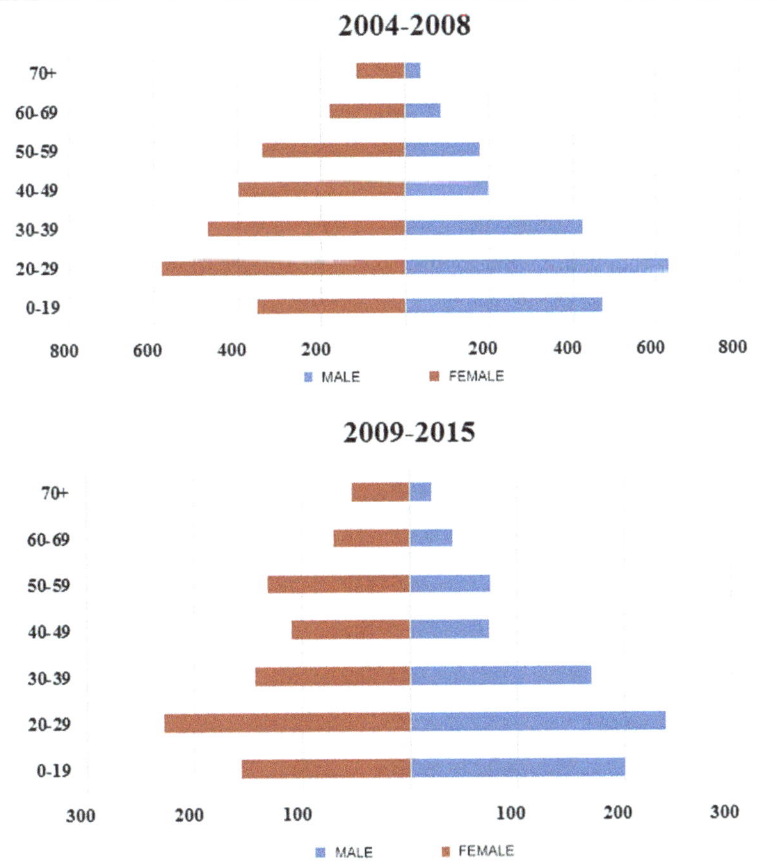

Fig. 1 Age and gender distribution of newly Crohn's disease patients diagnosed in 2004–2008/2009–2015

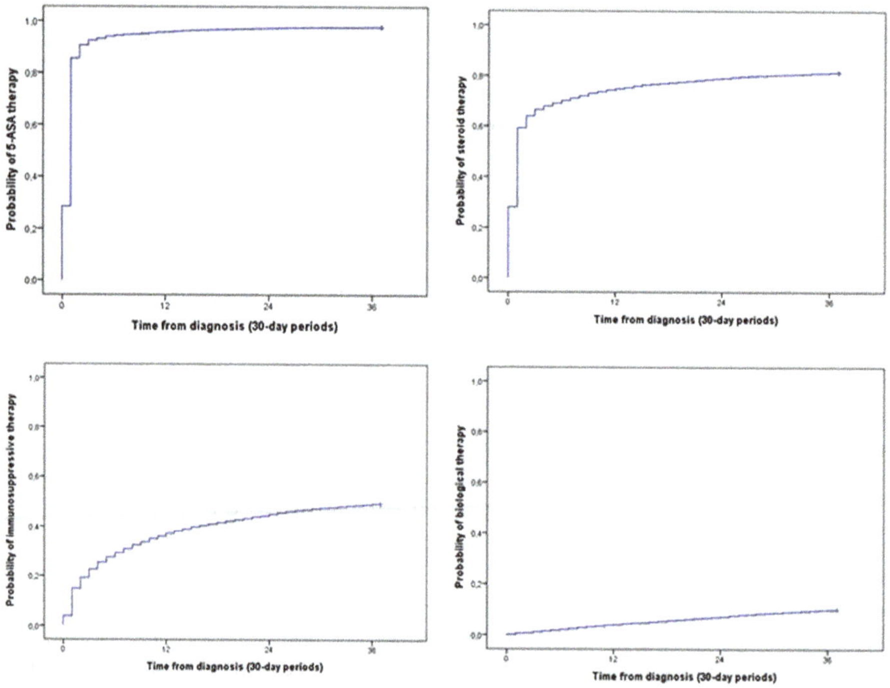

Fig. 2 The cumulative probability of 5-ASA, steroid, IS and biological therapy in the whole observation period

diagnosis: it was 48.9%/53.5% after the first 3 months from diagnosis in patients with steroids as maximum treatment step (pLogRank = 0.09), 74%/74.8% in patients with IS as maximum treatment step (pLogRank = 0.95) and 81.2%/78.7% in patients with biological therapy as maximum step (pLogRank = 0.31), in patients diagnosed before and after 2009 (Fig. 3).

Exposure to immunosuppressive therapy was frequent in both diagnostic eras, with higher probability (pLogRank < 0.001 for the max. IS group and $p = 0.007$ for the max. Biological group) and earlier initiation in the second period. Probability of immunosuppressive therapy was 17.5% vs. 22.9% at 3 months, 29.3% vs. 35.4% at 1 year and 39.9% vs. 45.2% at 3 years in 2004–2008 vs. 2009–2015 in patients with IS as maximum treatment step. Exposure of IS was higher in patients needing anti-TNF therapy: 31.5% vs. 40.3% at 3 months, 66.7% vs. 73.1% at 1 year and 86.7% vs. 91.8% at 3 years in 2004–2008 vs. 2009–2015 (Fig. 4).

The probability of biological therapy was significantly higher in patients diagnosed between 2009 and 2015 (pLogRank< 0.001). It was 1% vs. 1.2% after 3 months, 2.9% vs. 6.4% after 1 year and 8.4% vs. 13.7% after 3 years in 2004–2008 vs. 2009–2015 (Fig. 5).

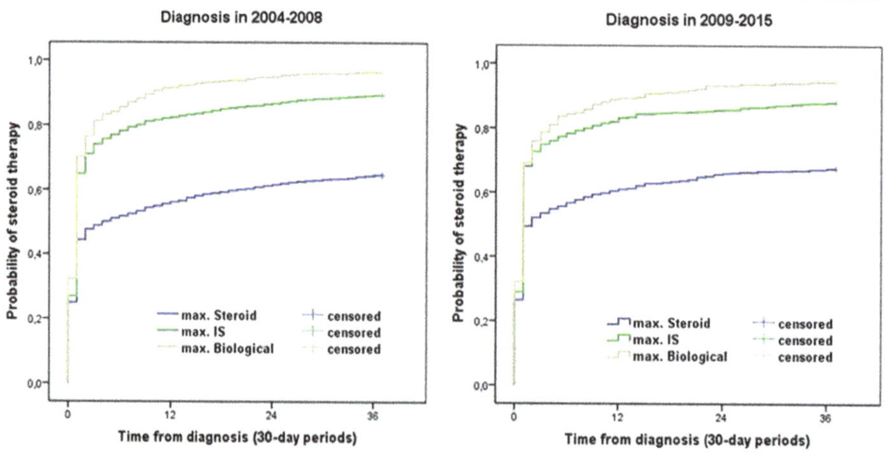

Fig. 3 Probability of steroid therapy according to the maximum treatment steps

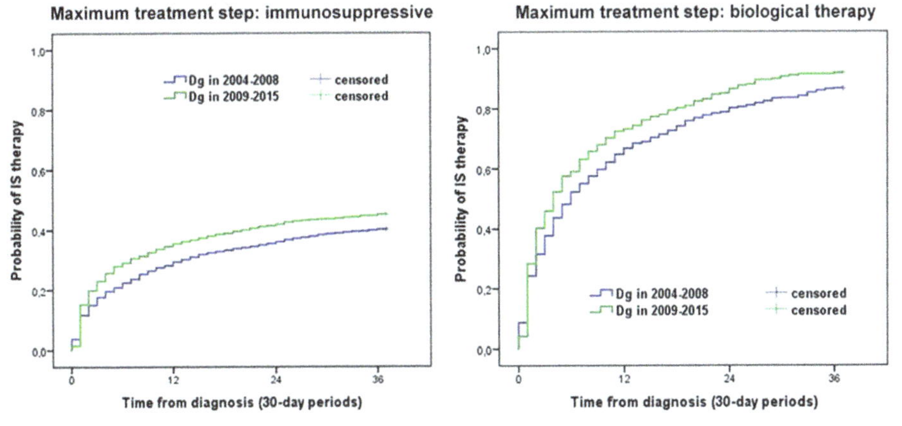

Fig. 4 Probability of immunosuppressive therapy according to the diagnostic period and the maximal treatment steps

Hospitalizations and surgery rates according to the maximal treatment steps in the biological era

Probability of hospitalizations in the first 3-years after the diagnosis was significantly lower in patients diagnosed in 2009–2015 than in patients diagnosed in 2004–2008 (total probability: 55.7% vs. 47.4% in patients diagnosed in 2004–2008 vs. in 2009–2015, pLogRank < 0.001 for the total cohort). When we analysed the hospitalization rates according to the maximal treatment steps, the difference was significant in the steroid and IS group (total probabilities: 5-ASA group: 32.6% vs. 26.7% pLogRank = 0.16, Steroid group: 44.2% vs. 36.8% pLogRank = 0.007, IS group: 64.6% vs. 56.1% pLogRank< 0.001, Biological group: 73% vs. 66.7% pLogRank = 0.10) (Fig. 6).

In contrast, surgery rates were altogether low and not significantly different in the two periods, but they were associated with the maximum therapeutic step. A proportion of patients underwent surgery at around the time of diagnosis (within 3 months from diagnosis) in both diagnostic eras, regardless of the maximum treatment step (9.1%/8.6% in the total cohort in 2004–2008/2009–2015). Thereafter the probability of surgery remained unchanged in patients with 5-ASA and steroid only, while it increased continuously in the IS and biological group (at 1 year: overall: 12% vs. 11.9%, biological therapy: 20.9% vs. 19.6%, IS: 17.4% vs. 17.3%, steroid 5.8% vs. 6%, 5-ASA 8.9% vs. 9.1%, at 3 years: overall: 16.0% vs. 15.3% (pLogRank = 0.672), biological therapy: 26,7% vs. 27.2% (pLogRank = 0.993), IS: 24.1% vs. 22.2% (pLogRank = 0.565), steroid 8.1% vs. 7.9% (pLogRank = 0.896), 5-ASA 10% vs. 11% (pLogRank = 0.816) in patients diagnosed in 2004–2008 vs. 2009–2015) (Fig. 7).

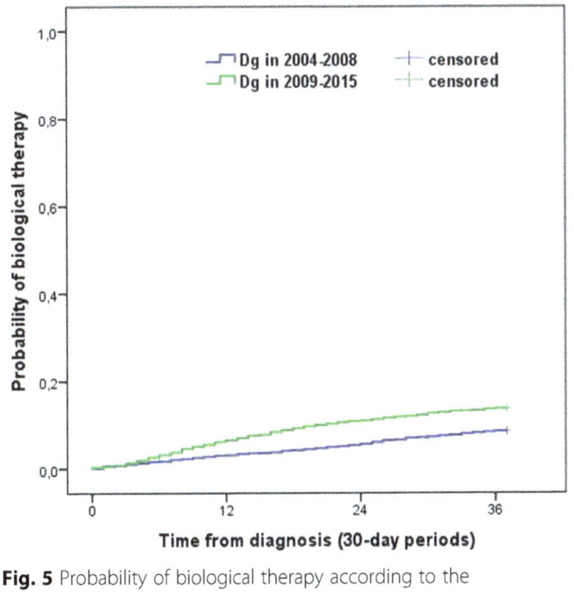

Fig. 5 Probability of biological therapy according to the diagnostic period

Discussion

The aim of the present study was to demonstrate a nationwide description about the therapeutic strategy and outcomes in newly diagnosed patients with Crohn's disease in the biological era in Hungary.

The main findings of the study were that hospitalization but not surgical rates differed significantly in patients diagnosed between 2004 and 2008 and between 2009 and 2015, along with the earlier and more frequent use of IS and biologicals in the second diagnostic period. Of note, surgery rates were altogether low. In addition, hospitalizations and surgeries were more frequent in the biological and the IS group compared to patients with steroids and 5-ASA only, suggesting that maximal therapeutic steps can be used as severity markers in patients with IBD when analysing health insurance databases.

In the present study, the overall probability of surgery was 9.1%/8.6% after 3 months, 12%/11.9% after 1 year and 16%/15.3% after 3 years from diagnosis among patients diagnosed in 2004–2008/2009–2015. This is in

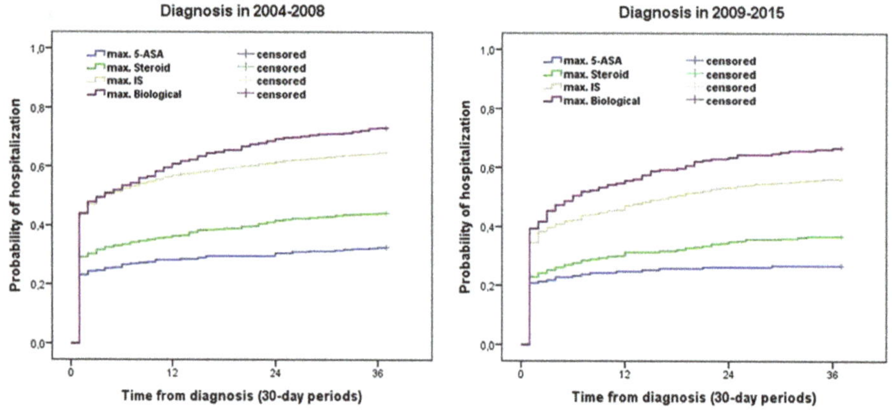

Fig. 6 Probability of hospitalization according to the maximum treatment steps in patients diagnosed in 2004–2008/2009–2015

line with new data reported after 2000 [6]. According to the meta-analysis of Frolkis et al. based on 30 population-based studies, the cumulative risk of surgery in CD-patients diagnosed in the 2000s was 12.6 and 24.2% after 1 and 5 years from diagnosis [19]. The study from Manitoba also reported that probability of surgery was 10% and 18% after 1 and 5 year from diagnosis in CD patients diagnosed after 2000 [8]. In contrast, ECCO-EpiCom 2011 inception cohort study showed that 24 and 7% of patients from Eastern Europe and Western Europe/Australia underwent surgery within the first year of diagnosis [13].

Interestingly, the present study demonstrated that a stable proportion of patients (app. 9%) had surgery at around the diagnosis (within 3 months from diagnosis) in both diagnostic eras, independently from the maximum treatment step and further disease course. Similarly, Solberg et al. reported that very early CD-related surgery rates remained unchanged and did not influence long term clinical remission rates or outcomes [20]. In contrast, a recent study from Portugal concluded that patients undergoing an early surgery after diagnosis have an increased reoperation rate [21]. Of note, the rate of early surgery within 1 year from diagnosis remained stable in most epidemiological cohorts suggesting that at least a propostion of early surgeries can be regarded as unavoidable [6, 19].

Furthermore, our results suggest that the earlier and more frequent use of biological therapy did not reduce the probability of early surgery during the first 3 years from diagnosis. Previous population-based studies reported that the need for surgery significantly decreased between the 1980s and 2000s, parallel with the increased use of immunosuppressives [7, 8, 22]. Similarly, a former study from Hungary demonstrated that increased and earlier azathioprine use was independently associated with significant change in the natural history of CD and reduced surgery rates [17]. However, only few population-based studies are available from the biological era, and it is still conflictive whether biological therapy further decreases surgical rates on a population-based level [6, 23]. A recent meta-analysis based on 7 randomized controlled trial studies concluded that anti-TNFs were efficacious in reducing hospitalization and

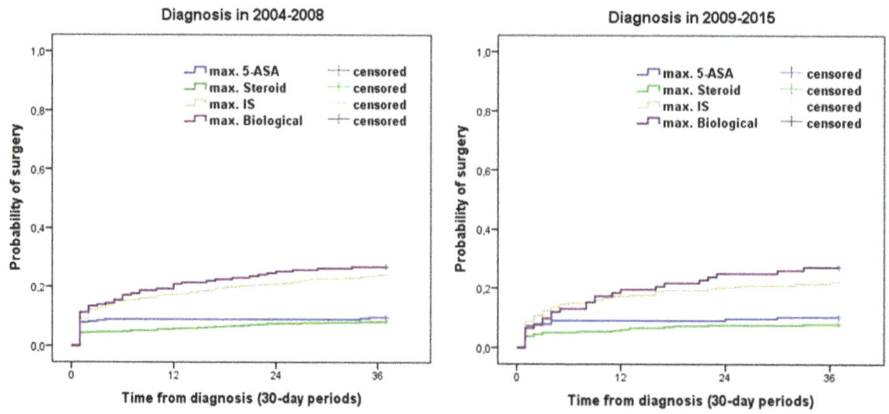

Fig. 7 Probability of surgery according to the maximum treatment steps in patients diagnosed in 2004–2008/2009–2015

surgery rates compared to placebo, while no statistically significant reduction was noted to azathioprine (AZA) and vedolizumab in moderate-to-severe CD patients [23]. Similarly to our findings, a Spanish study concluded that IFX availability did not reduce surgical requirements with a step-up therapeutic algorithm in newly diagnosed CD patients [24]. Moreover, a study based on the Manitoba-cohort suggested that decline in surgery was associated with the care by a gastroenterology specialist but not with the immunomodulatory use in multivariate analysis. This study also concluded that use of more aggressive medical therapy can be a severity marker in non-randomized trial settings [8]. Furthermore, the recent update of the 5-years follow-up of the 2010 ECCO-EpiCom inception cohort study also reported that similar surgery and hospitalization rates were shown in Eastern and Western Europe, despite of more early and aggressive treatment with biologicals in Western Europe [25]. A study from Northern California concluded that prevalence of prolonged steroid exposure and hospitalization rates declined, whereas surgery rates remained constant in parallel with the increasing use of IS and biologicals in CD [26].

The probability of hospitalization was frequent around the diagnosis, but thereafter the frequency of hospitalization was not associated with the maximal therapeutic steps in the present study. Frequency of hospitalization was lower in all treatment groups in the second diagnostic period (decrease was significant in the steroid and IS group), showing a change in the patient management and the possible role of the accelerated treatment strategy. These results are in concordance with previous data that hospitalization is frequent around the diagnosis but it declines significantly from the second year after the diagnosis [27, 28]. Nevertheless, hospitalization rates vary significantly between countries, depending on health care/reimbursement policy and ethnic differences [2, 6].

The other primary aim of the study was to analyse the therapeutic strategy in the two diagnostic eras. Surprisingly, almost every CD patient received 5-ASA therapy in Hungary at around the diagnosis. This result is in concordance with the result of the ECCO-EpiCom 2011 inception cohort study and with other nationwide studies [13, 14]. Possible explanations are that physicians prescribe 5-ASAs until the diagnosis is finally confirmed or patients with mild CD are given 5-ASAs for maintenance therapy. Similarly, a national survey from Germany showed that app. 40% of physicians followed "wait and see" management strategy without any medical therapy in mild CD patients as maintenance, while third of physicians preferred 5-ASA in these cases [29].

Interestingly, the use of steroids remained common in both periods. The majority of patient received steroid therapy as initial treatment at diagnosis and it increased slightly over time. Compared to other recent population-based studies, the use of steroids was more frequent in the present cohort. In previous population-based studies the half of the CD patients received steroids during the early disease course [8, 30, 31]. Other studies showed steroid sparing effect of the increased IS and biological use [7, 26]. In contrast, the ECCO-EpiCom 2011 inception cohort reported that 61 and 67% of patients from Eastern Europe and Western Europe/Australia received systemic steroids during the first year of disease course [13].

The use of immunosuppressives was more frequent in the second period with earlier initiation. This suggests an accelerated step-care strategy in Hungary, similarly to those reported from the Spanish Administrative Database [24]. In the first period, the probability of IS use after 1 year from diagnosis was similar to the previous data from Hungary from the same decade (35.5% vs. 34.8%), while rate of IS use in the second period was higher, similar to rates from Western-Europe (41.3% vs. 45%) [13, 16, 32].

Finally, the use of biologicals was more frequent with earlier initiation in the second period in accordance with the changes of the drug prescription guidelines of OEP allowing an earlier and more extensive availability of anti-TNFs after 2009 in Hungary. In a previous study by Rencz et al. Hungary had the best access to biologicals in IBD in Central-Eastern Europe [33]. However, the use of biological therapy was in line with the Eastern European data in the 2010 ECCO EpiCom inception cohort study, it remained less frequent compared to Western Europe [25, 32].

The authors are aware of the possible limitations of the present work including the limitations of administrative databases such as the lack of disease phenotype data, time bias due to patient stratification or possible bias of patient ascertainment. In contrast, the strength of the present study is the nationwide nature of the study. The administrative database of the National Health Fund is unique in many regards, as in Hungary this is the only insurance plan with a full coverage and it collects in-, outpatient visits, diagnostic procedures and drug prescription data. Thus, it offers an invaluable opportunity to study treatment practices and changes in outcomes representative for the full spectrum of IBD patients in Hungary. Moreover, earlier publications suggested that the first 3-years of the disease are the most sensitive and representative for the further disease course [16, 34]. Thus, results from the present study can be extrapolated in the prediction of the further disease course as well as may be generalizable to most administrative databases from countries with similar health insurance policies.

Conclusion

In conclusion, the present study, representing the nationwide practices in Hungary suggests, that there is an accelerated therapeutic strategy in CD in Hungary with IS and biological use becoming more frequent. Hospitalization decreased in the whole cohort, while surgery remained low but constant during the observation period.

Exposure to steroids and 5-ASA remained high. The association between maximal treatment step and hospitalization and surgery rates suggests that maximal treatment steps can be regarded as proxy severity markers in patients with IBD.

Abbreviations

5-ASA: 5-Aminosalicylic Acid; Anti-TNF: Anti - tumor necrosis factor; AZA: Azathioprine; CD: Crohn's disease; ECCO-EpiCom: European Crohn's Colitis Organization Epidemiology Committee; IBD: Inflammatory bowel disease; ICD-10: 10th revision of the International Statistical Classification of Diseases and Related Health Problems; IS: Immunosuppressives,; OEP: National Health Insurance Fund,

Acknowledgments

Gimesi-Orszagh J contributed in the study providing the data of the National Health Insurance Fund.

Funding

This work was supported by OTKA (Hungarian Scientific Research Fund) Research Grant 2015 (Grant ID: 115345).

Authors' contributions

ZK: data collection, data validation and draft of the article; AI, ZV, PAG, BDL, LG: data collection and article preparation; PFF, GK: statistical analysis, data collection. PLL: study design, data collection, supervising the collection and validation of patients, database construction, statistical analysis, and article preparation; All authors approved the final draft submitted.

Competing interests

No author reported any potential conflict of interest regarding the present study.

Author details

[1]1st Department of Medicine, Semmelweis University, Budapest H-1083, Hungary. [2]Strategic Analysis Department, National Health Insurance Fund (OEP), Budapest H-1139, Hungary. [3]Division of Gastroenterology, McGill University Health Centre, 1650 Ave. Cedar, D16.173.1, Montreal, QC H3G 1A4, Canada. [4]Faculty of Health Sciences, Department of Clinical Studies, Semmelweis University, Budapest H-1088, Hungary. [5]Division of Gastroenterology/Hepatology Unit and Endoscopy, Semmelweis University, Koranyi S 2A, Budapest H-1083, Hungary.

References

1. Molodecky NA, Soon IS, Rabi DM, Ghali WA, Ferris M, Chernoff G, Benchimol EI, Panaccione R, Ghosh S, Barkema HW, Kaplan GG. Increasing incidence and prevalence of the inflammatory bowel diseases with time, based on systematic review. Gastroenterology. 2012;142:46–54. [PMID: 22001864. https://doi.org/10.1053/j.gastro.2011.10.001.
2. Burisch J, Jess T, Martinato M, Lakatos PL, ECCO-EpiCom. The burden of inflammatory bowel disease in Europe. J Crohns Colitis. 2013;7:322–37. [PMID: 23395397. https://doi.org/10.1016/j.crohns.2013.01.010.
3. Vegh Z, Kurti Z, Lakatos P. The epidemiology of inflammatory bowel diseases from west to east. J Dig Dis. 2017;18:92–8. [PMID: 28102560. https://doi.org/10.1111/1751-2980.12449.
4. Peyrin-Biroulet L, Sandborn W, Sands BE, Reinisch W, Bemelman W, Bryant RV, D'Haens G, Dotan I, Dubinsky M, Feagan B, Fiorino G, Gearry R, Krishnareddy S, Lakatos PL, Loftus EV Jr, Marteau P, Munkholm P, Murdoch TB, Ordás I, Panaccione R, Riddell RH, Ruel J, Rubin DT, Samaan M, Siegel CA, Silverberg MS, Stoker J, Schreiber S, Travis S, Van Assche G, Danese S, Panes J, Bouguen G, O'Donnell S, Pariente B, Winer S, Hanauer S, Colombel JF. Selecting therapeutic targets in inflammatory bowel disease (STRIDE): determining therapeutic goals for treat-to-target. Am J Gastroenterol. 2015; 110:1324–38. [PMID: 26303131. https://doi.org/10.1038/ajg.2015.233.
5. Mandel MD, Balint A, Golovics PA, Vegh Z, Mohas A, Szilagyi B, Szabo A, Kurti Z, Kiss LS, Lovasz BD, Gecse KB, Farkas K, Molnar T, Lakatos PL. Decreasing trends in hospitalizations during anti-TNF therapy are associated with time to anti-TNF therapy: results from two referral centres. Dig Liver Dis. 2014;46:985–90. [PMID: 25156871. https://doi.org/10.1016/j.dld.2014.07.168.
6. Bernstein CN, Loftus EV, Ng SC, Lakatos PL, Moum B. Epidemiology and natural history task force of the International Organization for the Study of inflammatory bowel disease (IOIBD). Hospitalisations and surgery in Crohn's disease. Gut. 2012; 61:622–9. [PMID: 22267595. https://doi.org/10.1136/gutjnl-2011-301397.
7. Rungoe C, Langholz E, Andersson M, Basit S, Nielsen NM, Wohlfahrt J, Jess T. Changes in medical treatment and surgery rates in inflammatory bowel disease: a nationwide cohort study 1979–2011. Gut. 2014;63:1607–16. [PMID: 24056767. https://doi.org/10.1136/gutjnl-2013-305607.
8. Nguyen GC, Nugent Z, Shaw S, Bernstein CN. Outcomes of patients with Crohn's disease improved from 1988 to 2008 and were associated with increased specialist care. Gastroenterology. 2011;141:90–7. [PMID: 21458455. https://doi.org/10.1053/j.gastro.2011.03.050.
9. Mandel MD, Miheller P, Müllner K, Golovics PA, Lakatos PL. Have biologics changed the natural history of Crohn's disease? Dig Dis. 2014;32:351–9. [PMID: 24969279. https://doi.org/10.1159/000358135.
10. Gomollón F, Dignass A, Annese TH, Van Assche G, Lindsay JO, Peyrin-Biroulet L, Cullen GJ, Daperno M, Kucharzik T, Rieder F, Almer S, Armuzzi A, Harbord M, Langhorst J, Sans M, Chowers Y, Fiorino G, Juillerat P, Mantzaris GJ, Rizzello F, Vavricka S, Gionchetti P, ECCO. 3rd European evidence-based consensus on the diagnosis and Management of Crohn's disease 2016: part 1: diagnosis and medical management. J Crohns Colitis. 2017;11:3–25. PMID: 27660341 doi: https://doi.org/10.1093/ecco-jcc/jjw168
11. Burisch J, Pedersen N, Čuković-Čavka S, Brinar M, Kaimakliotis I, Duricova D, Shonová O, Vind I, Avnstrøm S, Thorsgaard N, Andersen V, Krabbe S, Dahlerup JF, Salupere R, Nielsen KR, Olsen J, Manninen P, Collin P, Tsianos EV, Katsanos KH, Ladefoged K, Lakatos L, Björnsson E, Ragnarsson G, Bailey Y, Odes S, Schwartz D, Martinato M, Lupinacci G, Milla M, De Padova A, D'Incà R, Beltrami M, Kupcinskas L, Kiudelis G, Turcan S, Tighineanu O, Mihu I, Magro F, Barros LF, Goldis A, Lazar D, Belousova E, Nikulina I, Hernandez V, Martinez-Ares D, Almer S, Zhulina Y, Halfvarson J, Arebi N, Sebastian S, Lakatos PL, Langholz E, Munkholm P, EpiCom-group. East–west gradient in the incidence of inflammatory bowel disease in Europe: the ECCO-EpiCom inception cohort. Gut. 2014;63:588–97. [PMID: 23604131. https://doi.org/10.1136/gutjnl-2013-304636.
12. Vegh Z, Burisch J, Pedersen N, Kaimakliotis I, Duricova D, Bortlik M, Avnstrøm S, Vinding KK, Olsen J, Nielsen KR, Katsanos KH, Tsianos EV, Lakatos L, Schwartz D, Odes S, Lupinacci G, De Padova A, Jonaitis L, Kupcinskas L, Turcan S, Tighineanu O, Mihu I, Barros LF, Magro F, Lazar D, Goldis A, Fernandez A, Hernandez V, Niewiadomski O, Bell S, Langholz E, Munkholm P, Lakatos PL, EpiCom-group. Incidence and initial disease course of inflammatory bowel diseases in 2011 in Europe and Australia: results of the 2011 ECCO-EpiCom inception cohort. J Crohns Colitis. 2014;8: 1506–15. [PMID: 24998983. https://doi.org/10.1016/j.crohns.2014.06.004.
13. Vegh Z, Burisch J, Pedersen N, Kaimakliotis I, Duricova D, Bortlik M, Vinding KK, Avnstrøm S, Olsen J, Nielsen KR, Katsanos KH, Tsianos EV, Lakatos L, Schwartz D, Odes S, D'Incà R, Beltrami M, Kiudelis G, Kupcinskap L, Jucov A, Turcan S, Barros LF, Magro F, Lazar D, Goldis A, de Castro L, Hernandez V, Niewiadomski O, Bell S, Langholz E, Munkholm P, Lakatos PL, EpiCom-group. Treatment steps, surgery, and hospitalization rates during the first year of follow-up in patients with inflammatory bowel diseases from the 2011 Ecco-EpiCom inception cohort. J Crohns Colitis. 2015;9:747–53. PMID: 26055976 doi: https://doi.org/10.1093/ecco-jcc/jjv099
14. Peyrin-Biroulet L, Harmsen WS, Tremaine WJ, Zinsmeister AR, Sandborn WJ, Loftus EV Jr. Surgery in a population-based cohort of Crohn's disease from Olmsted county, Minnesota (1970–2004). Am J Gastroenterol. 2012;10:1693–701. [PMID: 22945286. https://doi.org/10.1038/ajg.2012.298.

15. Shivashankar R, Tremaine WJ, Harmsen WS, Loftus EV Jr. Incidence and prevalence of Crohn's disease and ulcerative colitis in Olmsted County, Minnesota from 1970 through 2010. Clin Gastroenterol Hepatol. 2017;15: 857–63. [PMID: 27856364. https://doi.org/10.1016/j.cgh.2016.10.039.
16. Lakatos L, Kiss LS, David G, Pandur T, Erdelyi Z, Mester G, Balogh M, Szipocs I, Molnar C, Komaromi E, Lakatos PL. Incidence, disease phenotype at diagnosis, and early disease course in inflammatory bowel diseases in western Hungary, 2002–2006. Inflamm Bowel Dis. 2011;17:2558–65. [PMID: 22072315. https://doi.org/10.1002/ibd.21607.
17. Lakatos PL, Golovics PA, David G, Pandur T, Erdelyi Z, Horvath A, Mester G, Balogh M, Szipocs I, Molnar C, Komaromi E, Veres G, Lovasz BD, Szathmari M, Kiss LS, Lakatos L. Has there been a change in the natural history of Crohn's disease? Surgical rates and medical management in a population-based inception cohort from western Hungary between 1977–2009. Am J Gastroenterol. 2012;107:579–88. [PMID: 22233693. https://doi.org/10.1038/ajg.2011.448.
18. Kurti Z, Vegh Z, Golovics PA, Fadgyas-Freyler P, Gecse KB, Gonczi L, Gimesi-Orszagh J, Lovasz BD, Lakatos PL. Nationwide prevalence and drug treatment practices of inflammatory bowel diseases in Hungary: a population-based study based on the National Health Insurance Fund database. Dig Liver Dis. 2016;48:1302–7. [PMID: 27481587. https://doi.org/10.1016/j.dld.2016.07.012.
19. Frolkis AD, Dykeman J, Negrón ME, Debruyn J, Jette N, Fiest KM, Frolkis T, Barkema HW, Rioux KP, Panaccione R, Ghosh S, Wiebe S, Kaplan GG. Risk of surgery for inflammatory bowel diseases has decreased over time: a systematic review and meta-analysis of population-based studies. Gastroenterology. 2013;145:996–1006. [PMID: 23896172. https://doi.org/10.1053/j.gastro.2013.07.041.
20. Solberg IC, Vatn MH, Høie O, Stray N, Sauar J, Jahnsen J, Moum B, Lygren I, IBSEN Study Group. Clinical course in Crohn's disease: results of a Norwegian population-based ten-year follow-up study. Clin Gastroenterol Hepatol. 2007;5: 1430–8. [PMID: 18054751. https://doi.org/10.1016/j.cgh.2007.09.002.
21. Magro F, Dias CC, Coelho R, Santos PM, Fernandes S, Caetano C, Rodrigues Å, Portela F, Oliveira A, Ministro P, Cancela E, Vieira AI, Barosa R, Cotter J, Carvalho P, Cremers I, Trabulo D, Caldeira P, Antunes A, Rosa I, Moleiro J, Peixe P, Herculano R, Gonçalves R, Gonçalves B, Tavares Sousa H, Contente L, Morna H, Lopes S. Impact of early surgery and Immunosuppression on Crohn's disease disabling outcomes. Inflamm Bowel Dis. 2017;23:289–97. [PMID: 28107278. https://doi.org/10.1097/MIB.0000000000001007.
22. Chatu S, Saxena S, Subramanian V, Curcin V, Yadegarfar G, Gunn L, Majeed A, Pollok RC. The impact of timing and duration of thiopurine treatment on first intestinal resection in Crohn's disease: national UK population-based study 1989–2010. Am J Gastroenterol. 2014;109:409–16. [PMID: 24469612. https://doi.org/10.1038/ajg.2013.462.
23. Mao EJ, Hazlewood GS, Kaplan GG, Peyrin-Biroulet L, Ananthakrishnan AN. Systematic review with meta-analysis: comparative efficacy of immunosuppressants and biologics for reducing hospitalisation and surgery in Crohn's disease and ulcerative colitis. Aliment Pharmacol Ther. 2017;45:3–13. [PMID: 27862107. https://doi.org/10.1111/apt.13847.
24. Domènech E, Zabana Y, Garcia-Planella E, López San Román A, Nos P, Ginard D, Gordillo J, Martínez-Silva F, Beltrán B, Mañosa M, Cabré E, Gassull MA. Clinical outcome of newly diagnosed Crohn's disease: a comparative, retrospective study before and after infliximab availability. Aliment Pharmacol Ther. 2010;31:233–9. [PMID: 19832727. https://doi.org/10.1111/j.1365-2036.2009.04170.x.
25. Burisch J, Halfvarson J, Kupcinskas L, Hernandez V, Kaimakliotis I, Valpiani D, Pedersen N, Duricova D, Kievit L, Dahlerup JF, Fumery M, Salupere R, Arebi N, Nielsen KR, Giannotta M, Oksanen P, Katsanos KH, Vegh Z, Ellul P, Schwartz D, Čuković-Čavka S, D'Incà R, Turcan S, Magro F, Goldis A, Langholz E, Lakatos PL, Munkholm P, EpiCom Study Group. Disease course during the first five years following diagnosis in a prospective European population-based inception cohort – the ECCO-EpiCom cohort. J Crohns Colitis. 2017;11(suppl_1):S435–6. doi: https://doi.org/10.1093/ecco-jcc/jjx002.818
26. Herrinton LJ, Liu L, Fireman B, Lewis JD, Allison JE, Flowers N, Hutfless S, Velayos FS, Abramson O, Altschuler A, Perry GS. Time trends in therapies and outcomes for adult inflammatory bowel disease, northern California, 1998–2005. Gastroenterology. 2009;137:502–11. [PMID: 19445944. https://doi.org/10.1053/j.gastro.2009.04.063
27. Odes S, Vardi H, Friger M, Wolters F, Russel MG, Riis L, Munkholm P, Politi P, Tsianos E, Clofent J, Vermeire S, Monteiro E, Mouzas I, Fornaciari G, Sijbrandij J, Limonard C, Van Zeijl G, O'morain C, Moum B, Vatn M, Stockbrugger R, European Collaborative Study on Inflammatory Bowel Disease. Cost analysis and cost determinants in a European inflammatory bowel disease inception cohort with 10 years of follow-up evaluation. Gastroenterology. 2006;131: 719–28. [PMID: 16952541. https://doi.org/10.1053/j.gastro.2006.05.052.
28. Munkholm P, Langholz E, Davidsen M, Binder V. Disease activity courses in a regional cohort of Crohn's disease patients. Scand J Gastroenterol. 1995;30: 699–706. PMID: 7481535
29. Klag T, Stange EF, Wehkamp J. Management of Crohn's disease - are guidelines transferred to clinical practice? United European Gastroenterol J. 2015;3:371–80. [PMID: 26279846. https://doi.org/10.1177/2050640615580228.
30. Munkholm P, Langholz E, Davidsen M, Binder V. Frequency of glucocorticoid resistance and dependency in Crohn's disease. Gut. 1994;35: 360–2. PMID: 8150347
31. Peyrin-Biroulet L, Loftus EV Jr, Colombel JF, Sandborn WJ. The natural history of adult Crohn's disease in population-based cohorts. Am J Gastroenterol. 2010; 105:289–97. [PMID: 19861953. https://doi.org/10.1038/ajg.2009.579.
32. Ott C, Takses A, Obermeier F, Schnoy E, Salzberger B, Müller M. How fast up the ladder? Factors associated with immunosuppressive or anti-TNF therapies in IBD patients at early stages: results from a population-based cohort. Int J Color Dis. 2014;29:1329–38. [PMID: 25179426. https://doi.org/10.1007/s00384-014-2002-z.
33. Rencz F, Péntek M, Bortlik M, Zagorowicz E, Hlavaty T, Śliwczyński A, Diculescu MM, Kupcinskas L, Gecse KB, Gulácsi L, Lakatos PL. Biological therapy in inflammatory bowel diseases: access in central and Eastern Europe. World J Gastroenterol. 2015;21:1728–37. [PMID: 25684937. https://doi.org/10.3748/wjg.v21.i6.1728.
34. Munkholm P, Langholz E, Davidsen M, Binder V. Disease activity courses in a regional cohort of Crohn's disease patients. Scand J Gastroenterol. 1995;30: 699–706.

Uninvestigated dyspepsia and associated factors of patients with gastrointestinal disorders in Dessie Referral Hospital, Northeast Ethiopia

Abdurahaman Seid[1*], Zemenu Tamir[2] and Wondmagegn Demsiss[3]

Abstract

Background: Dyspepsia is a common problem in the community and clinical practice with symptom(s) considered arising from the gastroduodenal region. Dyspepsia burden and associated factors vary from country to country. The aim of this study was to determine the prevalence of uninvestigated dyspepsia (UD) using Rome III criteria, associated risk factors and self-reported dyspepsia symptoms' correlation with *H. pylori* infection.

Methods: A cross-sectional study was conducted among randomly selected 318 out patients with gastrointestinal complaints during the period from September 1 to December 30, 2015. All patients completed a questionnaire for collecting data regarding sociodemographic, lifestyle and functional gastrointestinal disorders. Diagnosis of dyspepsia was made according to the Rome III criteria. *H. pylori* infection was assessed using stool antigen test. SPSS version 20.0 statistical software package was used for data analysis.

Results: From a total of 318 patients, 48.4% had UD according to Rome III criteria; with 42.1% symptoms of epigastric pain/burning, 26.1% postprandial fullness and 22.6% early satiation. Epigastric pain/burning (AOR = 1.92, 95% CI 1.07–3.43), early satiation (AOR = 2.68, 95% CI 1.38–5.20) and belching (AOR = 4.7, 95% CI 1.54–14.40) were significantly correlated with *H. pylori* infection. *H. pylori* infection (AOR = 4.33, 95% CI 2.41–7.76) and aspirin/NSAIDs consumption (AOR = 5.29, 95% CI 2.82–9.93) were independent risk factors for UD. However, consumption of raw fruits/ vegetables at least once a week (AOR = 0.48, 95% CI 0.24–0.98) and taking two or more cups of tea a day (AOR = 0.339, 95% CI 0.17–0.70) were inversely associated with UD.

Conclusions: UD is highly prevalent among adults with gastrointestinal complaints. *H. pylori* infection is significantly associated with UD and correlates with its symptoms. Individuals with epigastric pain/burning, early satiation and belching should be primary focus of *H. pylori* infection diagnosis and treatment. The role of consumption of tea, raw fruits and vegetables on dyspepsia needs further large scale study.

Keywords: *H. pylori*, Uninvestigated dyspepsia, Rome III, Self-reported, Ethiopia

* Correspondence: nebat_abdurae2003@yahoo.com; gechdk2000@yahoo.com
[1]Department of Medical Laboratory Sciences, College of Medicine and Health Sciences, Wollo University, Po. Box 1145, Dessie, Ethiopia
Full list of author information is available at the end of the article

Background

Functional gastrointestinal disorders (FGIDs) are highly prevalent in the general population and are frequent cause for consultation of a general practitioner [1]. Individuals with FGIDs contribute heavily to healthcare utilization [2]. The Rome III criteria for diagnosis of FGIDs were developed in 2006 [3], and since then a few studies have estimated prevalence of FGIDs, described associated factors, signs and symptoms using this criteria [4].

Dyspepsia is one of a common symptom complex of FGIDs with an extensive differential diagnosis and a heterogeneous pathophysiology. According to Rome III definition, dyspepsia is "chronic or recurrent pain and/or discomfort thought to originate from the gastroduodenal region" and at least having one or more of the following symptoms: postprandial fullness (PPF), early satiation (ES), epigastric pain or burning [5–7]. Moreover, one symptom must be present for at least the last 3 months with an onset of symptoms at least 6 months prior to diagnosis [7].

Patients with symptoms of dyspepsia but didn't undergo any investigations such as upper gastrointestinal (GI) endoscopy and is not categorized as functional or organic in etiology are classified as having uninvestigated dyspepsia (UD), whereas those who undergo investigation and have no detectable cause for their symptoms are considered to have functional dyspepsia (FD) [6]. Numerous cross-sectional surveys reported different prevalence of dyspepsia in the community which varies from 7% to 54.6%, and globally estimated that 25% of the general populations suffer from dyspeptic symptoms [8–12]. High prevalence of UD (41.2%) was observed in the general population with 70–80% of patients with dyspepsia had no clinically significant findings at endoscopy [12]. Recently conducted systematic review and meta-analysis has demonstrated 21% pooled prevalence of UD, but varied among countries (1.8% to 57.0%) and according to the criteria used to define its presence [13].

Dyspepsia complaints are the most common reasons for outpatient visits to primary care providers [5, 14] and 20% to 40% gastroenterology appointments [14]. Both in an uninvestigated dyspeptic and FD patients, the most prevalent symptoms are PPF (68–86%), upper abdominal bloating (68–84%), epigastric pain (68–74%), ES (49–72%) [15, 16], belching (50–60%), epigastric burning (35–57%), nausea (39–65%) and vomiting (23–31%) [16].

The causes of dyspepsia remain uncertain as being females and underlying psychological disturbances contribute to FD, whilst environmental/lifestyle factors such as poor socio-economic status, smoking, increased caffeine intake and ingestion of non-steroidal anti-inflammatory drugs (NSAIDs) appear to be more related to UD [17]. Moreover, the role of *H .pylori* infection in dyspepsia is still unclear. Some authors indicated no association between *H. pylori* infection and dyspepsia [18–21], whereas others indicated that dyspepsia may be a sign of acute or chronic *H. pylori* infection as evidenced from population-based study conducted in UK [22].

In Ethiopia, many hospital-based studies reported different prevalence rates of *H. pylori* infection among dyspeptic patients [21, 23–26], but have not estimated the burden of dyspepsia. Moreover, Rome III criteria have not been widely applied for diagnosis and classification of FGIDs. Thus, the proportion of dyspeptic patients and their frequent typical symptoms of individuals presented with FGIDs were not documented according to Rome III criteria. Furthermore, no study has been conducted concerning potential risk factors of dyspepsia.

The determination of dyspepsia burden along with its associated symptoms and potential risk factors is important to increase physicians' ability of symptoms-based approach of sufferers to provide more precise diagnosis, treatment and prevention of the disorder particularly in resource limited settings like Ethiopia. Therefore, the aim of this study is to assess the prevalence of UD using Rome III criteria and its major symptom types of adults with FGIDs complaining patients. Furthermore, the present study is designed to assess associated risk factors of UD and correlation of *H. pylori* infection with self-reported functional upper GI symptoms.

Methods

Study patients and setting

This cross-sectional study was conducted at Dessie Referral Hospital, Dessie town, Northeast Ethiopia, from September 1 to December 30, 2015. The sample size was estimated to be 384 by taking 50% prevalence since there was no previous similar study in Ethiopia. The study population consisted of randomly selected new adult patients fulfilling the inclusion criteria at the outpatient department of the hospital.

We assessed the number of GI symptomatic patients who visited the hospital of previous comparative months of the study period. An average of 15 new GI symptomatic patients attended the outpatient department each day. In our country, working day of the month are Monday to Friday (5 days) giving a total of 22 days per month. The total expected new symptomatic patients attending the hospital during the study period were estimated to be 1320. The average number of study participants included per day, obtained by dividing the sample size to total working day of study period, was approximately 5. When the total population was divided by the sample size, the sample interval was found 3. The first person was selected by lottery method and then systematic random sampling method was used for selecting the patients at an interval of every 3 patients using the sequential order of their card number as a sampling frame.

Inclusion criteria

The presence of at least one of the following GI complaints existing for at least 3 months with the onset of symptom at least 6 months before clinical visit. These includes abdominal pain, bloating, nausea, vomiting, ES, PPF, heartburn, regurgitation, epigastric pain/burning and belching.

Exclusion criteria

GI symptomatic patients less than 18 years of age, and who took treatment against *H. pylori* infection within 3 months prior to this study, those who used proton pump inhibitors or H2-blockers for more than two weeks before study enrollment, presence of confirmed systemic disease such as congestive heart failure, coronary heart disease, liver failure, diabetes mellitus, thyroid disease, hematological diseases (for all case it is obtained by reviewing their medical documents), presence of major psychiatric disorders and pregnant mothers were excluded. Patients who were unable to communicate, and at emergency were also excluded.

Questionnaires

Study participants were asked to complete the dyspepsia questionnaire consisting FD modules of FGIDs and scored using Rome III algorithm [27]. Sociodemographic data (age, gender, schooling level, residence, occupational and marital status) and life style (consumption of tea, coffee, spice food, raw fruits and vegetables, alcohol, and NSAIDs) related factors were also collected. We adapted a previously validated FD module of FGIDs questionnaire (English version) [27] and translated in to the local language, "Amharic" version, through a process of translation and back translation before data collection. "Amharic" is mother tongue of population in the study area.

The translation process was as follows: Two medical professional who were native speakers of" Amharic" and fluent in English, undertook translations independently. One professional translated the English version to "Amharic" and the other translated the "Amharic" version back to English. The original and back-translated (English) versions were compared to detect any misunderstandings, mistranslations, or inaccuracies in the "Amharic" draft questionnaire. Feed backs about the "Amharic" version of the FD module of FGIDs questionnaire was obtained from experts in gastroenterology. The translated questionnaire was administered to 19 participants with FGIDs to assess the clarity, understandability, and appropriateness of the translation's wording so that the final version which contains 30 questions was used to collect required information. Similar procedure was followed for preparing "Amharic" version of the socio-demographic and life style related questionnaire. For participants who can't read and write, interview was employed. The clinical residents explained the question and queries regarding the meaning of medical terms and elaboration of symptoms when asked by the patients.

Dyspepsia was assessed according to the Rome III criteria as having one or more of the following: PPF, ES, epigastric pain, and/or epigastric burning for the past three months with onset at least six months before diagnosis [3]. However, UD was not directly addressed by the Rome III criteria. We depended on the symptoms that were defined for FD by the Rome III criteria in order to recognize those with dyspepsia and since no upper GI endoscopy was performed, patients who fulfill the symptomatic criteria were diagnosed as UD. Therefore, individuals were classified as having UD if they have reported experiencing at least one of the following symptoms: (1) bothersome postprandial fullness happening after ordinary sized meals; (2) early satiation that prevents finishing a regular meal; (3) epigastric pain/burning localized to the epigastrium.

Evaluation of *H. pylori* status and ABO blood group

About 20 g of fresh stool was collected from each participant in sterile and screw caped containers. The presence of *H. pylori* antigen was determined using monoclonal anti-*H.pylori* antibody conjugated with colloid gold nitrocellulose membrane strip (Rapid stool antigen test) based on a lateral flow chromatographic immunoassay technique. Specimens were tested using one step stool antigen test (Zhejiang Orient Gene Biotech CO., LTD, China) with 94.9%–100% sensitivity and 95–100% specificity [28]. Test results were read and interpreted according to the manufacturer's instructions. This test kit is validated and approved by the ministry of health of the country and currently employed for the diagnosis of *H.pylori* infection in the country. Five ml of venous blood was collected and ABO blood grouping was performed by slide agglutination test using monoclonal anti-A, anti-B, anti-AB and anti-D (Rho) antibodies.

Statistical analysis

All completed questionnaires were coded. Data analysis was performed using SPSS version 20 in four major steps. First, descriptive statistics were used to summarize the participant characteristics. The chi square ($\chi 2$) test was used to test the association between socio-demographic and lifestyle factors and dyspepsia. Possible risk factors for dyspepsia were initially examined using univariate analyses. Risk factors with $p < 0.25$ were entered to logistic regression model using stepwise backward logistic regression analysis to identify the risk factors independently associated with dyspepsia. All tests were two-tailed and the level of statistical significance was set at $p < 0.05$ along with the corresponding odds ratio (OR) and 95% confidence intervals (CI) in cases of significant associations.

Ethical consideration

The study was commenced after ethically approved by the research ethics committee of Wollo University. Permission to conduct the study was also obtained from the hospital administration. Written informed consent was obtained from each study participant and the results were kept confidential. Any result that was necessary for the patient was communicated with the physician for appropriate management.

Results

Sociodemographic and life style characteristics

Among 383 randomly selected participants with GI complaints, 24 were not eligible (10 were below 18 years old, 14 were with symptom onset less than 6 months), and 41 returned incomplete questionnaire. Therefore, a total of 318 participants with complete information were included in the final analysis.

The mean (± SD) age of participants was 37.84 ± 12.41 years ranged from 18 to 77 years old, and 54.4% were females. Out of 318 participants, 46.9% were in the age group 30 to 49 years old, 67.4% were married and 61% were urban dwellers. Almost half of study participants had a habit of drinking alcohol, and 31.1% were actively infected with *H. pylori*. Sociodemographic and life style factors of study participants are described in Table 1.

Dyspepsia and its associated factors

Of 318 participants with complaints of GI symptoms, according to Rome III criteria, 63.5% had at least one self-reported functional GI symptom with the prevalence of UD being 48.4%. Commonly reported upper GI symptoms were epigastric pain or burning, PPF, complain of ES and belching (Table 2).

Chi-square test showed that *H. pylori* infection was significantly associated with UD ($\chi2 = 21.33$, $p < 0.001$) as were habit of taking aspirin and/or NSAIDs ($\chi2 = 30.27$, $p < 0.001$), consumption of tea ($\chi2 = 18.23$, $p < 0.001$) and raw fruit and/or vegetables ($\chi2 = 8.71$, $p =$

Table 1 Socio-demographic and lifestyle characteristics of functional gastrointestinal symptomatic adult patients in Dessie Referral Hospital, Northeastern Ethiopia, 2015 ($n = 318$)

Variable		Freq	%	Variables		Freq	%
Age (year) mean ± SD	37.84 ± 12.41			Eating spicy food	Yes	269	84.6
					No	49	15.4
Age group	< 30 years	105	33.01				
	30 to 49 years	149	46.9	Tea consumption	Never	106	33.3
	≥50 years	64	20.12		One cup/day	96	30.2
Sex	Male	145	45.6		>one cup/day	116	36.5
	Female	173	54.4	Coffee consumption	Never	114	35.8
Marital status	Married	214	67.4		One cup/day	53	16.7
	Single	63	19.8		>one cup/day	151	47.5
	Divorced/widowed	41	12.9	Raw fruits and/or Vegetable consumption	Never	78	24.5
Residence	Rural	73	23		at least once/day	53	16.7
	Urban	194	61		at least once/week	187	58.8
	Suburban	51	16	Alcohol drinking	Yes	156	49.1
Occupation	Gov,t	108	34		No	162	50.9
	Student	29	9.1	Recent drug consumption	Never	187	58.8
	Farmer	66	20.8		Aspirin/NSAIDs	87	27.4
	Merchant	51	16.0		Other drugs	44	13.8
	Housewife	51	16.0	Blood group	Group A	82	25.8
	Others	13	4.1		Group B	89	28.0
Education	No legal education	50	15.7		Group AB	21	6.6
	Grade 1–8	74	23.3		Group O	126	39.6
	Grade 9–12	72	22.6	*H. pylori* infection	Yes	99	31.1
	College and above	122	38.4		No	219	68.9

Table 2 Frequency and distribution of self-reported functional gastrointestinal symptoms in study population using Rome III criteria, Dessie Referral Hospital, Northeastern Ethiopia, 2015(n = 318)

Functional gastrointestinal symptoms			Freq	%	Functional gastrointestinal symptoms		Freq	%
At least one symptom		Yes	202	63.5	UD & HB	Yes	78	24.5
		No	116	36.5		No	240	75.5
UD		Yes	154	48.4	Belching	Yes	80	25.2
		No	164	51.6		No	238	74.8
UD typical symptoms	PPF	Yes	83	26.1	vomiting	Yes	18	5.7
		No	235	73.9		No	300	94.3
	ES	Yes	72	22.6	Nausea	Yes	11	3.5
		No	246	77.4		No	307	96.5
	Epigastric burning/pain	Yes	134	42.1	UD & belching	Yes	66	20.8
		No	184	57.9		No	252	79.2
	PPF and ES	Yes	62	19.5	UD, HB & belching	Yes	43	13.5
		No	256	80.5		No	275	86.5

Key: UD = uninvestigated dyspepsia, PPF = postprandial fullness, ES = early satiation, HB = heart burn

0.01) (Table 4). However, no significant association observed between sex, age, residence, educational level, occupational and marital status (Table 3), ABO blood group, consumption of coffee and spicy foods, drinking of alcohol and UD (Table 4).

Table 3 The prevalence of uninvestigated dyspepsia in relation to demographic variables among study participants in Dessie Referral Hospital, Northeastern Ethiopia, 2015 (n = 318)

Variable		Total (N)	UD n (%)	χ 2	*p*-value
Sex	Male	145	67(46.2)	0.53	0.468
	Female	173	87(50.3)		
Age	< 30 years	105	47(44.8)	0.96	0.618
	30 to 49 years	149	76(51.0)		
	≥ 50 years	64	31(48.4)		
Marital status	Married	214	99(46.3)	3.00	0.223
	Single	63	30(47.6)		
	Divorced/widowed	41	25(61.0)		
Residence	Rural	73	38(52.1)	2.83	0.242
	Urban	194	87(44.8)		
	Suburban	51	29(56.9)		
Occupation	Gov,t	108	48(44.4)	9.96	0.076
	Student	29	16(55.2)		
	Farmer	66	38(57.6)		
	Merchant	51	20(39.2)		
	Housewife	51	29(56.9)		
	Others	13	3(23.1)		
Education	No legal education	50	25(50.0)	0.62	0.893
	Grade 1–8	74	38(51.4)		
	Grade 9–12	72	35(48.6)		
	College and above	122	56(45.9)		

Exploring independent risk factors in a logistic regression model showed that *H. pylori* infection [AOR = 4.33, 95% CI 2.41–7.76, $p < 0.001$] and consumption of aspirin and/or NSAIDs [AOR = 5.29, 95% CI 2.82–9.93, $p <$ 0.001] were independent predictors of UD. However, consumption of raw fruit and/or vegetables at least once a week [AOR = 0.48, 95% CI 0.24–0.98, $p = 0.042$] and tea consumption at least two cups a day [AOR = 0.34, 95% CI 0.17–0.70, $p = 0.003$] showed a protective effect against UD. No association was distinguished between consumption of one cup of tea a day, marital status, ABO blood group, type of occupation and UD (Table 5).

Correlation of *H. pylori* infection to self-reported dyspepsia symptoms

Univariate analysis showed that *H. pylori* infection is significantly correlated with upper GI complaints such as PPF, ES, Epigastric burning/pain, nausea as well as their overlaps (Table 6).

Constructing a multivariate logistic regression model in which the *H.pylori* (+)/(−) variable taken as the dependent variable, and upper GI symptoms which were found to be significantly correlated in the univariate analysis as independent variables showed that *H. pylori* infection rate were significantly correlated with ES [AOR = 2.68, 95% CI 1.38–5.20], epigastric burning/pain [AOR = 1.92, 95% CI 1.07–3.43], belching [AOR = 4.7, 95% CI 1.54–14.40] and nausea [AOR = 3.91,95%CI 1.03–14.87] (Table 6).

Discussion

In the present study, 63.5% of study participants had at least one GI symptom. Park et al. in Korea reported that

Table 4 The prevalence of uninvestigated dyspepsia in relation to lifestyle and other factors of study participants in Dessie Referral Hospital, Northeastern Ethiopia, 2015 (n = 318)

Variables		Total	UD = n/%	χ 2	P-value
Eating spicy food	Yes	269	132(49.1)	0.29	0.591
	No	49	22(44.9)		
Tea consumption	Never	106	59(55.7)	18.23	<0.000
	One cup/day	96	57(59.4)		
	>one cup/day	116	38(32.8)		
Coffee consumption	Never	114	54(47.4)	0.19	0.911
	One cup/day	53	27(50.9)		
	>one cup/day	151	73(48.3)		
Raw fruits and/or Vegetables consumption	Never	78	49(62.8)	8.71	0.013
	Eat at least once/day	53	22(41.5)		
	Eat at least once/week	187	83(44.4)		
Alcohol drinking	Yes	156	79(50.6)	0.60	0.438
	No	162	75(46.3)		
Recent drug consumption	Never	187	67(35.8)	30.27	<0.000
	Aspirin/NSAIDs	87	61(70.1)		
	Other drugs	44	26(59.1)		
Blood group	Group A	82	37(45.1)	6.51	0.089
	Group B	89	35(39.3)		
	Group AB	21	12(57.1)		
	Group O	126	70(55.6)		
H. pylori infection	Yes	99	67(67.7)	21.33	<0.000
	No	219	87(39.7)		

among new consecutive patients presented with chronic GI symptoms 73.9% had upper gastroduodenal symptoms [4]. This variation could be due to differences in socioeconomic and life style factors contributing for gastrointestinal disorders.

In our study, using Rome III diagnostic criteria, the prevalence of UD was 48.8% which is higher than study conducted in African countries such as Nigeria (37.5%) [29] and Uganda (38.9%) [30], but the diagnostic criteria (Rome II) are quite different from current study. Our result is also higher than study conducted in Asian countries such as Korea (13.4%) [11], China (5.67%) [31], Taiwan (32.4%) [32], west part of Iran (41.2%) [12]; and European countries like UK (38%) [22] and Italy (15.1%), where Rome II criteria is employed as main diagnostic criteria [20]. However, our result is lower than another study conducted in Nigeria with 69.1% prevalence of UD among upper gastrointestinal symptomatic patients [33].

The observed variable proportion of UD may be partly explained with variation in geographical location, use of variable definitions and criteria for diagnosis of dyspepsia, study design and population. For instance, some studies employed Rome III criteria for diagnosis of dyspepsia [31–33] which is comparable to our work, but the design of most mentioned studies, whether employed Rome II or III criteria, [12, 20, 22, 29–32] are population based surveys involving asymptomatic patients. However, the high proportion of UD in our and Nigerian [33] study is due to being hospital based study where clinically suspected patients involved. Moreover, in our and other African studies [29, 30, 33] the prevalence of UD is higher as compared to studies conducted in Asia. This might be delayed presentation of patients to health care provider in African countries and the result of variation in dietary factors, socio-cultural and psychological issues, rate of gastrointestinal infection mainly caused by *H. pylori.* As a result eastern life styles may be a factor related to the lower prevalence dyspepsia.

The most common symptoms associated with UD was found to be epigastric pain/burning (42.1%), PPF (26.1%), ES (22.6%) and belching (25.2%) (Table 2). Similarly, among Ugandan patients presenting with upper GI symptoms the most common presenting complaint was epigastric pain (51.6%) [34]. Our result is also in line with study in Iran as epigastric pain or burning (58.3%) being dominant complaint of dyspeptic patients followed by PPF (37.3%) and ES (18.6%) [35]. Belching disorders (30.7%) was the dominant symptoms next to FD (46%)

Table 5 Regression analysis of different factors associated with uninvestigated dyspepsia of study participants in Dessie Referral Hospital, Northeastern Ethiopia, 2015 (n = 318)

Variable		Total	UD = n(%)	COR(95%CI)	AOR(95%CI)	p-value
Marital status	Married	214	99(46.3)	ref		
	Single	63	30(47.6)	1.06(0.60–1.85)	–	–
	Divorced/widowed	41	25(61.0)	1.82(0.92–3.59)	–	–
Residence	Rural	73	38(52.1)	ref	ref	
	Urban	194	87(44.8)	0.75(0.44–1.28)	2.32(0.73–7.34)	0.152
	Suburban	51	29(56.9)	1.21(0.59–2.49)	4.71(1.44–15.39)	0.010*
Occupation	Gov,t	108	48(44.4)	ref		
	Student	29	16(55.2)	1.54(0.68–3.51)	–	–
	Farmer	66	38(57.6)	1.70(0.91–3.15)	–	–
	Merchant	51	20(39.2)	0.81(0.41–1.59)	–	–
	Housewife	51	29(56.9)	1.65(0.84–3.23)	–	–
	Others	13	3(23.1)	0.38(0.10–1.44)	–	–
Tea consumption	Never	106	59(55.7)	ref	ref	
	One cup/day	96	57(59.4)	1.16(0.67–2.04)	0.99(0.47–2.07)	0.975
	>one cup/day	116	38(32.8)	0.39(0.23–0.67)	0.34(0.17–0.70)	0.003*
Raw fruit/ Vegetable consumption	Never	78	49(62.8)	ref	ref	
	Eat once/day	53	22(41.5)	0.42(0.21–0.86)	0.31(0.13–0.77)	0.011*
	Eat once/week	187	83(44.4)	0.47(0.28–0.81)	0.48(0.24–0.98)	0.042*
Recent drug consumption	Never	187	67(35.8)	ref	ref	
	Aspirin/NSAID	87	61(70.1)	4.20(2.43–7.27)	5.29(2.82–9.93)	<0.001*
	Other drugs	44	26/59.1	2.59(1.32–5.06)	3.12(1.46–6.69)	0.003*
Blood group	Group A	82	37/45.1	ref		
	Group B	89	35/39.3	0.79(0.43–1.45)	–	–
	Group AB	21	12/57.1	1.62(0.62–4.27)	–	–
	Group O	126	70/55.6	1.52(0.87–2.66)	–	–
H. pylori infection	No	219	87/39.7	ref	ref	
	Yes	99	67/67.7	3.18(1.93–5.24)	4.33(2.41–7.76)	<0.001*

among functional gastroduodenal disorders in Korean patients with chronic GI complaints [4].

Correlation of *H. pylori* infection with each upper GI symptoms is shown in Table 6. There was no correlation between PPF, combination of UD and heart burn, and vomiting with *H. pylori* infection. However, significant correlation was found between ES, epigastric pain/burning, belching, and nausea with *H. pylori* infection. The proportion of belching is more among *H. pylori* infected patients as compared to *H. pylori* free patients. i.e., presentation of belching is 4.7 times more likely to be associated with *H.pylori* infection as compared to *H. pylori* free patients. Our result is in agreement to report of Shokrzadeh et al. in Iran where the prevalence of belching was significantly higher among *H. pylori* infected patients with no correlation of vomiting [36]. This significant likelihood association *H. pylori* infection to belching could be explained as *H. pylori* is known to produces urease which helps to metabolizes urea into ammonia and carbon dioxide resulting in belching and bloating. However, our result is found contrary to his report where no difference was observed in the prevalence of epigastric abdominal pain, nausea, and ES between *H. pylori*-positive and *H. pylori*-negative patients [36]. This may be due to variation in laboratory tests for diagnosis of *H. pylori* infection (stool antigen detection in our case where as histological examination in Iranian study), population variation and lifestyle factors.

The association of *H. pylori* infection with UD has been reported with inconsistent findings in several studies. In our study, however, *H. pylori* infection was found to be significantly associated with UD (AOR = 4.33, 95% CI 2.41–7.76, $p < 0.001$) which is similar to study conducted in Taiwan [32], Kenya [37] and Ethiopia [23]. A large population based study in Denmark also showed that *H. pylori* infection is a significant risk factor for

Table 6 Regression analysis on comparison of self-reported upper gastrointestinal symptoms between *H.pylori* (+) ($n = 99$) and *H.pylori* (−) ($n = 219$) patients, Dessie Referral Hospital, 2015

Self-reported Upper gastrointestinal symptoms		HP(+) = n (%)	HP(−) = n (%)	COR(CI)	p-value	AOR(CI)	p-value
PPF	Yes	41(41.5)	42(19.2)	2.98(1.76–5.02)	<0.001	–	–
	No	58(48.5)	177(80.8)	ref			
ES	Yes	39(39.4)	33(15.1)	3.66(2.12–6.33)	<0.001	2.68(1.38–5.20)	0.004*
	No	60(60.6)	186(84.9)	ref		ref	
Epigastric burning/pain	Yes	58(58.6)	76(34.7)	2.66(1.64–4.33)	<0.001	1.92(1.07–3.43)	0.028*
	No	41(41.4)	143(65.3)	ref		ref	
PPF & ES	Yes	34(34.3)	28(12.8)	3.57(2.01–6.33)	<0.001	–	–
	No	65(65.7)	191(87.2)	ref			
UD & HB	Yes	40(40.4)	38(17.4)	3.23(1.90–5.50)	<0.001	–	–
	No	59(59.6)	181(82.6)	ref			
Belching	Yes	40(40.4)	40(18.3)	3.47(1.05–12.57)	0.050	4.70 (1.54–14.4)	0.007*
	No	59(59.6)	179(81.7)	ref		ref	
vomiting	Yes	9(9.1)	9(4.1)	2.33(0.90–6.07)	0.082	–	–
	No	90(90.9)	210(95.9)	ref			
Nausea	Yes	7(7.1)	4(1.8)	4.09(1.17–14.31)	0.028	3.91(1.03–14.87)	0.045*
	No	92(92.9)	215(98.2)	ref		ref	
UD & bleaching	Yes	33(33.3)	33(15.1)	2.82(1.61–4.93)	<0.001	0.28(0.06–1.01)	0.051
	No	66(66.7)	186(84.9)	ref		ref	
UD, HB & bleaching	Yes	25(25.3)	18(8.2)	3.77(1.95–7.31)	<0.001	–	–
	No	74(74.7)	201(91.8)	ref			

Key: PPF = postprandial fullness, ES = early satiation, AOR = adjusted oddis ratio, COR = crude oddis ratio, HP = *H. pylori*, HB = heart burn, CI = confidence interval, UD = uninvestigated dyspepsia

dyspepsia although of less importance than NSAIDs use, unemployment and heavy smoking [38]. However, other authors indicated no association between *H. pylori* infection and dyspepsia [18–20, 39] as most *H. pylori* infected individuals didn't show dyspepsia [40–43].

Even though some surveys have indicated association of dyspepsia with alcohol consumption [44, 45], our result showed no significant association between coffee and alcohol consumption with UD which is in agreement with studies conducted elsewhere in the world reporting no association with dyspepsia [17, 19, 20, 39, 46, 47]. This discordance could be due to difference in type and amount of alcohol consumed as well as sociocultural practices of study population. Moreover, in our study in addition to small sample size we didn't determine the amount and type of consumed alcohol, as well as the type of coffee consumed so that further population-based study is needed to elucidate their association with dyspepsia.

Our result also showed that NSAIDs use is statistically associated with UD (AOR = 5.29, 95% CI 2.82–9.93, $p < 0.001$) which is in agreement with British and American populations based studies where NSAIDs use have been identified as an important independent risk factor for UD [22, 32, 46]. However, population based study in Italy and Sweden showed no association between use of NSAIDs/aspirin or corticosteroids and UD [20, 39]. Sex and age matched case control study conducted in Nigeria showed that NSAIDs user for a minimum of one week prior to 30 days before enrolment to the study did not show any association with UD [19].

Our study also showed that consumption of two or more cup of tea a day (AOR = 0.34, 95%CI 0.17–0.70, $p = 0.003$) and consumption of raw fruits and/or vegetables at least once a day (AOR = 0.31, 95% CI 0.13–0.77, $p = 0.011$) was protective against UD which is in agreement with reports of Khademolhosseini et al. in Iran, where inverse relationship was observed between dyspepsia and fruits as well as vegetables consumption [47]. However, Seyedmirzaei et al. in Iran, by controlling possible confounding factors, showed no protective effect of high fruit and vegetable consumption, and current tea-coffee consumption [35]. Hospital-based study in Taiwan also showed no significant association between consumption of tea, vegetable and UD, but consumption of coffee was protective against UD [32]. Contrary to above findings, Solomon et al. in Nigeria indicated significant association of high amount of tea consumption and UD [19]. This may depend on the type of tea, fruit and vegetables as well as type of biological molecules that can be found within it, which is not investigated in our study and others too. Thus, future well designed study is warranted to assess whether different kinds of tea as well as fruit and vegetables have different biological effects in the pathogenesis of dyspepsia.

The strength of our study is that we have included new patients by using randomized recruitment strategy to represent all patients with symptoms of GI disorders. However, the cross-sectional nature of this study has a limitation to show cause and effect associations between UD and associated factors, and the result cannot be representative of the general population. This study is a hospital based study involving subjects with symptoms who have had many underline disease conditions as a confounding factors that could not fully controlled so that it might have impact on the statistical correlations between dyspepsia and other variables of interest.

Conclusions

In conclusion, this is the first hospital-based study in Ethiopia for assessing UD among patients with FGIDs using Rome III criteria. The prevalence of UD in the study population was 48.4%, with epigastric pain/burning being the most prevalent symptom (42.1%). The observed high proportion of UD alerts health care providers and program planners about the disease, and suggesting a critical management issue of dyspepsia in the country. *H. pylori* infection is significantly associated with UD and habit of aspirin/NSAIDs consumption. However, consumption of raw fruit and/or vegetable at least once a day and more than one cup of tea a day showed inverse association with UD which needs further well designed study to ascertain the observed association. Upper GI symptoms such as early satiation, epigastric burning/pain, belching, and nausea showed strong likelihood association with *H. pylori* infection.

Abbreviations

ES: early satiation; FD: functional dyspepsia; FGIDs: functional gastrointestinal disorders; GI: gastrointestinal; NSAIDS: nonsteroidal anti-inflammatory drugs; PPF: post prandial fullness; UD: uninvestigated dyspepsia

Acknowledgements

We would like to express our special thanks to the staff of Dessie Referral Hospital for technical support in this study. Moreover, we would like to thank the study participants.

Funding

This study was supported by Wollo University. The funders had no role in study design, data collection and analysis, decision to publish, or preparation of the manuscript.

Authors' contributions

ASY: design of the study; acquisition of data, data management, analysis, interpretation of data and manuscript preparation. ZM: contributed to the design of the study, manuscript preparation and study supervision. WD: contributed to the design of the study, manuscript preparation and study supervision. All authors have read and approved the final manuscript.

Competing interests

The authors declare that they have no competing interests.

Author details

[1]Department of Medical Laboratory Sciences, College of Medicine and Health Sciences, Wollo University, Po. Box 1145, Dessie, Ethiopia. [2]Department of Medical Laboratory Sciences, College of Health Sciences, School of Allied Health Sciences, Addis Ababa University, Addis Ababa, Ethiopia. [3]Department of Medical Laboratory Sciences, College of Medicine and Health Sciences, Wollo University, Dessie, Ethiopia.

References

1. Talley NJ, Zinsmeister AR, Schleck CD, Melton LJ. Dyspepsia and dyspepsia subgroups: a population-based study. Gastroenterology. 1992;102:1259–68.
2. Nyrop KA, Palsson OS, Levy RL, Von Korff M, Feld AD, Turner MJ, Whitehead WE. Costs of health care for irritable bowel syndrome, chronic constipation, functional diarrhoea and functional abdominal pain. Aliment Pharmacol Ther. 2007;26(2):237–48.
3. Drossman DA, Corazziari E, Delvaux M, Spiller RC, Talley NJ, Thompson WG, et al. In: Drossman DA, Corazziari E, Delvaux M, Spiller RC, Talley NJ, Thompson WG, Whitehead WE, editors. The functional gastrointestinal disorders. 3rd edn. Virginia: Degnon associates, Inc., McLean; 2006. p. 963–90.
4. Park JM, Choi MG, Cho YK, Lee IS, Kim JI, Kim SW, Chung IS. Functional gastrointestinal disorders diagnosed by Rome III questionnaire in Korea. J Neurogastroenterol Motil. 2011;17(3):279–86.
5. Wallander MA, Johansson S, Ruigomez A, Garcia Rodriguez LA, Joqnes R. Dyspepsia in general practice: incidence, risk factors, comorbidity and mortality. Fam Pract. 2007;24:403–11.
6. Tack J, Talley NJ, Camilleri M, Holtmann G, Hu P, Malagelada J-R, Stanghellini V. Functional gastroduodenal disorders. Gastroenterology. 2006;130:1466–79.
7. Tepeš B. Subgroups of dyspepsia. In: Duvnjak M, editor. Dyspepsia in clinical practice. Springer; 2011. p. 9–18.
8. Boyce PM, Talley NJ, Burke C, Koloski NA. Epidemiology of the functional gastrointestinal disorders diagnosed according to Rome II criteria: an Australian population-based study. Intern Med J. 2006;36:28–36.
9. Drossman DA1, Li Z, Andruzzi E, Temple RD, Talley NJ, Thompson WG, Whitehead WE, Janssens J, Funch-Jensen P, Corazziari E,. U.S. householder survey of functional gastrointestinal disorders. Prevalence, sociodemography, and health impact. Dig DisSci.1993;38: 1569–80.
10. Hasan M. Dyspepsia in primary care practice in Bangladesh. Bangladesh Med J .2013; 42 (2):63–69. A review article.
11. Ghoshal UC, Singh R, Chang FY, Hou X, Wong BC, Kachintorn U. Epidemiology of uninvestigated and functional dyspepsia in Asia: facts and fiction. J Neurogastroenterol Motil. 2011;17(3):235–44. doi: https://doi.org/10.5056/jnm.2011.17.3.235.
12. Yazdanpanah K, Moghimi N, Yousefinejad V, Ghaderi E, Azizi A, Nazem SF. Dyspepsia prevalence in general population aged over 20 in the west part of Iran. J Pak Med Assoc. 2012;62(7):672–6.
13. Ford AC, Marwaha A, Sood R, Moayyedi P. Global prevalence of, and risk factors for, uninvestigated dyspepsia: a meta-analysis. Gut. 2015;64:1049–57.
14. Talley NJ, Ford AC. Functional dyspepsia. N Engl J Med. 2015;373:1853–63.
15. Piessevaux H, De Winter B, Louis E, Muls V, De Looze D, Pelckmans P, Deltenre M, Urbain D, Tack J. Dyspeptic symptoms in the general population: a factor and cluster analysis of symptom groupings. Neurogastroenterol Motil. 2009;21(4):378–88.
16. Tack J, Bisschops R, Sarnelli G. Pathophysiology and treatment of functional dyspepsia. Gastroenterology. 2004;127:1239–55.
17. Mahadeva S, Goh KL. Epidemiology of functional dyspepsia: a global perspective. World J Gastroenterol. 2006;12(17):2661–6.

18. Rejchrt S, Koupil I, Kopa ´cˇova´ M, Vor, ´sˇek V, Seifert B, Pozler O. Prevalence and sociodemographic determinants of uninvestigated dyspepsia in the Czech Republic. Eur J Gastroenterol Hepatol 2008; 20: 898–905.
19. Solomon OA, Ajayi AO. Risk factors for un-investigated dyspepsia among primary care patients in northern Nigeria. African health Science. 2013;13(4): 1007–11.
20. Zagari RM, Law GR, Fuccio L, Cennamo V, Gilthorpe MS, Forman D, Bazzoli F. Epidemiology of functional dyspepsia and subgroups in the Italian general population: an endoscopic study. Gastroenterology. 2010;138(4): 1302–11.
21. Tesfahun T, Yohannes M, Kassu D, Daniel A. Seroprevalence of helicobacter pylori infection in and its relationship with ABO blood groups. Ethiop.J. Health Dev .2005; 19(1):55–59.
22. Moayyedi P, Forman D, Braunholtz D, Feltbower R, Crocombe W, Liptrott M, Axon A. The proportion of upper gastrointestinal symptoms in the community associated with helicobacter pylori, lifestyle factors, and nonsteroidal anti-inflammatory drugs. Leeds HELP study group. The Am J Gastroenterol. 2000;95(6):1448–55.
23. Gizachew T, Abebe H, Kassu D, Samuel E, Abate B. Association of dyspepsia symptoms and Helicobacter pylori infections in private higher clinic, Addis Ababa, Ethiopia. Ethiop Med J. 2011; 49 (2). Abstract.
24. Moges F, Kassu A, Mengistu G, Adugna S, Andualem B, Nishikawa T, Ota F. Seroprevalence in dyspeptic patients and its relationship with HIV infection, ABO blood group and life style in a university hospital, north west Ethiopia. World J Gastroenterol. 2006;12(12):1957–61.
25. Wubejig A, Mulugeta K, Bayeh A. Prevalence and risk factors of H. Pylori from dyspeptic patients in Northwest Ethiopia: a hospital based cross-sectional study. Asian Pac J Cancer Prev. 2014;15(11):4459–63.
26. Asrat D, Nilsson I, Mengistu Y, Ashenafi S, Ayenew K, Al-Soud WA, Wadström T, Kassa E. Prevalence of helicobacter pylori infection among adult dyspeptic patients in Ethiopia. Trop Med Parasitol. 2004;98(2):181–9.
27. Rome Foundation, "Rome III: A self-reported integrated questionnaire to diagnose adults for one or more functional gastrointestinal disorders, including alarm symptoms/red flags," https://theromefoundation.org/products/copyright-and-licensing/.
28. Demiray E, Yilmaz O, Sarkis C, Soyturk M, Simsek I. Comparison of invasive methods and two different stool antigen tests for diagnosis of H. Pylori infection in patients with gastric bleeding. World J Gastroenterol. 2006; 12(26):4206–10.
29. Ogunmodede JA, Bojuwoye MO, Olokoba AB, Bolarinwa OA, Kolo PM. Self-reported symptoms of uninvestigated dyspepsia among university staff in Ilorin, Nigeria. Res. J. of Health Sci. 2016;4(4):296–303.
30. Bitwayiki R, Orikiiriza JT, Kateera F, Bihizimana P, Karenzi B, Kyamanywa P, Walker TD. Dyspepsia prevalence and impact on quality of life among Rwandan healthcare workers: a cross-sectional survey. S Afr Med J. 2015; 105(12):1064–9.
31. Li M, Lu B, Chu L, Zhou H, Chen M-Y. Prevalence and characteristic of dyspepsia among college students in Zhejiang province. World j gastronology. 2014;20(13):3649–54.
32. Lee J-Y, Hsu Y-C, Chen M-J, Tseng P-H, Chang C-Y, Yang T-H, Chang W-H, J-Y W, Wang H-P, Luo J-C, Lin J-T, Shun C-T, Distinct WM-S. Aetiopathogenesis in subgroups of functional dyspepsia according to the Rome III criteria. Gut. 2015;64:1517–28. https://doi.org/10.1136/gutjnl-2014-308114.
33. Nwokediuko SC, Ijoma U, Obienu O. Functional Dyspepsia: Subtypes, Risk Factors, and Overlap with Irritable Bowel Syndrome in a Population of African Patients. Gastroenterology Research and Practice, Article ID. 2012: 562393, 5 pages. doi: https://doi.org/10.1155/2012/562393.
34. Obayo S, Muzoora C, Ocama P, Cooney MM, Wilson T, Probert CS. Upper gastrointestinal diseases in patients for endoscopy in south-western Uganda. Afri Health Sci. 2015;15(3):959–66. https://doi.org/10.4314/ahs.v15i3.33.
35. Seyedmirzaei S M, Haghdoost AA, Afshari M; Dehghani A. Prevalence of Dyspepsia and its Associated Factors Among the Adult Population in Southeast of Iran in 2010. Iran Red Crescent Med J. 2014; 16(11): e14757. doi: https://doi.org/10.5812/ircmj.14757.
36. Shokrzadeh L, Baghaei K, Yamaoka Y, Shiota S, Mirsattari D, Porhoseingholi A, Zali MR. Prevalence of helicobacter pylori infection in dyspeptic patients in Iran. Gastroenterology Insights. 2012;4:e8. doi: https://doi.org/10.4081/gi.2012.e8.
37. Shmuely H, Samson O, Douglas J, Abuksis G, Yahav J, Fraser G, Pitlik S, Niv Y. yspepsia symptoms and *Helicobacter pylori* infection, Nakuru, Kenya. Emerging Infectious Diseases. 2003;9(9):1103–7.
38. Wildner-christensen M, Hansen J M & Schaffalitzky de muckadell O B. Risk factors for dyspepsia in a general population: non-steroidal anti-inflammatory drugs, cigarette smoking and unemployment are more important than helicobacter pylori infection. Scand J Gastroenterol 2006; 41: 149–154.
39. Aro P, Talley NJ, Ronkainen J, Storskrubb T, Vieth M, Johansson SE, Bolling-sternevald E, Agréus L, Anxiety I. Associated with uninvestigated and functional dyspepsia(Rome III criteria) in a Swedish population-based study. Gastroenterology. 2009;137:94–100.
40. Suzuki H, Matsuzaki J, Hibi T. What Is the Difference between *Helicobacter pylori* Associated Dyspepsia and Functional Dyspepsia?. J Neurogastroenterol Motil. 2011; 17(2):124–30. Review article.
41. Mohammad MA, Altayar M, Toboli AB, Bakk A. Characteristics of helicobacter pylori infection in libyan healthy peoples in two teaching hospitals in benghazi. Medical Journal of Islamic World Academy of Sciences. 2011;19(1):27–32.
42. Aguemon BD, Struelens MJ, Massougbodji A, Ouendo EM. Prevalence and risk factors for helicobacter pylori infection in urban and rural Beninese populations. Clin Microbiol Infect. 2005;11:611–7.
43. Khan MA, Ghazi HO. Helicobacter pylori infection in asymptomatic subjects in Makkah Saudi Arabia. *JPMA*. 2007;57(3):114–7.
44. Shah SS, Bhatia SJ, Mistry FP. Epidemiology of dyspepsia in the general population in Mumbai. Indian J Gastroenterol. 2001;20:103–6.
45. Haque M, Wyeth JW, Stace NH, Talley NJ. Prevalence, severity and associated features of gastro-oesophageal reflux and dyspepsia: a population-based study. N Z Med J. 2000;113:178–81.
46. Shaib Y, El-Serag HB. The prevalence and risk factors of functional dyspepsia in a multiethnic population in the United States. Am J Gastroenterol. 2004; 99:2210–6.
47. Khademolhosseini F, Mehrabani D, Zare N, Salehi M, Heydari ST, Beheshti M, Saberi-Firoozi M. Prevalence of dyspepsia and its correlation with demographic factors and lifestyle in shiraz, southern Iran. Middle East Journal of Digestive Diseases. 2010;2(1):24–30.

Permissions

All chapters in this book were first published in GASTROENTEROLOGY, by BioMed Central; hereby published with permission under the Creative Commons Attribution License or equivalent. Every chapter published in this book has been scrutinized by our experts. Their significance has been extensively debated. The topics covered herein carry significant findings which will fuel the growth of the discipline. They may even be implemented as practical applications or may be referred to as a beginning point for another development.

The contributors of this book come from diverse backgrounds, making this book a truly international effort. This book will bring forth new frontiers with its revolutionizing research information and detailed analysis of the nascent developments around the world.

We would like to thank all the contributing authors for lending their expertise to make the book truly unique. They have played a crucial role in the development of this book. Without their invaluable contributions this book wouldn't have been possible. They have made vital efforts to compile up to date information on the varied aspects of this subject to make this book a valuable addition to the collection of many professionals and students.

This book was conceptualized with the vision of imparting up-to-date information and advanced data in this field. To ensure the same, a matchless editorial board was set up. Every individual on the board went through rigorous rounds of assessment to prove their worth. After which they invested a large part of their time researching and compiling the most relevant data for our readers.

The editorial board has been involved in producing this book since its inception. They have spent rigorous hours researching and exploring the diverse topics which have resulted in the successful publishing of this book. They have passed on their knowledge of decades through this book. To expedite this challenging task, the publisher supported the team at every step. A small team of assistant editors was also appointed to further simplify the editing procedure and attain best results for the readers.

Apart from the editorial board, the designing team has also invested a significant amount of their time in understanding the subject and creating the most relevant covers. They scrutinized every image to scout for the most suitable representation of the subject and create an appropriate cover for the book.

The publishing team has been an ardent support to the editorial, designing and production team. Their endless efforts to recruit the best for this project, has resulted in the accomplishment of this book. They are a veteran in the field of academics and their pool of knowledge is as vast as their experience in printing. Their expertise and guidance has proved useful at every step. Their uncompromising quality standards have made this book an exceptional effort. Their encouragement from time to time has been an inspiration for everyone.

The publisher and the editorial board hope that this book will prove to be a valuable piece of knowledge for researchers, students, practitioners and scholars across the globe.

List of Contributors

Cristina Canova, Gisella Pitter, Renzo Zanotti and Lorenzo Simonato
Laboratory of Public Health and Population Studies, Department of Molecular Medicine, University of Padua, via Loredan 18, 35131 Padua, Italy

Jonas F. Ludvigsson
Department of Medical Epidemiology and Biostatistics, Karolinska Institutet, 17177 Stockholm, Sweden
Department of Pediatrics, Örebro university Hospital, Örebro 70185, Sweden

Pierantonio Romor
Friuli-Venezia Giulia Regional Health Information System, Informatica per il Sistema degli Enti Locali (INSIEL) S.p.A., Udine, Italy

Loris Zanier
Epidemiological Service, Health Directorate, Friuli Venezia-Giulia Region, Udine, Italy

Ji Eun Kim, Jun Go, Ji Eun Sung, Hyun Ah Lee, Woo Bin Yun and Dae Youn Hwang
Department of Biomaterials Science, College of Natural Resources & Life Science/Life and Industry Convergence Research Institute, Pusan National University, 50 Cheonghak-ri, Samnangjin-eup Miryang-si, Gyeongsangnam-do 627-706, Korea

Jin Tae Hong
College of Pharmacy, Chungbuk National University, Chungju 361-763, Korea

Tom G. S. Williams and Simon J. Griffin
School of Clinical Medicine, University of Cambridge, Cambridge, UK

Joaquín Cubiella
Department of Gastroenterology, Complexo Hospitalario Universitario de Ourense, Instituto de Investigación Biomédica Ourense-Vigo-Pontevedra, Ourense, Spain

Griffin, Fiona M. Walter and Juliet A. Usher-Smith
The Primary Care Unit, Department of Public Health and Primary Care, University of Cambridge, Cambridge CB1 8RN, UK

D. Lundgren and P. Karling
Department of Public Health and Clinical Medicine, Division of Medicine, Umeå University, SE-90187 Umeå, Sweden

J. Rutegård
Department of Surgery and Perioperative Science, Surgery, Umeå University, SE-90187 Umeå, Sweden

V. Eklöf and R. Palmqvist
Department of Medical Biosciences, Pathology, Umeå University, SE-90187 Umeå, Sweden

Yoo Mi Park, Jae Jun Park, Young Hoon Youn, Jie-Hyun Kim and Hyojin Park
Department of Internal Medicine, Gangnam Severance Hospital, Yonsei University College of Medicine, 211 Eonjuro, Gangnam-gu, Seoul 135-720, South Korea

Hee Sun Kim, Su Jung Baik and Yoo Mi Park
Health Promotion Center, Gangnam Severance Hospital, Yonsei University College of Medicine, Seoul, South Korea

Wencheng Kong, Rongchao Ying and Huicheng Jin
Department of Gastroenterological Surgery, Hangzhou First People's Hospital, School of Clinical Medicine, Nanjing Medical University, Hangzhou 310006, China

Jian Wang, Yousheng Li, Qi Mao and Danhua Yao
Intestinal Rehabilition and Transplant Center, Jinling Hospital, School of Medicine, Nanjing University, Nanjing 210002, China

Mingxiao Guo
Department of Gastroenterological Surgery, Linyi People's Hospital, Shandong 276000, China

Yousheng Li
Department of Surgery, Jinling Hospital, School of Medicine, Nanjing University, 305 East Zhongshan Road, Nanjing 210002, China

Andrea Smarrazzo and Luigi Greco
Department of Translational Medical Sciences, School of Medicine, University "Federico II", Naples, Italy
European Laboratory for Food Induced Diseases, Naples, Italy

Zrinjka Misak
Children's Hospital Zagreb, Zagreb, Croatia

Stefano Costa and Giuseppe Magazzù
Celiac Regional Centre, Pediatric Gastroenterology and Cystic Fibrosis Unit, University of Messina, Via Consolare Valeria 1, 98125, Messina, Italy

Dušanka Mičetić-Turk
Paediatric Department, University Medical Centre, Maribor, Slovenia

Mona Abu-Zekry
Cairo University Children Hospital, El Cairo, Egypt

Aydan Kansu
Department of Pediatric Gastroenterology, School of Medicine, Ankara University, Ankara, Turkey

Abdelhak Abkari
Centre Hospitalier Universitaire Ibnou Rochd, Casablanca, Morocco

Karim Bouziane-Nedjadi
Faculté de Médecine d'Oran, Oran, Algeria

Mongi Ben Hariz
Pediatric Unit, Mongi SLIM's Hospital of Tunis, Marsa, Tunisia

Eleftheria Roma
First Department of Pediatrics, University of Athens, Athens, Greece

Virtut Velmishi
Service of Pediatric Gastroenterology "Mother Teresa" Hospital, Tirana, Albania

Maria Legarda Tamara
Paediatric Gastroenterology Unit, Cruces University Hospital, Bilbao, Spain

Thomas Attard
University of Malta, Msida, Malta

Veselinka Djurisic
Clinical Center of Montenegro, Podgorica, Montenegro

Massimo Bellini
Gastrointestinal Unit, Department of Gastroenterology, University of Pisa, Via Paradisa, 2, 56127 Pisa, Italy

Paolo Usai-Satta
Brotzu Hospital, Gastroenterology Unit, Cagliari Italy

Antonio Bove
AORN "A. Cardarelli", Naples, Italy

Renato Bocchini
Malatesta Novello, Private Hospital Cesena, Italy

Francesca Galeazzi
Division of Gastroenterology, Department of Surgery, Oncology and Gastroenterology, University of Padua, Padua, Italy

Edda Battaglia
Cardinal Massaia Hospital, Gastroenterology Unit, Asti, Italy

Pietro Alduini
San Luca Hospital, Digestive Endoscopy Unit, Lucca, Italy

Elisabetta Buscarini
Gastroenterology and Digestive Endoscopy Unit, Maggiore Hospital, Crema, Italy

Gabrio Bassotti
Gastrointestinal and Hepatology Section, Clinical & Experimental Medicine, Perugia, Italy

Chen Si, Zhu Xiuli, Xie Li, Jia Yong and Zhang Kaiguang
Department of Gastroenterology, Affiliated Provincial Hospital of Anhui Medical University, Hefei, China

Zhou Ying
Department of Obstetrics, Affiliated Provincial Hospital of Anhui Medical University, Hefei, China

David Díaz-Jiménez, Marjorie De la Fuente, Karen Dubois-Camacho, Glauben Landskron and Marcela A. Hermoso
Programa Disciplinario de Inmunología, Instituto de Ciencias Biomédicas, Facultad de Medicina, Universidad de Chile, Santiago, CL 8380453, Chile

Daniela Simian
Subdirección de Investigación, Dirección Académica, Clínica Las Condes, Santiago, CL 7591018, Chile

Janitza Fuentes and Tamara Pérez
Unidad de Hígado y Gastroenterología, Instituto Chileno-Japonés de Enfermedades Digestivas, Hospital San Borja-Arriarán, Santiago, CL, Chile

María Julieta González
Programa disciplinario de Biología Celular, Instituto de Ciencias Biomédicas, Facultad de Medicina, Universidad de Chile, Santiago, CL 8380453, Chile

Rodrigo Quera
Servicio de Gastroenterología, Clínica Las Condes, Santiago, CL 7591018, Chile

Hye Ryoung Sul, Hyun Woong Lee and Jeong Wook Kim
Department of Internal Medicine, Chung-Ang University College of Medicine, 224-1 Heuk Seok-Dong, Dongjak-Ku, Seoul 156-755, Republic of Korea

Sung Jae Cha and Yoo Shin Choi
Department of Surgery, Chung-Ang University College of Medicine, Seoul, Republic of Korea

Gi Hyeon Kim and Byung Kook Kwak
Department of Radiology, Chung-Ang University College of Medicine, Seoul, Republic of Korea

Daisuke Yamaguchi, Yuki Takeuchi, Takahiro Yukimoto, Kei Ikeda, Kosuke Matsumoto, Rikako Kinoshita, Saori Kamachi, Tomohito Morisaki, Keisuke Ario and Seiji Tsunada
Department of Gastroenterology, National Hospital Organization Ureshino Medical Center, Ureshino 843-0301, Japan

Naoko Yamaguchi, Kyosuke Sugiyama and Ryo Katsuki
Department of Anesthesiology, National Hospital Organization Ureshino Medical Center, Ureshino 843-0301, Japan

Daisuke Yamaguchi, Yuki Takeuchi and Kazuma Fujimoto
Department of Internal Medicine and Gastrointestinal Endoscopy, Saga Medical School, Saga 849-8501, Japan

Hisako Yoshida
Clinical Research Center, Saga Medical School, Saga 849-8501, Japan

Bunchorn Siripongpreeda, Navara Dusitanond, Tassanee Sriprayoon, Bunlung Muyphuag, Thaniya Sricharunrat, Narongchai Teerayatanakul, Watanya Chaiwong, Wipra Worasawate, Prassanee Sattayarungsee, Juthamas Sangthongdee, Jirapa Prarom, Gaidganok Sornsamdang, Kamonwan Soonklang and Kasiruck Wittayasak
Chulabhorn Hospital, Bangkok, Thailand

Chulabhorn Mahidol
Chulabhorn Research Institute, Bangkok, Thailand

Chirayu U. Auewarakul
Faculty of Medicine Siriraj Hospital, Mahidol University, Bangkok, Thailand

Michał Bulsa
Pediatrics and Pediatric Nursery Unit of The Pomeranian Medical University in Szczecin, ul. Żołnierska 48, 71-210 Szczecin, Poland

Grażyna Czaja-Bulsa
Division of Paediatrics, Gastroenterology and Rheumatology of The "Zdroje" Hospital in Szczecin, Szczecin, Poland

Aneta Gębala
Independent Laboratory of Propaedeutics in Paediatrics of The Pomeranian Medical University in Szczecin, Szczecin, Poland

Zhidong Gao, Chao Wang, Zhanlong Shen, Kewei Jiang, Kai Shen, Bin Liang, Xiaodong Yang, Qiwei Xie, Shan Wang and Yingjiang Ye
Department of Gastrointestinal Surgery, Peking University People's Hospital, Beijing 100044, People's Republic of China

Qian Xue and Jingtong Wang
Department of Gastroenterology and Endoscopy, Peking University People's Hospital, Beijing 100044, People's Republic of China

Kousaku Kawashima, Shunji Ishihara, Takafumi Yuki, Nobuhiko Fukuba, Naoki Oshima, Hiroki Sonoyama, Noritsugu Yamashita, Yasumasa Tada, Ryusaku Kusunoki, Akihiko Oka, Yoshiyuki Mishima and Yoshikazu Kinoshita
Department of Internal Medicine II, Shimane University Faculty of Medicine, 89-1, Enya-cho, Izumo, Shimane 693-8501, Japan

Hideaki Kazumori
Division of Internal Medicine, Matsue Seikyo General Hospital, 8-8-8, Nishitsuda, Matsue 690-8522, Japan

Ichiro Moriyama
Cancer center, Shimane University Hospital, 89-1, Enya-cho, Izumo, Shimane 693-8501, Japan

Andrea Cikova, Anna Dobisova, Andrea Gebhardtova Zora Flassikova and Aktham Yaghi
University Hospital Bratislava, Nemocnica Ruzinov, ICU, KAIM, Clinic of Anesthesiology and Intensive Care Medicine, Faculty of Medicine, Comenius University in Bratislava, Bratislava, Slovakia

Diana Vavrincova-Yaghi and Peter Vavrinec
Department of Pharmacology and Toxicology, Faculty of Pharmacy, Comenius University in Bratislava, Bratislava, Odbojarov 10, 832 32 Bratislava, Slovakia

Mark A. Seelen
Department of Internal Medicine, University of Groningen, University Medical Center Groningen, Groningen, the Netherlands

Robert H. Henning
Department of Clinical Pharmacy and Pharmacology, University of Groningen, University Medical Center Groningen, Groningen, the Netherlands

Stefano Costa, Giovanni Currò, Salvatore Pellegrino, Maria Cristina Lucanto and Giuseppe Magazzù
Celiac Regional Centre, Pediatric Gastroenterology and Cystic Fibrosis Unit, University of Messina, Via Consolare Valeria 1, 98125 Messina, Italy

Giovanni Tuccari and Antonio Ieni
Department of Human Pathology of Adult and Evolutive Age 'Gaetano Barresi', University of Messina, Messina, Italy

Giuseppina Visalli
Department of Biomedical and Dental Sciences and Morphofunctional Imaging, University of Messina, Messina, Italy

Domenico Santoro
Department of Clinical and Experimental Medicine, Unit of Nephrology and Dialysis, University of Messina, Messina, Italy

Maraci Rodrigues
Department of Gastroenterology, Hospital das Clínicas, School of Medicine, University of Sao Paulo (SMUSP), Av. Dr Eneas de Carvalho Aguiar, 255, 05403-000, Sao Paulo, Brazil

Glauce Hiromi Yonamine and Carla Aline Fernandes Satiro
Department of Pediatric, Instituto da Criança, Division of Nutrition, Hospital das Clínicas, School of Medicine, University of Sao Paulo (SMUSP), Sao Paulo, Brazil

Satu Oltedal, Kjersti Tjensvoll, Bjørnar Gilje, Rune Smaaland and Oddmund Nordgård
Department of Hematology and Oncology, Stavanger University Hospital, 4068 Stavanger, Norway

Ivar Skaland and Emiel A. M. Janssen
Department of Pathology, Stavanger University Hospital, 4068 Stavanger, Norway

Jodi Maple-Grødem
The Norwegian Centre for Movement Disorders, Stavanger University Hospital, 4068 Stavanger, Norway
Centre for Organelle Research, University of Stavanger, 4036 Stavanger, Norway

Reino Heikkilä
Oslo University Hospital, 0424 Oslo, Norway

Elizabeth Ann Forrest, Mark Wong, Srinivasa Nama and Siddharth Sharma
Diagnostic, Emergency and Medical Services, Gold Coast Hospital and Health Service, Gold Coast University Hospital, 1 Hospital Blvd, Southport, Gold Coast, Queensland 4215, Australia

M. C. Valenzano and E. Rybakovsky
Lankenau Institute for Medical Research, 100 Lancaster Avenue, Wynnewood, PA 19096, USA

J. M. Mullin
Division of Gastroenterology, Lankenau Medical Center, Wynnewood, PA 19096, USA

K. M. DiGuilio
Philadelphia College of Osteopathic Medicine, 4170 City Avenue, Philadelphia, PA 19131, USA

Yong juan Wang and Hui qing Jiang
Department of Gastroenterology and Hepatology, The Second Affiliated Hospital of Hebei Medical University, Hebei, China

Yu ming Wang, Yan min Zheng and Jie Zhang
Department of Gastroenterology and Hepatology, The General Hospital of Tianjin Medical University, Tianjin, China

Thorbjørn Søren Rønn Jensen, Badar Mahmood, Morten Bach Damm and Mark Berner Hansen
Digestive Disease Center K, Bispebjerg Hospital, DK-2400 Copenhagen, NV, Denmark

Marie Balslev Backe, Mattias Salling Dahllöf, Steen Seier Poulsen and Niels Bindslev
Department of Biomedical Sciences, Faculty of Health Sciences, University of Copenhagen, DK- 2200 Copenhagen N, Denmark

N. ZP. Ng, Y. D. Chen, Y. H. M. Chee and C. L. Tang
Department of Colorectal Surgery, Singapore General Hospital, 20 College Road, Academia Level 5, Singapore 169856, Singapore

W. J. Tan and F. J. Foo and M. H. Chew
Department of General Surgery, Sengkang General Hospital, 110 Sengkang East Way, Singapore 544886, Singapore

Zsuzsanna Kurti, Akos Ilias, Lorant Gonczi, Zsuzsanna Vegh, Petra A. Golovics and Barbara D. Lovasz
Department of Medicine, Semmelweis University, Budapest H-1083, Hungary

Petra Fadgyas-Freyler and Gyula Korponay
Strategic Analysis Department, National Health Insurance Fund (OEP), Budapest H-1139, Hungary

Peter L. Lakatos
Division of Gastroenterology, McGill University Health Centre, 1650 Ave. Cedar, D16.173.1, Montreal, QC H3G 1A4, Canada
Division of Gastroenterology/Hepatology Unit and Endoscopy, Semmelweis University, Koranyi S 2A, Budapest H-1083, Hungary

Barbara D. Lovasz
Faculty of Health Sciences, Department of Clinical Studies, Semmelweis University, Budapest H-1088, Hungary

Abdurahaman Seid
Department of Medical Laboratory Sciences, College of Medicine and Health Sciences, Wollo University, Dessie, Ethiopia

Zemenu Tamir
Department of Medical Laboratory Sciences, College of Health Sciences, School of Allied Health Sciences, Addis Ababa University, Addis Ababa, Ethiopia

Wondmagegn Demsiss
Department of Medical Laboratory Sciences, College of Medicine and Health Sciences, Wollo University, Dessie, Ethiopia

Index

www.ingramcontent.com/pod-product-compliance
Lightning Source LLC
LaVergne TN
LVHW080727210926
848485LV00003B/526
* 9 7 8 1 6 3 9 2 7 1 4 1 2 *